Experiences of Depression

International Perspectives in Philosophy and Psychiatry

Series editors: Bill (K.W.M.) Fulford, Lisa Bortolotti, Matthew Broome, Katherine Morris, John Z. Sadler, and Giovanni Stanghellini

OXFORD
UNIVERSITY PRESS

Great Clarendon Street, Oxford, OX2 6DP,
United Kingdom

Oxford University Press is a department of the University of Oxford.
It furthers the University's objective of excellence in research, scholarship,
and education by publishing worldwide. Oxford is a registered trade mark of
Oxford University Press in the UK and in certain other countries

First Edition published in 2015

Impression: 6

Published in the United States of America by Oxford University Press
198 Madison Avenue, New York, NY 10016, United States of America

British Library Cataloguing in Publication Data

Data available

Library of Congress Control Number: 2014948993

ISBN 978-0-19-960897-3

Printed and bound in Great Britain by
CPI Group (UK) Ltd, Croydon, CR0 4YY

Experiences of Depression
A Study in Phenomenology

Matthew Ratcliffe

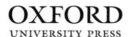

This book is dedicated to the memory of Jonathan Lowe. Our many conversations over the years hugely enriched the space of intellectual possibilities I inhabit. It was a privilege to be his friend.

Acknowledgements

The research for this book was carried out as part of the project 'Emotional Experience in Depression: A Philosophical Study'. I am very grateful to all my project colleagues, especially Achim Stephan, Jan Slaby, Hannah Bowden, Benedict Smith, Kerrin Jacobs, Somogy Varga, and Angela Woods, for all the time we spent discussing the phenomenology of depression and related topics. I would also like to thank the UK Arts and Humanities Research Council and the Deutsche Forschungsgemeinschaft (German Research Foundation) for funding our research. My work on the phenomenology of depression owes a great deal to the many conversations I have had with philosophers, psychiatrists, psychologists, anthropologists, and others about this and related topics. They include Gwen Adshead, Havi Carel, Jonathan Cole, Giovanna Colombetti, Rachel Cooper, Tom Csordas, Owen Earnshaw, Thomas Fuchs, Bill Fulford, Shaun Gallagher, Philip Gerrans, Peter Goldie (1946–2011), George Graham, Robin Hendry, Peter Hobson, Gail Hornstein, Daniel Hutto, Ian Kidd, Laurence Kirmayer, Jonathan Lowe (1950–2014), Wayne Martin, Nick Medford, Gareth Owen, Elizabeth Pienkos, Jennifer Radden, Giovanni Stanghellini, Fredrik Svenaeus, Amanda Taylor Aiken, Henrik Walter, Mark Wynn, and many others. I am especially grateful to Matthew Broome and Louis Sass, for many long and illuminating discussions and also for their comments on draft chapters. Thanks to three anonymous referees for their insightful comments on an outline of this book and, in particular, to two further referees who kindly read and commented on the whole manuscript. I would also like to thank my wife, Beth, and our children, Samuel and Thomas, for putting up with the irritable and despondent moods that sometimes accompanied my writing.

Material from the book was presented at conferences, workshops or seminars hosted by the Tavistock Clinic, Institute of Psychiatry, and Institute of Philosophy, all in London, the Free University of Berlin, the Brocher Centre in Switzerland, the University of the West of England, Birkbeck College London, and the Universities of Central Florida, Cardiff, Copenhagen, Durham, Exeter, Heidelberg, Hull, Lancaster, Manchester, Memphis, Osnabrück, Rutgers, Södertörn, and Sussex, at a meeting of the International Society for Phenomenological Studies at Asilomar in California, and at conferences organized by the mental health charity SANE and the Gloucestershire Survivors of Bereavement by Suicide group. Thanks to participants in all these events for their many helpful comments, suggestions and criticisms. This book draws on some of my recently published articles and chapters. Chapter 6 is a revised version of Ratcliffe (2013a), Chapter 7 elaborates on Ratcliffe (2012a), and the final part of Chapter 10 is adapted from Ratcliffe (2014b). All three papers were published by Oxford University Press. Chapters 5 and 9 are loosely based on Ratcliffe (2010a) and Ratcliffe (2012b), published by Taylor and Francis Ltd (<http://www.tandf.co.uk/journals>). Sections of Chapters 4 and 8 are adapted from Ratcliffe (2013b) and Ratcliffe (2014a), published by Springer Science + Business Media. Chapter 3 is an expanded and revised version of my contribution to Ratcliffe, Broome, Smith and Bowden (2013), published by Imprint Academic. I am grateful to all of the publishers concerned for granting me permission to re-use material.

I learned a great deal from my lengthy collaboration with a research team that was—until recently—employed by the mental health charity SANE, for which I would especially like to thank Outi Benson, Sarah Brand, and Susanne Gibson. Amongst other things, they helped me and my colleagues at Durham University to design a questionnaire on the first-person experience of depression, which was then posted on the SANE website. My greatest debt of gratitude is to all those who completed this lengthy questionnaire. Their detailed accounts of what it is like to be depressed proved invaluable, and have had a significant influence on my thinking. I hope this book succeeds in casting at least some new light on the kinds of experience they described.

Contents

Introduction

Describing Depression

This book is a philosophical exploration of what it is like to be depressed. I develop a detailed account of depression experiences by drawing on work in phenomenology, philosophy of mind and psychology, and several other disciplines. In the process, I show how phenomenological research can contribute to psychiatry, by facilitating a better understanding of patients' experiences, as well as informing classification, diagnosis, and treatment. I also make clear the relevance of depression to several different areas of philosophical enquiry. By reflecting on how experiences of depression differ from 'healthy' forms of experience, we can refine our understanding of both. Hence this kind of enquiry can be integrated into our phenomenological method, facilitating discoveries that have wider applicability. However, the philosophical relevance of depression is not limited to phenomenology. As I show, the study of depression experiences can feed into philosophical debates concerning a wide range of topics, including the structure of intersubjectivity, the nature of empathy, our sense of free will, temporal experience, the ingredients of emotion and feeling, what it is to believe something, and what it is to hope. In addition to informing philosophy and psychiatry, I hope my discussion will be of interest, and perhaps also of use, to people who suffer from depression and those in supporting roles.

Although much has been written about the phenomenology of schizophrenia, there has been comparatively little phenomenological research on depression. Perhaps this neglect is due to the assumption that depression involves intensification or proliferation of commonplace feelings, emotions and moods, such as sadness, hopelessness, and guilt. So all one need do in order to appreciate the phenomenology of depression is imagine having unusually pronounced experiences of familiar kinds. Experiences of schizophrenia, by contrast, are utterly alien to most of us. But I will argue that experiences of depression likewise differ radically from many people's mundane, everyday experience. This is indicated by the consistent complaint in first-person accounts that depression falls outside the normal range of human experiences and is therefore difficult or even impossible to describe. For instance, the novelist William Styron

(2001, p.5, p.14) writes that depression is 'close to being beyond description' and later that it is like 'being engulfed by a toxic and unnameable tide that obliterated any enjoyable response to the living world', something 'close to, but indescribably different from, actual pain'. Others maintain that no linguistic resources are adequate to the task: 'I have no words to describe this thing that was totally alien to my life experience' (quoted by Whybrow, 1997, p.23). A number of different indescribability claims can be distinguished. It might be that depression or some aspect of it resists all attempts at description, that the sufferer is herself unable to describe it, that it can only be described metaphorically, that even metaphorical accounts are somehow lacking, that it cannot be conveyed to those who have not themselves experienced it, or that only certain media, such as art, music, or poetry, are adequate to the task. So it is not clear what exactly the problem consists of or whether everyone faces the same problem. However, we can at least take it as given that many people find it extremely hard to convey their experiences of depression to others, and that this difficulty is often attributed to a radical difference between depression and more familiar kinds of experience.

One of the main tasks of this book is to emphasize the often-profound difference between the 'world' of the depressed and the non-depressed, and to provide a detailed account of what this difference consists of. Drawing on themes in the work of phenomenologists such as Husserl, Heidegger, Merleau-Ponty and Sartre, I argue that human experience incorporates an ordinarily pre-reflective sense of 'belonging to a shared world', which is altered in depression. This accounts—in part—for why depression is so hard to describe: it involves an aspect of experience that is seldom an object of explicit reflection or discussion and that is consequently hard to articulate. I suggest that the phenomenology of depression can be further illuminated by appealing to a kind of feeling that I call 'existential feeling'. Existential feelings have a distinctive phenomenological role; they constitute a variable sense of the possibilities that the world incorporates. Depression, I maintain, involves a change in the kinds of possibility that are experienced as integral to the world and, with it, a change in the structure of one's overall relationship with the world. To describe this in detail, I focus on more specific themes that are consistently emphasized in first-person accounts: altered bodily experience, loss of hope, feelings of guilt, a diminished sense of agency and self, altered experience of time, and isolation from other people. All of these are to be conceived of as inextricable aspects of a unitary experience—a shift in existential feeling or 'existential change'.

As the discussion progresses, I build up a case for the view that the label 'depression' accommodates a range of different kinds of existential change, and that differences between them are often obscured by their being conveyed in much the same terms. This heterogeneity exacerbates the problem of communicating and understanding experiences of depression. Importantly, it is not just first-person narratives that struggle to convey these experiences. The descriptions we find in psychiatry and other contexts are also lacking, although they seldom include the confession of inadequacy that so often features in depression memoirs. There is considerable uncertainty and disagreement in psychiatry over what depression actually is, where its boundaries lie, and what its subtypes are, thus making my object of study unclear. So, to constrain and simplify my enquiry, I focus specifically on kinds of experience that are consistent with the diagnostic criteria for a 'major depressive episode' or, where it recurs, 'major depressive disorder', as described in the fourth and fifth editions of the *Diagnostic and Statistical Manual of Mental Disorders* (DSM-IV-TR, p.356; DSM-5; p.163).[1]

Now, it would be naïve and dogmatic to assume the legitimacy of this diagnostic category from the outset, accept that a distinctive kind of experience is uniquely associated with it, and proceed to describe the experience in question. Things are too messy for that. Conceptions of depression are historically changeable, and diagnostic categories have undergone numerous revisions (Radden, 2000; Glas, 2003; Callahan and Berrios, 2005; Horwitz and Wakefield, 2007). There is every reason to believe that current conceptions of depression and its subtypes will be found lacking in various ways and undergo further revision. Phenomenological research has the potential to guide and motivate such revisions. It can serve to reveal profound differences between kinds of experience that were previously assumed to be much the same, as well as similarities between kinds of experience that were assumed to be very different. So it can be critical rather than just descriptive, leading us to challenge categories of 'mental disorder', at least insofar as these categories are phenomenologically motivated. Hence, although I focus principally on 'major depression', I do not take it as given that this diagnosis is associated with a distinctive kind of experience, that there is such a thing as 'the experience' of major depression, or of depression more generally. I continue to use the term 'experience/s of depression' as a convenient shorthand, but in a non-committal way. A depressed person does not have an experience *of* something called 'depression'. Rather, those with diagnoses of depression have certain kinds of experience, and my object of study is simply 'whatever experiences turn out to be consistent with and relevant to a major depression diagnosis, however varied they might be'.

----

[1] DSM-5 (p.168) also recognizes 'persistent depressive disorder', which consolidates DSM-IV's 'chronic major depressive disorder' and 'dysthymia'.

Although DSM-5 (2013) differs significantly from its predecessor in many respects, the diagnostic criteria for major depression are unchanged. According to both editions, it involves the following:

> ...there is either depressed mood or the loss of interest or pleasure in nearly all activities. In children and adolescents, the mood may be irritable rather than sad. The individual must also experience at least four additional symptoms drawn from a list that includes changes in appetite or weight, sleep, and psychomotor activity; decreased energy; feelings of worthlessness or guilt; difficulty thinking, concentrating or making decisions; or recurrent thoughts of death or suicidal ideation or suicide plans or attempts.
>
> (DSM-5, p.163; see also DSM-IV-TR, p.349)

So, one of two core symptoms must be present (depressed mood or loss of interest), along with at least four others from a list of seven (weight and/or appetite changes; sleep disturbance; activity changes; fatigue; worthlessness and/or guilt; lack of concentration; thoughts of death or suicide). It is added that these symptoms must be present for at least two weeks and affect the ability to function socially or professionally. Importantly, with the exception of changes in appetite or weight, all of the symptoms either make explicit reference to experience or imply something about experience.[2] Little is offered by way of supplementary aetiological criteria. In DSM-5 (p.161, p.164), there are some cautionary remarks to the effect that depression should not be confused with appropriate reactions to significant loss but can be present in such circumstances (remarks that part company with DSM-IV, where those who have suffered a recent bereavement are automatically excluded from a depression diagnosis). It is also stated that symptoms attributable to a general medical condition should not count towards a depression diagnosis. But that is all, and an understanding of what major depression consists of therefore depends largely on a grasp of the associated phenomenology.

Books and articles on depression tend to list various facts and figures concerning the rising number of people affected by depression, along with the huge personal and socio-economic costs of the disorder. Perhaps the most popular of these is the World Health Organization statement that depression is already the world's 'leading cause of disability' (measured by 'years lived with disability'), that it is also the 'fourth leading contributor to the global burden of disease' (measured by 'years of potential life lost due to premature mortality and the years of productive life lost due to disability'), and that it is

---

[2] It might be objected that observable 'psychomotor agitation or retardation' is non-phenomenological in character (DSM-5, p.161). However, in practice, it is doubtful that behaviour is interpreted and described without some reference to the associated experience.

predicted to rise to second place by 2020, for all ages and both sexes.[3] Given the substantial number of people who are directly or indirectly affected by depression, and the consequent volume of research that has been dedicated to it, one might expect the kinds of *experience* associated with depression diagnoses to have been comprehensively described by now, and to be well understood by clinicians and researchers. After all, without a clear and shared sense of what the term 'depression' actually refers to, it is difficult to determine whether or not claims about its prevalence and socio-economic costs are true.

However, the DSM description is remarkably cursory. For example, the suggestion that we identify something called 'depression' by identifying something else called 'depressed mood' is uninformative, as it is unclear what a depressed mood is. Furthermore, several themes that are routinely emphasized in first-person accounts hardly feature at all. Prominent aspects of depression, such as loss of hope and changes in bodily experience, are briefly acknowledged, but altered experience of time is not mentioned. Most first-person accounts also convey the intimate relationship between depression and anxiety, a relationship that the DSM description does not make clear. DSM-5 (p.184) recognizes that major depression can occur 'with anxious distress', but this tells us nothing about how the two are related: is this a distinctive type of depression experience or a depression experience much like non-anxious depression, but accompanied by something extra? Other symptoms are described in ways that are not just cursory but misleading. For instance, it is noted that 'even the smallest tasks seem to require substantial effort' (DSM-IV-TR, p.350; DSM-5, pp.163–4). This does not accommodate those cases where action seems not merely difficult but impossible, in a way that is not attributable solely to the amount of actual or perceived effort required. Impaired social function is briefly mentioned as an effect of depression, and thus—it would seem—as something caused by it rather than integral to it. Yet this is in tension with the insistence, in almost every first-person account, that changes in social and interpersonal relations are absolutely central to experiences of depression and their development, rather than by-products of depression. More generally, it is unclear how the DSM symptoms relate to each other: are they separable experiential 'components' or aspects of a unified experience? There is also the issue of heterogeneity. One of two symptoms plus four of an additional seven allows for considerable variety. Further variety is accommodated by the inclusion of nine 'specifier codes', any number of which can be tagged onto a diagnosis of major depression (DSM-5, p.162).

---

[3] World Health Organization website: <http://www.who.int/mental_health/management/depression/definition/en/> Accessed 22nd June 2012.

Along with anxious distress, these include 'mixed', 'melancholic', 'atypical' and 'psychotic' features, 'catatonia', and non-phenomenological onset criteria ('peripartum' and 'seasonal').

What would an adequate understanding of depression experiences amount to? Where psychiatry is concerned, this surely need not be a comprehensive understanding. It is not the job of clinicians or their diagnostic criteria to fully *describe* depression; the aim is to diagnose it reliably and treat it effectively. By analogy, most medical practitioners lack the expertise required to produce a detailed phenomenological analysis of influenza, but this does not interfere with its diagnosis or treatment. The analogy is somewhat misleading though, as influenza can be identified in ways that are independent of the associated phenomenology, whereas depression currently cannot. Nevertheless, one could maintain that what is needed in order to diagnose depression is just the reliable *identification* of symptoms, which does not demand anything approximating a comprehensive phenomenological understanding of them. We can detect an instance of 'depressed mood' without having much insight into the nature of what we have detected. But I will argue that the level of phenomenological understanding needed to reliably identify a distinctive kind of experience is lacking. More problematic than the explicit heterogeneity admitted by the DSM is an implicit heterogeneity underlying it. Diagnostic criteria fail to distinguish a range of subtly different kinds of experience, where the differences are—in some cases at least—qualitative and quite profound. Most of the symptoms listed by diagnostic manuals arise in the context of what I will call an 'existential change', a shift in the person's overall sense of belonging to the world. And several different kinds of existential change are compatible with a major depression diagnosis. Symptoms are inextricable from their existential contexts and therefore turn out to be equally variable, but this variety is masked by brief and superficial descriptions. For instance, I will show how 'guilt' in depression takes several different forms, as does 'loss of hope'. DSM criteria and the like, I will suggest, are insensitive to an overarching distinction between what I will call 'existential'/'pre-intentional' and 'non-existential'/'intentional' variants of guilt and hopelessness, as well as to different forms that the existential variants can take. This applies equally to experiences of agency, time and other people.

Some have argued that current conceptions of 'depression' are overly broad, due in part to changes that have been made to diagnostic criteria. For example, Horwitz and Wakefield (2007) maintain that rising rates of depression are largely attributable to expansion of the category 'depression' since the publication of DSM-III, when a 'proportionality' criterion was removed. Before this, depression might not have been diagnosed where someone had just lost her job and gone through a divorce, given that her response could be deemed proportionate to the circumstances. But, with DSM-III, circumstances like these are no longer an explicit consideration. Ghaemi (2008) adopts a slightly different view, attributing over-diagnosis of major depression to removal of the category 'neurotic depression' from DSM-III. The result, he suggests, is a conception of major depression that embraces importantly different predicaments. My own approach is non-historical. I claim that the phenomenological understanding needed to reliably distinguish different kinds of depression experience is currently lacking, but this is not to suggest that it is something we once had and have since lost. Some of the distinctions I make may not have been made before, at least not explicitly. Even so, my position is compatible with the complaint that diagnostic categories have shifted, leading to an unprincipled widening of 'depression'. Indeed, the inevitable vagueness that stems from a lack of phenomenological sensitivity surely renders the category more susceptible to unprincipled shifts in scope, some of which may involve subtle changes in diagnostic practice that are not even reflected in explicit diagnostic criteria.

I should stress that this book is not principally a contribution to the fast-growing body of anti-DSM literature. The reason I emphasize the DSM here is that it is a prominent example of a much more widespread tendency to under-describe depression. Most of the concerns I raise about the DSM apply to diagnostic practices more generally. For instance, compare the ICD-10 criteria for depressive episodes. Here, a diagnosis of depression requires the presence of at least two symptoms from a list of three: depressed mood, loss of interest/enjoyment, and loss of energy/fatigue. Additional symptoms include lowered concentration, lack of self-esteem and self-confidence, feelings of guilt or worthlessness, pessimism over the future, thoughts of self-harm or suicide, sleep disturbance, and loss of appetite (1992, p.119). ICD-10 classifies depressive episodes as 'mild', 'moderate', or 'severe'. For a mild episode, two of these additional symptoms must be present, whereas a moderate episode involves three or four. For a diagnosis of severe depression, all three symptoms from the first list need to be present, plus at least four of the others. Again, most of the symptoms are phenomenologically based and, as with the DSM, they are described only briefly. Hence, although the DSM and ICD diagnostic categories differ (with the threshold for a 'major depressive episode' falling somewhere in between the ICD-10 'moderate' and 'severe' episodes), they are alike in their reliance on cursory descriptions of depression experience.[4]

---

[4] ICD-10 is, however, more tentative in some respects. It acknowledges that there is considerable interpersonal variation, with anxiety more noticeable than the depression in many cases. It also complicates diagnosis by bringing symptom 'intensity' into consideration, and places more emphasis on the role of clinical judgement.

My aim here is neither so specific nor so ambitious as to formulate a revisionary psychiatric classification system or a new set of diagnostic criteria for depression. I offer a way of thinking about experience that facilitates a clearer and more detailed understanding of the 'existential' character of most experiences of depression. I also draw distinctions between different kinds of depression experience, which have the potential to inform classification, diagnosis, and treatment. Whether and how this actually happens will be determined by some of the many different parties involved in the research, diagnosis, and treatment of psychiatric illness. So, although I maintain that phenomenological research has an important role to play, I do not wish to suggest that it can get the job done by itself. And I do not deny that some of the distinctions drawn here approximate distinctions that are already employed in certain areas of theory and practice. (The specific shortcomings of the DSM do not apply universally.) But my aim is not just to make phenomenological distinctions. I also supply a detailed account of *what* those distinctions consist of, one that is currently lacking.

Despite the heterogeneity of depression, most depression experiences have in common a number of broad themes, including a feeling of being disconnected from the world and other people, a sense that depression is timeless and therefore inescapable, an experience of inability, and—more generally—a sense of the world as devoid of certain kinds of possibility that are more usually taken for granted. At a very general level, the majority of depression experiences are characterized by some kind of 'existential change', the variants of which all involve an impoverishment of self and world. Furthermore, some or even all of the experiences I describe could turn out to feature at different stages during the same 'episode' of depression, and/or fit into longer-term patterns involving recurrent episodes. The ability to discriminate between them could thus lead to a better appreciation of the dynamics of depression. Hence, although there is considerable variety amongst depression experiences, this does not rule out a level of description or, indeed, a classification system that unites many of them. It should be added that the purpose of psychiatric classification is not exclusively or even principally to identify phenomenological types. All sorts of criteria could be invoked to determine whether or not a classification system is legitimate. Even so, given that current conceptions of depression are heavily reliant upon phenomenology, the ability to make more refined phenomenological distinctions surely has the potential to inform classification.

My object of study is therefore more wide-ranging than the 'melancholia' (and associated melancholic disposition) that has been a primary focus for the small body of phenomenological work so far done on depression (e.g. Tellenbach, 1980, 1982; Fuchs, 2003, 2005; Stanghellini, 2004; Sass and Pienkos, 2013a, b). The difference is principally one of emphasis, and the reasons for my departure are threefold. First of all, the majority of depression diagnoses will not conform to this subtype (which corresponds roughly to the DSM category of 'major depression with melancholic features'). A phenomenological study focusing on experiential changes consistent with 'major depression' has much broader applicability, without being so broad in scope as to render the task impossible. Second, rather than accepting and describing a particular subcategory of depression, I emphasize the heterogeneity of depression experiences and develop ways of making clearer distinctions between them. Third, the phenomenological account offered here is more abstract and does not commit us to specific subcategories of depression, although the distinctions that I draw can be employed to guide and critique attempts to identify and distinguish subcategories. Those who seek to find a distinctive, melancholic subtype will be able to locate it somewhere within the framework I supply, and will hopefully find that framework informative.

On the other hand, my discussion is not so wide-ranging as to address various other proposed subtypes of depression, such as borderline depression and types of 'mixed state', at least not in any detail. Neither do I offer a fully developed account of the relationship between mania and depression in bipolar disorder. Given that major depression turns out to be heterogeneous, the project of comparing and contrasting *the* phenomenology of major depression with *the* phenomenology of something else would be a hopeless one. Furthermore, the task of describing several other kinds of experience, on top of all those associated with major depression diagnoses, would be too much for one book. That said, I should stress that my aim here is not just to offer a phenomenological account of major depression. In so doing, I also seek to formulate an interpretative framework with much wider applicability, one that can be employed to understand experiences associated with other proposed subtypes of depression and with psychiatric illness more generally.

As well as identifying types of experience, the phenomenological account developed here can be used to understand particular cases. Many sufferers remark that an inability to convey their experiences to others exacerbates an all-pervasive and painful feeling of estrangement from other people that is already so central to depression. For example, John Stuart Mill, in his *Autobiography*, says of friends that 'I had at that time none to whom I had any hope of making my condition intelligible' (1873, pp.135–6). The theme of social estrangement is equally prominent in more recent accounts, such as this:

> I could not reach other human beings. There was just an unfathomable distance between me and any other human being and it was desperately important to be able to bridge that gap, to seek a true human word between two people, you know.
>
> (Quoted by Hornstein, 2009, p.222)

A person's experience of depression cannot be cleanly separated from her ability or inability to understand it and communicate it to others, and so an enhanced appreciation of what depression is like offers the potential to mitigate distress. The point applies equally to those who are attempting to understand someone else's depression, whether medical practitioners, therapists, family, or friends. Another person's understanding, especially when recognized as such, can itself prove therapeutic.

Summary of the Argument

I begin in Chapters 1 and 2 by developing a phenomenological framework for understanding depression experiences. Chapter 1 elaborates on what I have outlined in this introduction, to emphasize how depression involves a transformation of the person's world, a change in the overall structure of experience. I suggest that talk of inhabiting a different 'world' when depressed approximates the conception of world advocated by phenomenologists such as Edmund Husserl. The 'world', in this sense, is not an explicit object of experience or thought but something we already 'find ourselves in', something that all our experiences, thoughts and activities take for granted. Depression thus involves disturbance of something so fundamental to our experience that it is seldom reflected upon and poorly understood. The chapter concludes by addressing some methodological issues we face when attempting to draw phenomenological conclusions from first-person narratives of depression. In the process, it introduces the reader to a questionnaire study, the results of which I draw on extensively in the chapters that follow. Chapter 2 then develops a more refined phenomenological analysis of the 'world' of depression. I start by introducing the term 'existential feeling', which I use to refer to variants of and changes in a 'sense of reality and belonging' that shapes all experience and thought (Ratcliffe, 2005, 2008). I go on to show how existential feelings can be understood in terms of experienced possibility: experience incorporates many different kinds of possibility, and changes in existential feeling are changes in the *kinds* of possibility one is open to. I further suggest that experiences of possibility are inextricable from bodily feeling. Although my account of how we experience possibilities takes its lead from the work of Husserl, I add that we can arrive at much the same position by starting from Heidegger. Having laid out my phenomenological approach, I make a general case for the view that depression centrally involves disturbances of existential feeling. I focus on the theme of incarceration, which features in almost all first-person accounts, and show how it can be understood in terms of possibility. In short, the world is bereft of possibilities for significant change, or at least certain kinds of significant change, with the result that one's predicament seems inescapable, eternal. The chapter concludes by proposing that 'cognitive biases' in depression are symptomatic of existential changes.

Each of Chapters 3 to 8 focuses on a more specific aspect of the existential change sketched in Chapter 2. Together, they distinguish a number of different forms that this change can take. In Chapter 3, I turn to bodily experience and emphasize that depression is very much a bodily condition, to the extent that it is sometimes difficult to distinguish phenomenologically from somatic illnesses such as influenza. I then appeal to neurobiological and immunological research on the relationship between depression and inflammation, to further support the view that depression and somatic illness have much in common. However, I add that not all depression experiences are associated with inflammation and that this points to heterogeneity, with some depressions much more akin to influenza-type experiences than others. Chapter 4 picks up on the theme of heterogeneity, this time in relation to feelings of hopelessness. First of all, I distinguish between 'intentional' and 'existential' forms of hopelessness (where the former involves feeling hopeless *about* something while the latter involves partial or complete loss of the ability to hope). I argue that, although the two are very different, both are compatible with a diagnosis of major depression. However, depression more often involves existential hopelessness, something that comes in several different forms. Some losses of existential hope are 'deeper' or 'more profound' than others, and there are also qualitative differences that cannot be couched in terms of comparative depth. The relevant conception of 'depth' is further refined in Chapter 5, this time in relation to guilt. I suggest that, although it would be incorrect to maintain that some existential feelings are deeper than others, *changes* in existential feeling can sometimes be distinguished in terms of relative depth. I distinguish between intentional and existential forms of guilt, and argue that some but not all instances of guilt that arise in depression are existential. Matters are complicated by the fact that neither intentional nor existential guilt invariably feature in depression. Furthermore, when existential guilt does arise, it is plausibly construed as a contingent way of interpreting an existential feeling that is not an intrinsically 'guilty' one.

This leads into a more general discussion of the relationship between existential feeling and self-interpretation, which explores how existential feelings shape self-narratives and vice versa.

Chapter 6 turns to the experience of inability, something that is closely associated with loss of hope and also guilt. Contrary to orthodox approaches, I propose that the sense of 'agency' or 'free will' does not consist in an 'internal' feeling. Drawing on Sartre, I argue that it is instead embedded in the experienced world, in the form of certain kinds of possibility that the world offers. Hence a change in how the world appears can also be a change in the feeling of being able to act. I distinguish several forms this can take, all of which involve the absence (and sometimes felt absence) of certain kinds of possibility from the world, amounting to a variably diminished sense of agency and vitality. I add that some depression experiences also involve other kinds of possibility becoming more salient; an all-encompassing feeling of dread can stifle activity even where some degree of experienced ability remains. Diminished agency is closely linked to changes in the structure of temporal experience, which I address in Chapter 7. Drawing on some work by Thomas Fuchs, I first distinguish implicit from explicit experiences of time. Then I challenge Fuchs' view that altered temporal experience in depression is attributable to diminution or absence of what he calls 'conative drive', a kind of active orientation towards the future. Although his account applies to some cases, I maintain that others involve—in addition or instead—a loss of significance from the world that differs from loss of conation. In the process, I offer some remarks on the phenomenology of mania and mixed states. I also further consider anxiety and guilt. The chapter teases out several different kinds of temporal experience that can be associated with a diagnosis of major depression. These map onto the different forms of hopelessness and diminished agency distinguished in earlier chapters.

Chapter 8 focuses on interpersonal experience, something that is centrally implicated in most, if not all, kinds of depression and permeates every aspect of the experience. I begin by sketching a phenomenological account of what it is to experience and relate to someone *as a person*, after which I show how depression involves a change in the structure of that relation I emphasize how relations with others can serve to 'expand' or 'contract' one's world, by changing the possibilities to which one is receptive. 'Depression', I suggest, encompasses a range of different changes in the structure of interpersonal experience. For instance, one might be indifferent to others, painfully cut off from them or experience them only in terms of threat. In all cases, though, there is loss of dynamism and openness, something that is inextricable from how hope, agency, and time are experienced. Chapter 9 further pursues the theme of interpersonal experience by asking whether and how one might empathize with depression. I argue that empathy is not principally a matter of understanding someone else by experiencing, in the first-person, what she experiences. Hence one need not have a depression-like experience oneself in order to empathize with someone else's depression. More central to empathy is the recognition and collaborative exploration of phenomenological differences between self and other. I also show how a phenomenological understanding of depression can be incorporated into an empathic process, allowing one to acknowledge the possibility of existential differences between self and other that would otherwise be missed or misconstrued.

In Chapter 10, I begin by addressing the status of the categories 'depression' and 'major depression'. I suggest that both are best regarded as metaphysically non-committal 'ideal types'. If tightened up so as to exclude non-existential changes in experience, they can serve a useful methodological role in research and practice. I also raise the issue of cultural differences and concede that the existential structure of depression may be historically and culturally variable. Then I offer some tentative remarks on whether and how depression experiences might differ from the kinds of experience associated with other diagnoses, with an emphasis on schizophrenia and depersonalization. Following this, I consider whether and why depression should be regarded as pathological, and suggest that the distinction be drawn pragmatically. I bring the discussion to a close by addressing the question of whether depression embodies an accurate or distorted evaluation of what human life has to offer. To do so, I focus on a distinctive form of 'existential despair', as described by Tolstoy. After showing that several different arguments fail to arbitrate, I identify a more promising line of enquiry, which points to the conclusion that existential despair offers an impoverished view of human life.

Chapter 1

The World of Depression

Throughout this book, I draw on work in the phenomenological tradition of philosophy in order to illuminate the nature of depression experiences. My aim in this chapter is largely methodological. I explain how what I call a 'phenomenological stance' can help us to understand and describe what it is like to be depressed, after which I outline the phenomenological method to be adopted in the chapters that follow. I begin by turning to a theme that is central to many first-person accounts: depression is somehow like being in 'a different world'. Then I suggest that what depressed people often refer to, when they use 'world' or other terms with similar connotations, is an aspect of experience that some phenomenologists similarly describe in terms of the 'world'. It is something that many who reflect on the nature of human experience overlook altogether, including many philosophers. As disturbances of world cannot be understood unless 'world' is first acknowledged as a phenomenological achievement, I suggest that a phenomenological stance (conceived of in a fairly permissive way) can be fruitfully integrated into the study of depression experiences. Following this, I describe the specifics of my own approach, which involves employing a phenomenological stance to interpret numerous first-person accounts of depression, drawing out common themes and subtle differences in the process. This is not just a matter of applying pre-formed phenomenological insights to a specific subject matter. It is also a way of doing phenomenology, which can involve making phenomenological discoveries, as well as refining, elaborating, and revising established phenomenological claims.

A Different World

I will argue that most experiences of depression involve a change in the overall structure of experience, in terms of which a variety of symptoms—including despair, bodily discomfort, inability to act, guilt, worthlessness, anxiety, and estrangement from other people—are to be understood. I refer to this as an 'existential change', by which I mean an all-enveloping shift in one's sense of 'belonging to a shared world', in something that all of one's thoughts, experiences, and activities more usually take for granted.[1] We can start to get an idea of what it amounts to by turning to a theme that is central to many first-person accounts of depression. One might think that certain kinds of familiar experience are heightened in depression while others are diminished: one feels less happy, more tired, less hopeful, more anxious, less enthusiastic, and so on. However, as I noted in the Introduction, sufferers consistently indicate that depression is qualitatively different from what many of us regard as 'everyday' experience. The depressed person finds herself in a different 'world', in an isolated, alien realm that is cut off from the consensus reality where people have more mundane experiences of feeling 'more x' or 'less y' than usual. As I also mentioned, sufferers often emphasize that the experience is extremely difficult or even impossible to describe. Sometimes, this difficulty is no doubt partly attributable to effects that depression has on one's cognitive abilities. But people still struggle to convey the experience after recovering, and their accounts often suggest that the problem stems from its very nature. Depression involves a disturbance of something that is fundamental to our lives, something that goes unnoticed when intact. What is eroded or lost is a 'sense' or 'feeling' of being comfortably immersed in the world:

> You know that you have lost life itself. You've lost a habitable earth. You've lost the invitation to live that the universe extends to us at every moment. You've lost something that people don't even know is. That's why it's so hard to explain. (Quoted by Hornstein, 2009, p.213)

> Such feelings are not easy to describe: our vocabulary—when it comes to talking about these things—is surprisingly limited. The exact quality of perception requires the resources of poetry to express. [...] I awoke into a different world. It was as though all had changed while I slept: that I awoke not into normal consciousness but into a nightmare. (Quoted by Rowe, 1978, pp.268–9)

Again and again, people remark on the strangeness and profundity of what has happened to them. Various sub-themes can be discerned, including loneliness and isolation from others, vulnerability and insecurity, unfamiliarity, inescapability, heaviness, and general unpleasantness:

> Most of all I was terribly alone, lost, in a harsh and far-away place, a horrible terrain reserved for me alone. There was nowhere to go, nothing to see, no panorama. Though this landscape surrounded me, vast and amorphous, I couldn't escape the awful confines of my leaden body and downcast eye. (Shaw, 1997, p.40)

---

[1] I am not committed to the view that an existential change is involved in all cases where a person clearly meets the diagnostic criteria for 'depression' or even 'major depression'. As my discussion proceeds, it will become clear that diagnostic criteria are not sufficiently discriminating. 'Major depression' and other diagnoses most likely encompass many kinds of predicament that do involve existential changes, along with others that do not.

My task in this book is to describe, in detail, what these changes in a person's 'world' consist of, to distinguish some of the subtly different forms they can take, and to show how they differ from other—superficially similar—experiences that arise in the context of an undisturbed world. I will begin by explaining how adoption of a phenomenological method contributes to this task.

The Relevance of Phenomenology

The phenomenological tradition encompasses a range of different methods and claims. However, we can step back from the finer details of what phenomenologists have said in order to discern a common theme: a distinctive kind of perspectival shift is nurtured, which facilitates reflection upon a more usually implicit sense of belonging to a world. I will now describe this 'phenomenological stance' and, in so doing, convey at least something of what it reveals.[2] To begin with, it may be helpful to distinguish the charge that approaches to depression in psychiatry (and elsewhere too) fail to recognize the 'world' from two complementary but importantly different criticisms. One of these, which appears in several different guises, is that biologically oriented approaches to psychiatric illness sideline the 'psychological', the 'mental', or the 'mind'. For instance, Garner and Hardcastle (2004, p.368) refer to an entrenched division between 'psyche' and 'soma'. This, they say, is accompanied by a tendency to prioritize an understanding of the 'material world', with the result that the 'mind and the mental become marginalized, perhaps even erased entirely'.[3] Much of what I will say here complements that view, and I will stress throughout that one cannot understand depression if one neglects or trivializes human experience. Nevertheless, the point could be made just as easily without adopting the kind of stance advocated here. To adopt a phenomenological stance is not merely to emphasize that our mental lives and, more specifically, our 'experience' should not be ignored.

A second criticism is that certain attitudes towards psychiatric illness restrict themselves to an objective, impersonal standpoint and thus exclude the *personal*. One can adopt an impersonal attitude towards psyche just as well as to soma, treating it as a poorly understood ingredient of the objective, ultimately

---

[2] This section further develops my account of the 'phenomenological stance' in Ratcliffe (2009a).

[3] Such criticisms need not imply any metaphysical commitments regarding the relationship between mind and matter. The concern raised by Garner and Hardcastle is that those features of human beings we label as 'psychological' get sidelined, regardless of what the 'psychological' might ultimately turn out to consist of.

impersonal world. Responding to someone as a person involves a different kind of stance or attitude. A 'personal stance' does not consist in observing certain kinds of moving object and positing the existence of mental states inside them. It is a matter of experiencing and relating to others as *persons*, something that demands adoption (usually without thought or effort) of a perspective very different from that which a scientist might adopt when scrutinising an inanimate entity. R. D. Laing (1960) compares the movement between impersonal and personal perspectives to a gestalt switch; in adopting a personal stance towards another individual, one perceives that individual very differently. He also suggests that there are no grounds for regarding the impersonal stance as epistemically privileged over the personal, or as the only type of stance that is legitimate for scientific enquiry: 'The science of persons is the study of human beings that begins from a relationship with the other as person and proceeds to an account of the other still as person' (Laing, 1960, p.20).

Laing is not alone in claiming that impersonal perspectives in psychiatry miss something important. Binswanger (1975, p.210) similarly observes that, 'as soon as I objectify my fellow man, as soon as I objectify his subjectivity, he is no longer my fellow man'. The difference between impersonal and personal stances is also emphasized by several phenomenologists, including Edmund Husserl (1989) and Alfred Schutz (1967). Again, I am sympathetic to such concerns, and I will offer a detailed account of what it is to experience and relate to someone as a person in Chapter 8.[4] However, I will do this having already adopted a phenomenological stance, and so an emphasis on the personal is not what makes the stance distinctive either. To explain what does, I will draw on the work of Husserl, but will also suggest that we can detach ourselves from the specifics of his position to endorse a broader kind of attitude that characterizes phenomenological research more generally.

Husserl maintains that, when we experience or think about another human being in a personal or an impersonal way, we do so in the context of a world that is shared by interpreter and interpreted. A background sense of residing in the same world as one's object of study is itself part of one's experience. It is something we already take for granted when reflecting on how we or others experience things. This 'world' tends to be overlooked, not because it is inessential to our experience but because it is so habitually engrained that we fail to notice it: 'more than anything else the being of the world is obvious. It is so

---

[4] For recent defences of the view that understanding others involves experiencing them as persons through a distinctive kind of stance, and for discussion of what receptivity towards others as persons consists of, see also Hobson (2002) and Ratcliffe (2007, Chapter 6).

very obvious that no one would think of asserting it expressly in a proposition' (Husserl, 1931/1960, p.17). To experience the world, in this sense, is not to experience an entity (a very big one) in the way we might experience a coffee cup sitting on the table, and neither is it a matter of entertaining some thought along the lines of 'the world exists and I am part of it'. What Husserl seeks to convey is a sense of habitual dwelling, which shapes all of our experiences and thoughts:

> Waking life is always a directedness toward this or that, being directed toward it as an end or as means, as relevant or irrelevant, toward the interesting or the indifferent, toward the private or public, toward what is daily required or intrusively new. All this lies within the world-horizon; but special motives are required when one who is gripped in this world-life reorients himself and somehow comes to make the world itself thematic, to take up a lasting interest in it. (Husserl, 1954/1970b, p.281)

There are two inextricable aspects to this background acceptance of the world: (i) an experience of being 'there', part of some situation, and (ii) what I call a 'sense of reality'. Let us start with the latter. Consider the experience of seeing a cat in front of you—what does the appreciation that 'a cat is present' involve? Taking it to be the case that a cat is present is not ordinarily a matter of assenting to the truth of a proposition on the basis of evidence gained through perception. Instead, it at least seems that you are perceptually presented with an entity of the kind 'cat', and that the perceptual experience also includes a sense of that entity as *here, now*.[5] In another situation, you might judge that a particular cat exists and is currently located somewhere, without perceiving a cat at the time. Having a *sense of reality* is not a matter of experiencing however many entities as 'here, now' or of making however many non-perceptual judgments to the effect that some state of affairs is or is not the case. Rather, it is what enables us to distinguish 'here, now' from other possibilities, and to distinguish what is the case from what is not the case. Hence it is equally presupposed by our remembering that *x* really happened, believing *x* to be true, merely imagining *x*, expecting *x*, and so on. Without any appreciation of the *contrast* between *x*'s being 'here, now' and *x*'s not being 'here, now', or *x*'s being the case and *x*'s not being the case, we could not take things to be either way. The distinctions between perceiving, believing, remembering, imagining, and expecting would therefore break down. For instance, if we lost sense of the contrast between 'here, now' and other possibilities, the distinction between perceiving and remembering would be compromised, while erosion of the more general distinction between something's being and

---

[5] There is considerable disagreement amongst philosophers concerning what we are able to 'perceive'. I will further discuss the nature and limits of 'perceptual content' in Chapter 2, clarifying my own position in the process.

not being the case would weaken our grasp of the difference between imagining that p and believing that p.

The sense of reality is itself a *phenomenological* achievement, one that is inseparable from the experience of belonging to a shared world. The 'world', in the sense I am concerned with here, is not first and foremost the object of some attitude, but a backdrop against which we are able to adopt attitudes of whatever kind towards states of affairs within the world. So it is easily missed when we reflect on the nature of our experience, given a tendency to focus exclusively on acts of perception and thought with specific contents, such as 'the cat is on the chair' or 'Jupiter is bigger than Earth'. To put it another way, the world is presupposed by the *modalities* of experience and judgment. It is a phenomenological framework in the context of which perceiving, remembering, imagining, anticipating, doubting, believing, and so forth are intelligible possibilities for a person.

Although this 'world' or 'sense of reality and belonging' is not completely lost in depression, I will argue in the following chapters that it is profoundly *altered*—the person does not feel fully 'part of the world' and everything seems somehow different. Some first-person accounts state that things look 'unreal' when one is depressed. For instance, Kaysen (2001, p.43) describes depression as 'a trip to the country of nothingness', where reality 'loses its substance and becomes ghostly, transparent, unbelievable'. But depression usually involves something more subtle: things don't seem quite 'there' or 'the case' in the way they did, which is not to say they don't appear as 'there' or 'the case' at all. I will show that such experiences cannot be accounted for solely in terms of *what* the person perceives, feels, believes, or remembers. They involve a change in the *structure* of perceiving, feeling, believing, and remembering, attributable to a disturbance of 'world'.

According to Husserl, a perspectival shift is needed in order to recognize 'world' as a phenomenological achievement. To accomplish this, he instructs us to perform the 'epoché', a suspension or bracketing of the 'natural attitude' of believing in the existence of the world. This involves, he says, a 'universal depriving of acceptance, [an] "inhibiting" or "putting out of play" of all positions taken towards the already-given Objective world and, in the first place, all existential positions' (Husserl, 1960, p.20). It is not a matter of *doubting* that the world exists. Instead, one *abstains* from all judgments concerning what 'is' and what 'is not'. Right now, I see a cup in front of me, and I take it as given that the cup is actually there. However, I can bracket my acceptance of the cup's presence and instead treat my experience of its being there as a phenomenological achievement. In the process, I do not jettison my more usual acceptance that the cup is here in front of me, in a world of which I am also a part. I preserve that aspect of the experience intact, but I detach myself from it so as to study the experience's structure. What Husserl proposes is more radical than this though. He advocates a complete or universal epoché, a total suspension of the natural attitude and all that it encompasses. This facilitates the 'phenomenological reduction', a sustained attitudinal shift that enables us to scrutinize more usually presupposed aspects of experience without distorting them in the process. In Husserl's words, the world 'goes on appearing, as it appeared before' but without 'the natural believing in existence involved in experiencing the world—though that believing too is still there and grasped by my noticing regard' (1960, pp.19–20).

If belief is construed as a matter of taking something to be the case, our 'belief' in the world's existence is not really a belief. The 'natural attitude' that Husserl asks us to suspend operates as a backdrop to our various experiences and beliefs. What is interrogated through the phenomenological reduction is not just everything we take to be the case but also the sense of reality and belonging that is presupposed by our taking anything to be the case or otherwise, something that personal and psychological understandings continue to take for granted.[6] As we will see, disturbances in this sense of 'world' are central to experiences of depression. It follows that these experiences cannot be adequately understood if we focus exclusively on changes in experiences and thoughts that occur within a pre-given world.

We do not need to endorse the finer details of Husserl's method in order to adopt what I call a 'phenomenological stance'. Husserl is often criticized for demanding that a phenomenological reduction involve complete bracketing of the natural attitude, whereby the sense of inhabiting a world becomes an object of reflection for some mysterious, detached, observational consciousness. If the reduction is conceived of as a way of experiencing one's own experience, which allows the phenomenologist to keep the sense of belonging to a world wholly intact while at the same time withdrawing from it completely in order to gaze upon its structure, then it is doubtful that such a perspective is psychologically achievable. It seems unlikely that any attitude could facilitate suspension of the natural attitude in its entirety; we will always end up presupposing something or other. Furthermore, it is arguable that a reflective attitude

---

[6] A phenomenological stance is therefore quite different from introspection, where the latter is construed as a process of 'inner' reflection. What the phenomenologist attends to, amongst other things, is the experience of being part of a world *within which* one occupies a contingent and partial perspective. In focusing attention 'inwards' or 'outwards', one has already accepted world-experience as a backdrop against which some things are experienced as internal and others external.

cannot be adopted towards an experience without altering the experience in some way. But the kind of attitude I seek to nurture here does not require anything so extreme, and is something that other phenomenologists who criticize Husserl's approach themselves adopt. For instance, Merleau-Ponty (1945/1962, ix–xiv) states that the 'most important lesson which the reduction teaches us is the impossibility of a complete reduction'. However, he describes his own project as returning to a 'world which precedes knowledge', to a kind of experience that is 'not even an act, a deliberate taking up of a position' but 'the background from which all acts stand out', something that is 'presupposed by them'. He adds that, despite disagreements between Husserl and Heidegger, what Heidegger in *Being and Time* calls 'Being-in-the-world' is exactly what we gain reflective access to by performing the phenomenological reduction. This sounds right to me. For example, Heidegger (1927/1962, p.102) writes that 'the world itself is not an entity within-the-world; and yet it is so determinative for such entities that only in so far as "there is" a world can they be encountered and show themselves, in their Being, as entities which have been discovered'. This conveys much the same broad conception of 'world' that we find in Husserl and Merleau-Ponty: something that is seldom an explicit object of experience or thought; something that we are already practically, unreflectively immersed in when we experience something, think about it, or act upon it.

Instead of worrying any more about the nature of the phenomenological reduction and whether it is possible, I want to adopt a fairly permissive conception of it. A phenomenological stance, as I understand it here, is not a radical transformation of all experience, where the phenomenologist becomes, as Husserl puts it, 'the "non-participant onlooker" at himself' (1960, p.37). Rather, it is a methodological shift, through which one comes to appreciate that certain questions cannot be satisfactorily addressed from the standpoint(s) of empirical science or from any other perspective that takes a sense of reality and belonging as given. Such a stance does not require total removal of all existential commitment. What it involves is the *acknowledgement* that there is an experientially constituted sense of reality and belonging, coupled with a commitment to studying it further using whatever resources are at our disposal. I do not want to suggest that we *first* adopt a phenomenological stance and *then* apply it to depression. Depression is not just a subject matter to which I apply a pre-formed phenomenological method; reflection upon disturbances of world-experience is integral to my method. Although a complete removal of the sense of reality from experience is not needed for phenomenological enquiry, examination of changes in world-experience can play an important role. Aspects of experience that we ordinarily overlook sometimes become more salient to us when they are altered in some way; we glimpse them as they shift.[7] I also maintain that the study of 'existential changes'—shifts in the background sense of reality and belonging—need not restrict itself to one's own experiences. Indeed, reflecting on others' descriptions of existential changes can assist in orienting the enquirer towards a phenomenological stance in the first place. First-person descriptions of experience can help make it apparent that there is a genuine realm of enquiry here, one that calls for a distinctive kind of approach. The relevant experiences can then be described more clearly and in more detail as one comes to interpret them through a phenomenological stance. Approaches that continue to presuppose the world will not succeed in interpreting these experiences, as they will misconstrue existential changes as changes in experiences and/or thoughts that arise within a world.

So a phenomenological stance need not be an attitude that is adopted in its entirety before anything of the world is revealed. After all, it is unclear how one could adopt the stance without at least some sense of what one is re-directing one's attention towards. Instead, there is a progressive coming into focus of the world, and thus an ongoing commerce between a phenomenological stance and its subject matter. It follows that the stance is not an attitude with neatly defined boundaries. Nevertheless, we can offer a general characterization of what it involves. A phenomenological stance, however refined, includes (i) attentiveness to an aspect of experience that is more usually presupposed and overlooked; (ii) a commitment to reflect upon it; and (iii) at least some appreciation of *what* the relevant aspect of experience consists of. Having adopted the stance and thus suspended acceptance of what is more usually taken for granted as *our* world (which was never just *my* world), we can then contemplate our own experience and/or that of others. Whichever the case, the stance allows us to entertain the possibility of phenomenological differences and changes of a kind that would otherwise be unintelligible. I will argue that most of those predicaments diagnosed as 'depression' involve changes in world. I say 'most', as I acknowledge that some do not. However, we cannot make sense of the distinction between experiences that involve

---

[7] Heidegger (1962, p.232) makes this point in relation to a change in the structure of world-experience that he calls 'anxiety' [*Angst*]. Heideggerian anxiety is a total eradication of practical significance from the world, of something that is partly constitutive of our more usual sense of belonging. Anxiety plays an important role in Heidegger's method; how we ordinarily take the world for granted becomes conspicuous in its absence and thus amenable to phenomenological study. See Ratcliffe (2008, Chapter 9) for the claim that a wide range of 'wobbles' in the structure of experience can similarly facilitate phenomenological enquiry.

changes *within* one's world and others that involve changes *to* one's world until we have adopted a phenomenological stance. The reader need not start out convinced by all of this. With at least some appreciation of what it is to make the world an object of enquiry, along with a degree of openness to the possibility of profoundly different forms of experience, we can let our subject matter guide us and—in the process—progressively refine our understanding of the sense of reality and belonging.

Narratives of Depression

To study the phenomenology of depression, we need access to experiences of depression. Although I have experienced at least some of the predicaments that I will describe here, this book is not primarily an exercise in first-person phenomenology and instead turns a phenomenological stance towards the experiences of others.[8] As I will further emphasize in Chapter 9, one need not have 'experienced depression' oneself in order to study it phenomenologically or, indeed, to empathize with it (and, as I will also make clear, empathy is not quite the same thing as phenomenological understanding). In what follows, I will engage with various written accounts of what it is like to experience depression, an approach that raises a number of methodological issues. It would be a mistake to take first-person descriptions at face value, to construe them as neutral, unmotivated, wholly reliable phenomenological reports. The content of any given account will be shaped by a wide range of factors. I will draw on published depression memoirs, amongst other sources. There is thus a risk of selection bias—these accounts are often written by professional authors, whose depression experiences and ways of relating them might differ from those of many others. Another concern is that depression memoirs are edited selectively for publication, and consist of polished prose that may differ markedly in style and content from unrevised first-person reports that are obtained in other ways. A depression narrative of whatever kind is also situated in a social and cultural context, which will be reflected to some extent in how the author understands his depression. For instance, it might be shaped by culturally entrenched conceptions of gender.[9] More generally, narrative content is constrained by the concepts a person has at her disposal, and by

[8] Having said that, I do worry a bit about Nietzsche's remark in *Beyond Good and Evil* that a work of philosophy is an implicit 'confession on the part of its author and a kind of involuntary and unconscious memoir' (2003, p.37).

[9] For example, Emmons (2008, pp.111–12) argues that the stereotype of the 'excessively emotional woman' fuels a conception of depression as a radical disturbance of men's affective lives but an 'outgrowth' of the 'complex emotional lives' of women.

culturally variable canonical narratives that become engrained from an early age (e.g. Bruner, 1990). Depression memoirs are also influenced in more specific ways by established styles of writing about depression, which could have a considerable influence on which aspects of the experience are related and how. This influence most likely extends to narrative form, as well as content. Many recent accounts of depression take the form of a quest or journey narrative: depression is portrayed as something one gets through or overcomes, like sailing a boat through a stormy sea or finding one's way through a dark forest.[10] In the process, a somewhat formulaic 'confessional style' is often adopted. Published narratives also tend to impose some degree of closure, an end to the journey, which may not reflect the untidy realities of the person's situation. In contrasting his own experience with established narrative styles, one author remarks, 'I see, or feel, no conclusions but rather ambiguities, contradictions, and openings' (Smith, 1999, p.275).

Furthermore, depression narratives are not unmotivated. Although not all motives will be transparent to authors or to readers, some are explicitly mentioned. For example, Tim Lott writes that his interpretation of events is driven not so much by a desire to relate an experience to others as by a yearning for coherence, a felt need to impose some kind of meaningful structure on what has happened:

> Facts, there are so many facts. I have left such a lot out. There must be many more unremembered and still more unknown. If I had chosen differently, it would be a different story, but this is the story I have told myself and I must hold to it. It is a trick I am trying to learn. I need a story and that is the nub, that is what it *boils down to*, as my father always says. [...] It is dangerous not knowing the shape of your own life. (Lott, 1996, p.174)

First-person accounts are not just descriptions of experience; they can also play regulatory roles. How the relationship between one's illness and one's life is narrated and re-narrated, and—in the process—interpreted and negotiated with family, friends, colleagues, clinicians, and others, could well have a significant influence on one's social relations and, through them, on the course of a depression (Kangas, 2001, p.77; Beilke, 2008). For instance, in constructing a narrative around her depression, a person might assemble a selective account of herself, excluding various deeds from her biography by attributing them to the illness (Radden, 2009, Chapter 10). Hence it is likely

---

[10] The word 'journey' often features in the titles of published accounts, as does the word 'through'. For instance, the 2002 reprint edition of Thompson (1995) has the new subtitle *A Journey through Depression*.

that experiences of depression are presented in ways that are, in some respects at least, misleading.

The problem is not simply that of determining whether one thing, a 'narrative', adequately represents a completely separate thing, a 'depression'. According to some, narrative is integral to emotional experience rather than something imposed on pre-formed emotional episodes. For instance, Goldie (2000, pp.4–5) construes emotions not as brief events but, in many instances, as processes. Their unity and the ways in which they unfold over time are, he maintains, partly attributable to their narrative structure: 'it is the notion of narrative structure which ties together and makes sense of the individual elements of emotional experience—thought, feeling, bodily change, expression, and so forth—as parts of a structured episode'. It is similarly arguable that how depression is experienced cannot be cleanly separated from how it is interpreted. It is also difficult to distinguish cause from effect here, as the relationship between depression and its interpretation is not unidirectional. Depression most likely disposes authors towards certain narrative styles, a point that I will return to in Chapter 5. However, even if the boundary between experience and its interpretation is blurred, this does not rule out a degree of mismatch between an experience and a written account of it. There may also be various competing narratives shaping the person's experience, thought and conduct, not all of which are represented in her written account.

Another concern is that depression memoirs are usually written after rather than during periods of depression, potentially compromising their reliability. Then again, narratives written while the person is depressed could be unreliable as well, due to the effects of cognitive biases and impairments that are symptomatic of depression. The line between depression and recovery is not, however, a clear one, and many people describe a process of recovery that involves occasional lapses into depression. Published accounts also often include letters or other writings that were composed while depressed (e.g. Shaw, 1997, pp.28–30). The fact that what people describe when depressed is largely consistent with what they describe after recovering offsets the worry that depression or recovery has a significant distorting effect. Even so, when taken together, the concerns I have raised suggest that first-person testimonies should be approached with caution. This is not to advocate distrust and suspicion; there is a difference between 'respect' and 'credulity' (Pies, 2013). We can respect a person's narrative, seek to interpret it in the light of a phenomenological theory and draw phenomenological insights from it, without naively taking its content at face value or ruling out the possibility of alternative interpretations.

Some of the issues I have raised apply specifically to published memoirs, and so it is important not to over-rely on them as a source of testimony. Another source, which I will draw on extensively in the chapters that follow, is an Internet questionnaire study that I conducted with colleagues in 2011. (All numbered quotations are from responses to this depression questionnaire, which I refer to hereafter as 'DQ'.) The choice of questions was guided by themes that feature prominently in depression memoirs, as well as in conversations I have had with depressed people, interview transcripts, self-help guides, and diagnostic manuals:

- Describe your emotions and moods during those periods when you are depressed. In what ways are they different from when you are not depressed?
- Does the world look different when you're depressed? If so, how?
- Do other people, including family and friends, seem different when you're depressed? If so, how?
- How does your body feel when you're depressed?
- How does depression affect your ability to perform routine tasks and other everyday activities?
- When you are depressed, does time seem different to you? If so, how?
- How, if at all, does depression affect your ability to think?
- In what ways, if any, does depression make you think differently about life compared to when you are not depressed?
- If you have taken medication for depression, what effect did it have?
- Are there aspects of depression that you find particularly difficult to convey to others? If so, could you try as best you can to indicate what they are and why they are so hard to express.
- What do you think depression is and what, in your view, caused your depression?
- Who and/or what have you consulted in order to try to understand your depression? (E.g., medical practitioners, friends, books, Internet sources, etc.).

Participants were asked to provide free text responses with no word limit. An introductory section requested background information, including age, gender, country of residence, year of diagnosis, details of diagnosis, any other psychiatric diagnoses, any treatment received, and whether they were depressed at the time of writing.[11] Within three months of posting the questionnaire on

---

[11] The study went through an ethical approval process conducted by the Durham University Department of Philosophy. It included a consent form and detailed guidance notes.

the website of the mental health charity SANE, 145 complete responses had been received, at which point it was closed to new entrants. Most responses included detailed descriptions of experience and, together, they added up to several hundred pages of testimony. Age range of participants was 16 to 76, and many more women than men participated, with 119 describing themselves as 'female', 24 as 'male', one as 'gender-queer' and one as 'confused'. 104 respondents stated that they were depressed at the time of writing and, in other cases, time since the last period of depression varied considerably. Several different depression diagnoses were listed. The most common were 'major depression', 'severe depression', 'clinical depression', and just 'depression'. Others included 'chronic depression', 'mild depression', 'major seasonal affective disorder', and 'dysthymia'. Additional psychiatric diagnoses appeared in 100 responses. 'Anxiety', 'anxiety disorder', or 'generalized anxiety disorder' was explicitly mentioned in 38 and implied by several others. In some instances, it was unclear whether separate diagnoses had been received: 'Anxiety, or is that part of the depression?' (#155).[12] In others, depression and anxiety diagnoses were given at different times. Other frequently mentioned diagnoses included 'borderline personality disorder', 'hypomania', 'bipolar disorder' (sometimes specified as bipolar I or II), 'obsessive compulsive disorder', and 'eating disorders'. Several respondents reported a succession of different diagnoses over several years, which were, in some instances, attributed to changes or differences in clinical opinion, rather than changes in their own experience of illness: 'I have had many possible diagnoses discussed with me over the years. [...] It has seemed hard for psychiatrists to agree on which category I am in' (#280).[13]

At a very general level of description, responses were fairly consistent and most of them pointed to an 'existential change', the nature of which I will describe

[12] Some people registered for the study but did not ultimately submit their questionnaires, which is why questionnaire identification numbers exceed 145.

[13] The issue of how to understand the relationship between depression and other psychiatric conditions that are 'comorbid' with it is complicated by the heterogeneity of depression. It can be difficult to distinguish 'an experience of one or another type of depression' from 'an experience of depression plus something else'. In the terms of my own analysis, what is described as 'x plus y' might instead be conceived of as a unitary existential change, z, one that differs from both x and y. In Chapters 6 and 7, I will argue that 'depression plus anxiety' should be understood as a unitary existential change, as should various 'mixed states' that include features of both mania and depression. In Chapter 10, I will make similar points about depression, schizophrenia, and depersonalisation. However, I do not wish to suggest that all cases of 'comorbidity' should be construed in the same way.

in Chapter 2. As I will show in Chapters 3 to 8, this existential change takes a number of different forms. But, for the most part, the specific diagnoses listed in questionnaires had little or no bearing on the kinds of experience described, the only obvious exceptions being a few responses that mentioned mania, psychosis, or eating disorders. All of the experiences I will describe here are consistent with a diagnosis of 'major depression' and, as differences in diagnosis were not phenomenologically informative, I will seldom mention them when drawing on questionnaire responses. However, I have added an appendix, with includes diagnoses for all those questionnaires I quote from. Another factor to consider is medication. DQ respondents mentioned several different prescribed medications (mostly selective serotonin re-uptake inhibitors [SSRIs]), as well as non-prescribed drugs such as alcohol. In those cases where the distinctive side-effects of medication were discussed, respondents tended to distinguish them from their experiences of 'depression'. Some stated that medication made them feel better, some worse, and others that it made no difference. No doubt, many different substances can play roles in causing, intensifying, altering, prolonging, or lessening depression experiences. And I do not wish to dismiss the plausible view that some prescribed medications and patterns of substance abuse are causally associated with certain *kinds* of depression experience. Nevertheless, the kinds of experience I discuss here are all wider-ranging; they are not *uniquely* associated with the effects of medication, prescribed or otherwise.[14]

Most DQ respondents offered detailed and nuanced descriptions of their experiences, even though some who self-identified as 'currently depressed' also wrote that they were barely able to think or act.[15] What those who were depressed at the time of writing described was entirely consistent with the

---

[14] There are many different phenomenological and causal stories to be told about the relationships between depression, medication, and substance abuse. Take the example of alcohol abuse. The kinds of experience related by some 'alcoholic memoirs' are difficult to distinguish from those found in some memoirs of depression. Indeed, it could be that the difference is sometimes one of narrative emphasis. Flanagan (2013, p.869) suggests that certain depression memoirs amount to 'recessive alcoholic memoirs'; the depression narrative takes centre-stage while alcoholism, which may be equally implicated in the events and experiences described, remains largely implicit.

[15] One might wonder why someone who feels barely able to act at all would complete a lengthy, anonymous questionnaire. In a few instances, participants expressed relief or gratitude that someone was asking these kinds of question, or stated that they found the exercise therapeutic. It is possible that engaging with the questionnaire fulfilled, to at least some degree, a need to connect with others (of a kind I will discuss in Chapter 8) and to communicate one's predicament. But this is just speculation. Of course, many people probably just wanted to help; depression seldom completely eradicates all cares, concerns, and commitments.

accounts of those who were not. Testimonies were also consistent with what published memoirs describe, serving to dispel some of the concerns raised about the latter. The only notable difference in content was that DQ respondents were often more openly hostile towards themselves and/or others. There was more anger, resentment, and hate: 'Negative. Self hate. Angry.' (#8); 'veer from being completely numb to anger and hatred and self-hatred' (#61); 'I am very aggressive and abusive' (#85). It is easy to see why some such themes might be edited out of published accounts or at least toned down in the absence of anonymity, given that the narrative is also a way for others to interpret its author and her actions.

Of course, the questionnaire study does not avoid all of the problems mentioned earlier, and we should be sensitive to its limitations. The risk of a sampling bias remains, as respondents were limited mostly to those who visited the SANE website and then decided to participate in an anonymous questionnaire study. Hence they had to be well enough to write, and they may also have over-represented a distinctive subset of the depressed population. All but five respondents were UK residents. Although this does not rule out the presence of considerable social and cultural diversity, it could well be that the kinds of experience described and ways of describing them were, in certain ways, population-specific. Gender is another issue. 82% of respondents were female (for this reason, I use the third-person pronoun 'she' more often than 'he' in the chapters that follow), and so the overall body of testimony may well reflect experiences and/or understandings of depression that are more typical of women than men.[16] It may well be that depression itself is more 'typical' of one gender than another, and it is routinely reported that around twice as many women as men suffer from depression.[17] That view is questionable though. For any number of reasons, it could be that women are more likely to receive depression diagnoses than men who have similar kinds of experience. Then again, it is at least possible that men are more likely to be diagnosed as depressed than women, and that the gender difference is even

---

[16] See Ussher (2010) for a wide-ranging discussion of women's depression. Ussher considers a number of hypothesized causes for higher prevalence of depression in women, as well as the possibility that it is a social construction involving the pathologisation of femininity. She adopts a 'critical-realist' approach, which acknowledges the reality of distress but maintains that it is 'only discursively constructed as "depression" within a specific historical and cultural context' (2010, p.23).

[17] See Nolen-Hoeksema (1990) for a detailed study of reported rates of depression in women and men (which takes account of age, social circumstances, and culture), as well as for a consideration of methodological issues and several candidate explanations.

more pronounced than it seems.[18] For current purposes, I set this issue aside. I am concerned not with whether or why more women than men become depressed but with what depression experiences consist of. And I am confident that none of the forms of experience I describe here are *exclusive* to women or men (unless post-partum depression is recognized as a distinctive *phenomenological* subtype), at least not at the level of description I adopt.

Use of questionnaires also has more general limitations. Any one response supplies us with less information than—say—a single, well-conducted interview, and the former is also more likely to be vague or ambiguous.[19] Interviews give one the opportunity to ask follow-up questions and seek clarification, to challenge and revise one's interpretations. As Jaspers (1963, p.55) emphasizes, sustained one-to-one dialogue can facilitate a kind of exploratory process that is essential to phenomenological work within psychiatry. Nevertheless, a questionnaire study has advantages too. One of these is breadth. When scrutinizing a substantial number of testimonies, broader patterns emerge and common themes are more readily discernible. I concede that it is easy to misinterpret any one response, and that I will have done so on occasion. But this does not detract from my overall aim, which is to distinguish the *types* of existential change associated with diagnoses such as 'major depression', something that does not require assigning every respondent to the right type with complete confidence. As I will emphasize in Chapter 9, the phenomenological framework developed here can then be integrated into a dialogical, empathetic process, so as to interpret the experiences of specific individuals with greater confidence.

When quoting from questionnaires, I have corrected spelling and typing errors, as well as some of the punctuation. One might object that some apparent 'mistakes' or 'anomalies' are expressive or otherwise informative and, in a few instances, presentation is indeed revealing. For example:

#65.
I feel:
black

---

[18] There are cultural differences to consider as well. For example, Kitanaka (2012, Chapter 8) discusses the male-oriented 'psychiatric master narrative' of depression in contemporary Japan and the impoverished appreciation of women's suffering that arises as a result. In conjunction with this, she notes, recorded rates of depression in Japan are as high in men as in women.

[19] In addition, I cannot exclude the possibility of respondents supplying deliberately misleading information. However, it is very unlikely that this would apply to more than a small minority. Furthermore, the consistency or responses and lack of any obvious anomalies suggests otherwise.

empty
dark
hopeless
worthless
unimportant
i think about dying
troubled
traumatized
like a shroud of darkness has descended on me

Here, the fragmented, unpunctuated list of adjectives itself conveys something of the emotions involved. It has been suggested that certain depression narratives, especially published ones, are misrepresentative. In contrast to the raw accounts that can be found on Internet chat rooms and elsewhere, they tidy up the prose and erase the expressiveness of textual structure (Benzon, 2008). However, the majority of DQ responses were written in clear, fairly conventional prose, and I very much doubt that sanitizing of structure poses a major challenge. That we can gain different insights from other modes of expression does not imply that conventional prose *misrepresents* depression or irrevocably excludes some aspect of the experience.

At no point do I treat first-person descriptions of depression as *data* to be *analysed* by an impartial spectator. Instead, I regard them as *testimony* to *interpret*. This book is an exercise in hermeneutic phenomenology: first-person testimonies are interpreted through a phenomenological stance, and both the stance and its subject matter increasingly resolve themselves as the discussion progresses. So what I am doing here is not a poor substitute for the scientific analysis of data. It is something different, something that is equally indispensable if we are to understand the nature of depression. One cannot adequately appreciate experiences of depression unless one adopts an interpretative stance along the lines I have described, thus directing enquiry towards a sense of belonging to the world that empirical scientific enquiry presupposes. A shift in this sense of belonging is a salient and consistent theme in DQ responses, as well as in published accounts. It is almost always described as a kind of 'feeling', often one of 'disconnection'. The person is cut off from the world and, most importantly, from habitual forms of interaction with other people:

#17. Often, the world feels as though it is a very long way away and [...] it takes an enormous amount of effort to engage with the world and your own life. It feels as though you're watching life from a long distance. At times it felt as though I was looking through a fish eye lens, and couldn't see clearly around the periphery, or even very well at all. I felt slightly pulled back from reality, as though there were cotton wool between my brain and my senses. A feeling of exhaustion often prevented me from being able to interact with the world, adding to the inability to process what was going on around me.

#20. When I'm depressed it is like I have become separated from the rest of the world.

#84. I feel disconnected from the rest of the world, like a spectator. I only see I was depressed when it stops. It's like dust, you don't notice it until you wipe it off and see the difference.

#138. I feel like I am watching the world around me and have no way of participating.

#282. It feels as if I am a ghost—I cannot touch or see the world clearly and it all becomes grey and transparent.

Several sub-themes can be discerned already: perception is somehow altered; the depressed person is cut off from everyone and everything; she feels exhausted, passive, and incapable of action. The theme of separation is often mirrored by that of incarceration—the person is adrift from the consensus world *and* imprisoned somewhere else: 'I feel as if I am in a bubble' (#143). She finds herself somewhere inescapable, eternal, and often threatening. However, the emphasis varies, and the theme of belonging to a world that is frightening, cruel,or even evil often features without reference to that of detachment or incarceration: 'the world seems scarier and more hateful' (#61); 'It seems a very unwelcoming place' (#168). Such differences in emphasis are, I will show, phenomenologically informative.

One might think that 'feeling' is just bodily, and therefore something that is distinct from how the world looks and whether one experiences oneself as part of it. However, I will argue that bodily feeling, how the world appears and how one relates to it are all inextricable aspects of a unitary phenomenological structure, a felt sense of reality and belonging. Chapter 2 will offer a general analysis of this structure and the kinds of existential shift that it is susceptible to, focusing on the theme of incarceration. The chapters that follow will turn to more specific aspects of depression, further refining the analysis while at the same time emphasizing depression's heterogeneity. In the process, it will become increasingly evident that seemingly different depression 'symptoms', such as bodily discomfort, altered experience of time, inability to act, estrangement from other people and deep despair are not mere accompaniments to each other but inseparable aspects of a unitary shift in 'how one finds oneself in the world'.

Chapter 2

Experiencing the Possible

In Chapter 1, I introduced the theme of 'world', as conceived of by phenomenologists such as Husserl. I described it as a 'sense of reality and belonging', to be contrasted with an object of experience or thought. In this chapter, I offer a more detailed phenomenological analysis. I begin by observing that the sense of reality and belonging is changeable. Although 'world' is seldom explicitly acknowledged as part of our experience, it becomes more salient when it shifts from one form to another. One might think that these shifts are unfamiliar to many or most of us. However, I suggest that how we 'find ourselves in a world' undergoes all sorts of subtle variations in the course of everyday life. Variants and the transitions between them are often alluded to in conversation, but there is no neat, established vocabulary for expressing and communicating them. They consist of a distinctive kind of *feeling*, one that does not fit into established categories such as 'emotion' and 'mood'. I call this 'existential feeling', given that it amounts to a changeable sense of being 'there', 'part of the world'.

My previous book, *Feelings of Being*, was a wide-ranging survey of existential feelings. I cover some of the same ground in this chapter, but also refine and elaborate my earlier account. Then, in the remainder of the book, I develop a detailed account of the kinds of existential feeling that arise in depression. This account focuses on several more specific aspects of existential feeling in depression (bodily discomfort, hopelessness, guilt, diminished agency, and altered temporal and interpersonal experience), and the concept of existential feeling does not always feature explicitly. Even so, it serves as a unifying interpretive framework throughout, within which to locate the more fine-grained analyses (although they can also be read independently of it). In this chapter, I supply the details of that framework by construing 'existential feeling' in terms of the kinds of *possibility* that experience incorporates. Although my approach draws on the work of Husserl and, to a lesser extent, Heidegger, I do not want to suggest that we take their writings as gospel. The aim is to formulate a phenomenological analysis that is broadly *right*, by drawing inspiration from the work of others (as I have interpreted it) and doing so critically. Towards the end of the chapter, I show how my analysis of existential feeling gives us the conceptual tools needed to understand existential changes in depression. To do so, I focus on the theme of feeling somehow 'confined' or 'incarcerated', and argue that it is attributable to the loss of certain kinds of possibility from experience. The chapter concludes by briefly addressing the shortcomings of cognitive approaches to depression, which either ignore or misconstrue the existential changes underlying depressive 'cognitive styles'.

Existential Feelings

Depression is said to be a 'mood disorder'. So, in order to understand the experience, we might turn to the fast-growing philosophical and interdisciplinary literature on emotions and moods. But something is missing from that literature, something essential to an understanding of depression experiences. Emotions are generally treated as intentional states, bodily feelings, or a combination of the two, and moods as generalized emotions. When one is angry, the anger has intentionality: it is directed at something, *about* something.[1] Along with this, one *feels* angry: there is an experience of bodily arousal that may or may not be specific to anger. Hence, when it is asked what emotions such as anger *are*, the central issue is often taken to concern the respective roles of feelings and intentional states: do emotions consist of one, the other, or both? Whereas one might be angry about something specific, such as being insulted, and often for a only a short time, moods are often construed as longer-term states that are directed at more encompassing states of affairs, perhaps even at the world as a whole.[2] For instance, Solomon (1993, p.71) claims that moods are just 'generalized emotions', with the level of generality varying from case to case. Goldie (2000, p.141) similarly proposes that the difference between moods and emotions is attributable primarily to the 'degree of specificity of their objects'.[3] Alternatively, it could be argued that moods lack intentionality altogether, that they are not about anything at all.

I accept that some moods are probably intentional experiences with very general objects and I also concede that, in some instances, it is unclear

---

[1] I adopt a phenomenological conception of intentionality throughout, treating it as a directedness that is integral to experience. In recent years, intentionality has been reinvented by some philosophers as a non-phenomenological relation of 'aboutness'. There is no philosophical disagreement here; it is just a terminological matter. I am using the term in its traditional sense, whereas they are using it to talk about something else.

[2] See Ratcliffe (2008, Chapter 1; 2010b) for a more detailed discussion of such views.

[3] Roberts (2003, p.115) adds that mood is analogous to a colour or tone: 'depression and elation color the objects of our experience in hues of value'.

what the intentional object is or whether there is an intentional object at all. However, this does not exhaust our options. Some of those experiences we call 'moods' are not generalized emotions or feelings without intentionality; they are 'ways of finding oneself in the world'. As such, they are what we might call 'pre-intentional', meaning that they determine the kinds of intentional states we are capable of having, amounting to a 'shape' that all experience takes on. (In what follows, I will use the terms 'pre-intentional' and 'existential' interchangeably and will, for the most part, adopt the latter. But the former is helpful for some purposes, in emphasizing what it is that distinguishes the 'existential' from the 'intentional'.) Not all moods fit this characterization, and so it is important to distinguish a pre-intentional subset of moods (Ratcliffe, 2010a; 2010b).[4] The point applies to emotions too. Some emotional experiences fall into the category 'pre-intentional', but others do not. For example, Brampton (2008, p.3) states that her experience of depression involved a 'paralysis of hope'. What she goes on to describe is not a matter of her ceasing to hope that *p* and hope that *q*, for however many hopes. The loss is more profound than that—her world is bereft of the possibility of hoping. Hence certain established emotion types, such as 'hope' (and 'hopelessness'), have both pre-intentional and intentional variants, a point I will return to in Chapters 4 and 5.

The aspect of experience to be addressed here is not restricted to 'some instances of some established types of mood and emotion'. There is a tendency in the philosophical literature and elsewhere to focus on standard inventories of emotions, which include the likes of anger, sadness, fear, joy, grief, jealousy, guilt, and so on.[5] Consequently, a range of other affective experiences, some of which do not even have established names, are overlooked. Although the category 'neglected feelings' is not phenomenologically unitary, many of these experiences do have something in common. Whenever we are happy, sad, or angry about something, we already *find ourselves in the world*, a phenomenological achievement that can vary in structure. Its variants, as well as the transitions between them, are most often described as 'feelings'. Such feelings feature prominently in first-person accounts of depression and other kinds of psychiatric illness, as well as in a range of other contexts. As I observed in my book *Feelings of Being*:

---

[4] See also Strasser (1977, Part 3) for a distinction between intentional and pre-intentional feelings. The term 'pre-intentional' is also used in a similar way by Searle (e.g. 1983, p.156).

[5] For an exception, see Roberts (2003, p.181), who lists many kinds of emotion, including some that seldom feature in scholarly discussions.

> People sometimes talk of feeling alive, dead, distant, detached, dislodged, estranged, isolated, otherworldly, indifferent to everything, overwhelmed, suffocated, cut off, lost, disconnected, out of sorts, not oneself, out of touch with things, out of it, not quite with it, separate, in harmony with things, at peace with things or part of things. There are references to feelings of unreality, heightened existence, surreality, familiarity, unfamiliarity, strangeness, isolation, emptiness, belonging, being at home in the world, being at one with things, significance, insignificance, and the list goes on. People also sometimes report that 'things just don't feel right', 'I'm not with it today', 'I just feel a bit removed from it all at the moment', 'I feel out of it' or 'it feels strange'. (Ratcliffe, 2008, p.68)

Some such experiences take the form of brief episodes, while others are more enduring. Indeed, they can persist for so long that they amount to character traits—a person can be habitually 'detached', 'distant', or 'out of touch'. Changes in the existential structure of experience are noticed to varying degrees and in different ways. They need not incorporate insight; one might look back and only then come to realize 'I was in a bad place at the time', 'I was somehow out of touch with things', or 'I was so alone that I didn't even realize it'. On occasion, other people are better able to detect a change in one's 'world', and increased first-person insight may then arise through dialogue. However, there is often first-person awareness of an 'existential change' as it occurs: the world *looks* somehow different, novel, or lacking; a feeling of strangeness is very much part of the experience. Talk of these experiences is actually quite commonplace, as we come to appreciate once we acknowledge them as a distinctive phenomenological type and are thus able to 'look out' for them. There is no tension between this and my claim in Chapter 1 that 'world' is an aspect of experience we seldom reflect upon. There is a difference between our gesturing towards a particular experience that we find puzzling, and our explicitly referring to, and then describing, a *type* of experience. Furthermore, although all of us are susceptible to subtle existential changes, fewer people experience profound disturbances of the kind that feature in major depression, which are not as easily conveyed through everyday discourse.

If we are to identify and then analyse the group of feelings that comprise pre-intentional ways of 'finding oneself in the world', a technical term is appropriate for two reasons. First of all, some established emotion and mood types accommodate pre-intentional and intentional experiences, and the differences between these experiences are eclipsed by use of the same terms to refer to both. Second, a term is needed to accommodate all those 'feelings' that do not currently fall under established categories. Hence I have adopted the term 'existential feeling' (Ratcliffe, 2005; 2008). Variants of existential feeling are often described as 'the feeling of *x*', where *x* can be a single word, such as 'unfamiliarity', 'strangeness', or 'detachment'. People also talk of 'the feeling of being *x*', where *x* might be 'cut off from everyone', 'behind a glass wall', 'suffocated', or, in contrast, 'at home in the world'. However, they are also conveyed in more elaborate ways, as illustrated by the many detailed and nuanced descriptions that can be found in literature. Take the famous lines:

> I have of late—but wherefore I know not—lost all my mirth, forgone all custom of exercises; and indeed it goes so heavily with my disposition that this goodly frame, the earth, seems to me a sterile promontory. This most excellent canopy, the air, look you, this brave o'erhanging firmament, this majestical roof fretted with golden fire, why, it appears no other thing to me than a foul and pestilent congregation of vapours. (*Hamlet*, Act 2, Scene 2)

Although Hamlet describes how something specific appears to him, the predicament conveyed by this passage is much more encompassing. It is a way of experiencing himself, his world, and the relationship between them, something that all of his intentionally directed experiences and thoughts presuppose. Hamlet has not lost his mirth in relation to states of affairs *p, q,* and *r,* and retained it in relation to *s, t,* and *u.* He has lost *all his mirth*; his world has changed in appearance insofar as the possibility of pleasure, curiosity, and motivation are drained from it. There remains a sense of contingency to the experience though. What Hamlet has lost is *his* mirth, and the act of conveying the experience to others indicates recognition of the phenomenological difference between speaker and listener. There is also an intra-personal contrast to be drawn; there remains an appreciation that 'the world was not like this for me in the past', that something has changed and things are somehow not right. This is not just a matter of having experience *p* and contrasting it with one's remembered experience *q,* along with other people's current experience *r.* A consistent theme of my discussion is that the feeling of strangeness, of difference, is often integral to the experience—the difference, the wrongness of it all, is very much *present*.

The various descriptions of existential feeling that appear in literature convey a range of subtly different predicaments. Consider the following:

> Meanwhile, the whole outside world disclosed itself as treacherously subjective. Neither good nor sinister, dull nor fascinating, luminous nor black, the exterior universe possessed no innate qualities, but was nightmarishly reliant on the grind of her interior lens. That the Boat Basin in Riverside Park would not, at least, remain a sublime and halcyon copse atrot with friendly dogs unnerved her, for the same Hudson walkway could transmogrify into a bleak and trashy strip, its dogs ratty and hostile, the vista of New Jersey grim and aggressively overfamiliar. Sweetspot as well could flip-flop overnight from tasteful clapboard haven to slick, elitist preserve for the spoiled rotten. Willy resented having responsibility for the fickle landscape outside her mind as well as in; there was no resort. As the seafarer craves dry land, she yearned for anything ineluctable and true, immutably one way or another. Instead Willy was smitten with the awful discovery that even the color of a lamppost was subject to her own filthy moods. (Shriver, 2006, pp.247–8)

I do not propose to account for everything in this passage in terms of existential feeling, and I will further discuss the relationships between existential feeling, conceptualization of experience, and self-narrative in Chapter 5. But what we have here is clearly something *felt*, which at the same comprises a way of relating to the world as a whole. It differs from Hamlet's loss of mirth. In place of a fairly consistent feeling that the world is bereft of something (a feeling that could be associated with inconsistent and indecisive *behaviour*, such as Hamlet's), there is an unstable self-world relationship. Willy's sense of reality and belonging 'wobbles' from moment to moment in quite pronounced ways, but it would be wrong to think of her as having one kind of existential feeling, then another, and then another. Her sense that she lacks grounding is itself an enduring feeling; her experience as a whole is characterized by a sense of instability, changeability, uncertainty, impermanence. (It resembles, in some respects, a loss of trust in the world and in other people that I will address in Chapters 4 and 8.) The passage thus draws attention to the temporal structure of existential feeling. Existential feelings unfold in time, arising, changing, and disappearing, but they are also ways of experiencing time, of inhabiting time. Willy's world is bereft of the confident anticipation and sense of consistency that permeates many people's temporal experience. In its place, there is an all-pervasive feeling of contingency and instability that is inseparable from how she relates to the future.

Existential feelings are not specific to our relationship with the impersonal world, and are also ways of finding ourselves with other people. The interpersonal is not to be construed as an 'add-on' to an already experienced impersonal world. 'The world' is 'our world', and changes in the structure of interpersonal experience are inseparable from more enveloping disturbances in the sense of reality and belonging. Consider this passage from a novel about the poet John Clare, who was admitted to High Beach Asylum in 1837:

> Stands in the wilderness of the world, stands alone, [...] surrounded by strangers, trembling, unable, the sun heating him, his will breaking inside him, until he bursts out, 'what can I do?' As though it were possible, he searches again the strangers' faces to find Mary or Patty or one of his own children or anyone, but there is no warm return from them. They are alien, moulded flesh only, and they frighten him. (Foulds, 2009, p.142)

The experience described here does not involve however many people looking strange and distant. It is a shape that all interpersonal experiences take on. The protagonist inhabits a world from which the possibility of interpersonal connection is absent; even those closest to him look strangely impersonal, distant, and frightening. This is inextricable from his experience of the world more generally, which has become an isolated, threatening place that he cannot engage with.[6]

I have already stated that depression is difficult to describe, largely because the experience involves something that is seldom an explicit object of study or discussion. It should now be clear that this point applies to existential feelings more generally. We seldom notice them, and they become salient to us only when they shift or take on a form that involves strangeness, novelty, unpleasantness, and/or lack. So one might think that depression does not present us with a particular problem, but that would be a mistake. When existential feelings are not disruptive, the need to describe them is not pressing. However, existential feeling is itself a problem in depression, and something that one may feel a *need* to share with others. Furthermore, the task is not just that of conveying one's own existential feeling *p*, which differs from someone else's existential feeling *q*, but of conveying the difference between *p* and *q*. Where that difference is more extreme, as it is when someone with depression addresses someone who is habitually and comfortably immersed in the world, the task is more difficult. What many first-person accounts struggle to communicate is not 'the experience of depression' but 'how different depression is from some other form of experience'. The contrast is not a simple one, involving a single, *typical* way of belonging to the world, along with occasional deviations from it in the guise of psychiatric illnesses and other 'anomalous' experiences. As I have already noted, existential feelings shift in subtle ways during the course of everyday life, and there is most likely considerable interpersonal variation too.[7] Furthermore, as later chapters will make clear, depression experiences themselves involve various different kinds of existential change.

Although the difficulties involved in describing existential feelings do not imply that they are seldom discussed, first-person accounts do tend to be vague and/or metaphorical. For example, one author writes of his depression that 'I felt like I'd been found incompetent and fired from my own life' (Steinke, 2001, p.64). This is far from uninformative, and surely succeeds in

---

[6] Depression is not the only psychiatric diagnosis that can be plausibly associated with existential feeling, or the only one that resonates with descriptions in literature. Experiences of people as 'alien', oddly inanimate, or 'flesh only' are more typical of schizophrenia than depression. I will turn to the comparative phenomenology of schizophrenia and depression in Chapter 10.

[7] There are many potential sources of variation. How one generally 'finds oneself in the world' will be influenced to an extent by cultural, social, and developmental factors. Furthermore, it is likely to shift as one ages (in ways that will vary from person to person), as well as in response to life events and significant changes in life circumstances.

conveying something of what the author experienced. But many people who attempt to describe their experiences of depression also complain that their metaphors fall short. Even when metaphors (and similes and analogies too) are to some degree effective, metaphorical language alone does not amount to a comprehensive phenomenological understanding of the kind that would allow us to (a) reliably distinguish one form of depression experience from another and (b) distinguish existential forms of depression from other kinds of experience. One person who emphatically endorses the statement 'I feel like I've been fired from my life' might well have an experience quite different from someone else who endorses it just as emphatically. And what do we say to someone who complains that he doesn't really understand such descriptions, just doesn't 'get' what is going on?[8]

Another way of conveying existential feelings is by referring to causes they are often associated with, rather than describing the feelings themselves. For example, a 'bad case of jetlag', a 'terrible hangover', and a 'feeling of grief' can all involve the world looking strangely distant, somehow different. Metaphors often rely on this technique too. When depression is described as an experience of 'being fired from one's life', the comparator experience, that of 'being fired from one's job', is not described but instead conveyed through reference to its cause. Once reference is achieved, the reader can entertain something along the same lines but somehow more profound. This is highly effective for certain purposes, but the task of describing a depression experience differs from that of somehow conveying or evoking it. And a phenomenological description is something that researchers, clinicians, therapists, sufferers, family members, friends, and professional colleagues may all find useful in some contexts. Even so, by reflecting on how people do convey wobbles in their sense of reality and belonging, we can 'bring something of the world to light' and gradually nurture a phenomenological stance of the kind that then facilitates phenomenological analysis.

So far, I have indicated that existential feelings are centrally implicated in experiences of depression, and I have construed them as 'ways of finding oneself in the world and with other people' that are—in some way—*felt*. However, one might object that this does not get us very far. The claim that something is 'a way of finding oneself in the world' may be evocative but it is also vague. What exactly is it to 'find oneself in the world'—haven't I just said that metaphor alone does not add up to phenomenological description? The

---

[8] This is not to imply that a phenomenological analysis should be free of metaphor, and mine is certainly not. The point is that metaphor cannot do all of the required work; something more is needed.

'felt' character of existential feelings requires clarification too. They are surely not 'bodily feelings', as they constitute a background sense of belonging to the world rather than an awareness of all or part of one's body. So what do I mean by calling them 'feelings'? An appeal to certain familiar experiences, first-person descriptions of psychiatric illness, and excerpts from literature might well draw attention to a neglected aspect of experience. And a technical term like 'existential feeling' might well help us *refer* to it more reliably. But reference is not description, and I have not yet supplied a phenomenological account. In the next four sections, I will do so. First of all, I will draw on Husserl's concept of a 'horizon' in order to describe how *possibilities* are integrated into human experience. Changes in existential feeling, I will then propose, are shifts in the *kinds of possibility* that experience incorporates. Following this, I will briefly indicate how we can arrive at much the same view by starting from Heidegger's description of 'mood', after which I will show how an experience of possibility can at the same time be an experience of the feeling body.

Horizons

Perhaps, one might think, existential feelings are difficult to describe *because* they have been neglected, but there is also something intrinsically elusive about them. In fact, some existential changes are seemingly paradoxical: everything looks just as it did before and yet utterly different. Consider Jaspers' description of the delusional 'atmosphere' or 'mood' that sometimes precedes full-blown schizophrenia, an experience that conforms to my description of existential feeling: 'perception is unaltered in itself but there is some change which envelops everything with a subtle, pervasive and strangely uncertain light' (Jaspers, 1963, p.98). If one were to classify all of the entities in one's vicinity and describe all of their perceived physical properties—such as shape and colour—in meticulous detail, there would be no difference between 'before' and 'after'.[9] In this respect, delusional atmosphere is unexceptional; existential changes in general are difficult to pin down. Almost all first-person accounts of depression similarly emphasize the profound gulf between the world of depression and where the person once was, where the exact nature of the difference remains quite unclear. A crucial first step in understanding it, I will now suggest, is the acknowledgement that we experience *possibilities*. The next step is to

---

[9] See Chapter 10 and also Ratcliffe (2013e) for further discussion of Jaspers on delusional atmosphere.

appreciate that depression involves a change in the *kinds* of possibility that are experienced.

The concept of a 'horizon', as employed by Husserl (e.g. 1948/1973, 1952/1989, 2001), and subsequently by Merleau-Ponty (1962), is a good place to start, and I will focus primarily on Husserl's later work here. His description of the 'horizonal' structure of experience begins with the observation that, when perceiving an entity such as a cup, we experience it as fully present even though only part of it is perceptually available at any given time. Along with this, we are able to experience it as persisting unchanged, despite the fact that its appearance changes markedly as our physical relationship with it changes. How, asks Husserl, do we experience a complete, enduring entity, when all we perceive are momentary and partial appearances? His answer is that, as well as presenting what actually appears to us at a given time, perceptual experience includes a sense of what is perceivable from other vantage points:

> In the noema of the act of perception, i.e., in the perceived, taken precisely as characterized phenomenologically, as it is therein an intentional Object, there is included a determinate directive for all further experiences of the object in question. (Husserl, 1989, p.38)

A cup appears *as* something that could be accessed visually from different angles, touched, or manipulated. These and other possibilities together comprise a structured system, which Husserl calls the entity's 'horizon':

> Everywhere, apprehension includes in itself, by the mediation of a 'sense', empty horizons of 'possible perceptions'; thus I can, at any given time, enter into a system of possible and, if I follow them up, actual, perceptual nexuses. (Husserl, 1989, p.42)

A horizon is not something that we perceive *in addition to* the actual; we do not experience possibilities floating around an already given object. Husserl maintains that an organized system of possibilities is integral to our sense of *what an entity is*, as well as our sense *that it is*. So the possible partly constitutes, rather than accompanies, the actual. We do not sense the possibility of *p*, plus the possibility of *q*, and so forth; horizons are not clusters of disparate possibilities but cohesive systems (Husserl, 2001, p.42). These systems are central to the achievement Husserl calls 'passive synthesis', meaning—roughly— a harmonious integration of appearances that enables us to experience the presence of enduring objects without conscious effort.

For current purposes, the importance of Husserl's approach is in the details. We can distinguish various different *kinds* of possibility, some (but perhaps not all) of which are implicated in our ability to experience an entity as 'here, now'. Husserl emphasizes possibilities for sensory access and maintains that horizons have an intersensory structure. For instance, visual perception of something includes tactual possibilities and vice versa: 'the thing is not split apart by the two groups of appearances; on the contrary, it is constituted in unitary apperception' (1989, p.75).[10] Take the experience of seeing a sharp carving knife sitting on a kitchen table, gleaming in the sunlight. On some such occasions, the possibility of its cutting you is *there*, integral to what you see; you can almost *feel* the knife sliding across your hand. In addition, horizons have an intersubjective structure. The cup that I currently see is experienced as potentially accessible to others as well. I may also recognize that my own possibilities for perceptual access differ from someone else's. Hence the interpersonal can contribute to the horizonal structure of an experience in different ways. For example, something might appear 'also available to other observers in this way', 'currently available to her or them but not to me or us', or 'currently available to me or us but not to her or them'.

Husserl makes clear that horizons are not to be construed solely in terms of what is available for detached, voyeuristic contemplation. I experience the cup as something I could see from another angle *by doing x* or as something that I could touch *by doing y*. Perception thus incorporates dispositions towards bodily movements. Husserl calls these movements 'kinaestheses', by which he means movements in the service of perception, as opposed to goal-directed action. Horizons, he says, are centrally but not solely a matter of *what I could do* and they involve a sense of active anticipation:

> The possibilities of transition are *practical* possibilities, at least when it is a question of an object which is given as enduring without change. There is thus a freedom to run through the appearances in such a way that I move my eyes, my head, alter the posture of my body, go around the object, direct my regard toward it, and so on. We call these movements, which belong to the essence of perception and serve to bring the object of perception to givenness from all sides insofar as possible, *kinaestheses*. (Husserl, 1973, pp.83–4)

Experienced possibilities have varying degrees of determinacy. When I look at an object, a possible perception could take the form 'if you turn me around, you will reveal a rough, red surface' or just 'if you turn me around, you will reveal a colour and texture'. Husserl (1973) calls this 'open uncertainty'. It is to be distinguished from 'problematic uncertainty', where there is a felt lack of confidence concerning the actualisation of some possibility, regardless of how determinate the possibility might be. When we anticipate seeing 'something red, smooth and curved' or 'something that has some shape, texture

---

[10] To quote Merleau-Ponty (1962, p.318), 'any object presented to one sense calls upon itself the concordant operation of all the others'.

and colour', we do so with varying degrees of confidence. Another way of putting it would be to distinguish the *content* of what is anticipated from the *mode* in which it is anticipated. The default mode of anticipation is, according to Husserl, that of certainty. Possibilities present themselves with a kind of affective force or allure that renders them sufficiently salient for other possibilities to be eclipsed altogether. He offers the example of watching a drinking glass fall and anticipating its breakage, where the breakage presents itself as inevitable—it is not that 'this might happen' but that 'this will happen'. This recognition of inevitability is not inferred from what is seen; the certainty of what will happen is *there*, embedded in one's experienced surroundings. In such a case, other possibilities are merely 'open', meaning that they are not ruled out but do not appear salient in any way: 'every event as a physical event is surrounded here by a horizon of possibilities—but they are open; nothing speaks in favor of them in this given moment; the expectations are straightforward certainties that are not inhibited' (Husserl, 2001, p.91). This applies equally to what we actively explore rather than passively witness. Here too, there are varying degrees of confidence.

Possibilities that are anticipated in the mode of certainty are usually harmoniously actualized, thus revealing further possibilities, which themselves appear certain, and so on. Hence the horizonal structure of perception is not to be conceived of in a static way; it involves a dynamic interplay of habitual expectation and fulfilment. As I walk across the street, I take for granted that the texture of the road will remain fairly constant and that I will not fall into a deep hole or sink into a bog. Alternative possibilities such as these do not feature in the experience at all. However, not all anticipation is in the guise of certainty. As I walk home during a dark night and see a person-like shape in the woods, there is a feeling of *uncertainty* over what it is. Then, as I approach and the shape seems to change and fragment, there is *doubt* over whether anything is there at all. This differs from open uncertainty, as it involves a sense of conflict: 'it might be a person but it might not be'. In such cases, an entity may subsequently resolve itself as what was originally anticipated or, alternatively, as something in conflict with it. So there can be an experience of 'disappointment', an awareness of things as somehow other than previously anticipated. Problematic uncertainty, where one feels that 'things might not turn out to be as they seem', is to be distinguished from a more determinate feeling of doubt, which involves competition between an original and a rival system of anticipation, such as 'it's a person' and 'it's a mannequin'. And, in both scenarios, disappointment of expectation is to be distinguished from experience of difference or change. We can anticipate both stability and change in the modes of certainty or conflict.

Experience of the possible is not restricted to variably determinate possibilities for perception by self and/or others, which present themselves with differing degrees of confidence. There is also a sense of how things are *significant*, where having significance is to be understood in terms of offering something that is relevant in one or another way to some set of concerns. So far as I know, Husserl does not state this explicitly, but he does at least refer to salient perceptual possibilities as 'enticing', meaning that they draw us in, calling upon us to act in such a way as to actualize them. These enticements are experienced as integral to entities but are, at the same time, felt bodily dispositions. Husserl describes the 'allure given to consciousness, the peculiar pull that an object given to consciousness exercises on the ego' (2001, p.196). There is, he suggests, a kind of 'striving' that belongs to 'normal perception', and a '*feeling*' that 'goes hand in hand with this striving' (1973, p.85). What we actually perceive *invites* us to actualize further perceptual possibilities, those that enhance our perceptual grasp on the object by reducing open uncertainty.[11] Hence the perceptual confidence that I described earlier does not take the conditional form 'if I do *x*, *y* will appear with certainty', where *y* is more or less determinate. It is more a case of 'do *x* now, to reveal *y*'. Possibilities invite us to realise them, and perception lays out a course for itself.

Husserl's account of enticing possibilities needs to be further complicated and also broadened. 'Enticement' does not distinguish between a number of different ways in which entities exert a practical pull on us; they may rouse our curiosity, fascinate us, offer pleasure, or appear immediately relevant to projects we care about. And there are other ways in which the world invites us to act; things can appear pressing, urgent, or required. The term 'enticing' is not appropriate for all of these, as a possibility need not 'entice' in a positive way for it to solicit action. For instance, we might have to 'deal with something' that presents itself as 'urgent' in order to avoid some occurrence, where not having to deal with it at all would have been preferable. As this suggests, possibilities for perception are not the only ones that draw us in; the account applies equally to goal-directed activities. Although Husserl emphasizes how possibilities entice us *perceptually* and does not explicitly implicate them in other activities, he does maintain that the world is not experienced as a realm of indifferent objects. Experienced entities are imbued with various kinds of value and utility, which reflect our concerns, commitments and ongoing projects:

> In ordinary life, we have nothing whatever to do with nature-Objects. What we take as things are pictures, statues, gardens, houses, tables, clothes, tools, etc. These

---

[11] This theme is further developed in Merleau-Ponty's writings (e.g. 1962, p.302).

> are all value-Objects of various kinds, use-Objects, practical Objects. They are not
> Objects which can be found in natural science. (Husserl, 1989, p.29)

This is consistent with the view that horizons incorporate various different kinds of significant possibility. There is more to 'significance' than just 'enticement'; a cup of water can appear significant in offering the possibility of drinking from but without currently soliciting action. Hence an immediate 'pull' (of whatever kind) that an entity may or may not have on us is to be distinguished from various other ways in which it might be encountered as significant. For instance, something could appear 'practically relevant in the context of a project' or 'threatening', and categories like these require further differentiation. Something that is practically significant could present itself more specifically as 'urgently required', 'appropriate for the task at hand', 'significant for others but not for me', 'significant for us', 'significant only for me', 'easy or difficult to use', or 'not needed yet'.[12] Threat similarly comes in a number of forms. A threat could be major, minor, imminent, self-directed, other-directed, directed more generally, avoidable, difficult to avoid, or unavoidable. And there are distinctively 'interpersonal' kinds of possibility too, which I will describe in Chapter 8. Types of significance relate to activity in different ways. What is anticipated might appear as something 'I could do now' or 'he/we could do at some variably determinate time', something 'easily achievable', 'potentially achievable', 'achievable in a specific way', or 'achievable through some not yet determinate course of action'. It could equally appear as 'something I can do nothing about'. For instance, a threat might be experienced as certain, as unstoppable, and the experience is thus one of passivity. There is also a distinction to be drawn between conditional and unconditional certainty: 'x will certainly happen unless I act' is to be distinguished from 'x will certainly happen regardless of what I do'.

As well as anticipation, the phenomenological structure that I have described includes experiences of fulfilment and lack of fulfilment. Recognition of a threat's failure to materialize usually takes the form of relief. In contrast, when we confidently anticipate something good happening, lack of fulfilment involves a feeling of disappointment—something is wrong, missing, or absent. We therefore experience something akin to 'negation', in a way that does not depend on a prior propositional appreciation that 'it is not the case that p'. What Husserl (1973, p.90) calls the 'original phenomenon of negation' consists of a *felt* discrepancy between what is anticipated and what is actualized: 'negation

---

[12] The theme of tool use and practical utility is more usually associated with the work of Heidegger (1962, Division One, III).

*is not first the business of the act of predicative judgment […] in its original form it
already appears in the prepredicative sphere of receptive experience'.* Here, a competing system of anticipation (which could be fairly inchoate or, in the case of a
concrete doubt, more specific) overrides its predecessor. Alternatively, what one
anticipates in the guise of certainty might fail to occur but without any prior
doubt, in which case there is a sense of surprise.

The theme of experienced negation is addressed in more detail by Sartre in
Being and Nothingness. Take the well-known example of going to meet Pierre
in a café and sitting there while he fails to show up. The possibility of meeting Pierre is integral to how the café is perceived; it becomes a backdrop to
the anticipated meeting, a meeting that is significant in however many different ways. As it becomes increasingly apparent that Pierre will not turn up, his
absence is very much *there* (Sartre, 1943/1989, pp.9–10). An unfulfilled system
of anticipation shapes experience of one's surroundings, in a way that cannot
be pinned down unless it is acknowledged that we experience the possible. To
apply Husserl's account, Pierre's absence first takes the form of anticipation
('this is the place where I am waiting for him; he is not here yet'), then problematic uncertainty or doubt ('he might not show up after all') and finally disappointment ('this is the place where I anticipated meeting him, and he never
came'). Once disappointed, the possibilities remain integral to the experienced
café, but *as* unfulfilled, as overridden by a competing system of anticipation.
Granted, some of this does take a propositional form. One contemplates the
proposition 'Pierre will not turn up' and takes it to be increasingly likely.
However, the experience is not exhausted by this, as illustrated by the contrast
between 'Pierre is not in the café' and 'Darth Vader is not in the café'. One
can equally reflect on and agree with both propositions but the experience of
absence only features in the former case and is not just a matter of propositional content. Sartre does not restrict his account of absence to experiences
of passive waiting. He also describes goal-directed action as the response to
an 'objective lack' in the world (1989, p.433). To experience something as significant, at least in a good way, is also to experience a current state of affairs as
somehow falling short in comparison with a potential or anticipated state of
affairs. In the context of a project, *p* appears not just as *possible* but as something *not yet done*. There is thus a sense of one's current situation as contingent,
as susceptible to significant changes of various kinds, which could be brought
about through one's own actions, the actions of others, or in some other way.[13]

---

[13] For the most part, Sartre's emphasis on how possibilities structure perception complements Husserl's account. However, he criticises Husserl for failing to appreciate that possibilities can be clustered around an entity that itself appears as 'absent', which differs
from their being deficiencies in an entity that appears as 'present' (Sartre, 1989, pp.26–27).

Hence it is clear how an experience can involve an unpleasant sense of absence or lack. There is a disappointed system of expectation, where what one anticipated had one or another kind of positive significance—it 'would have been a good thing'. J. H. van den Berg (1972, pp.34–5) offers the following description of how a bottle of wine looks after a dinner guest has cancelled at short notice:

> What I was seeing then was not a green bottle, with a white label, with a lead capsule, and things like that. What I was really seeing was something like the disappointment about the fact that my friend would not come or about the loneliness of my evening.

When a system of anticipation continues to be experienced but *as* negated, things *look* different from how they did before. In Chapters 4 to 8, I will describe various kinds of experienced absence that feature in depression.[14] These, I will show, involve anticipation without fulfilment and/or an absence of both anticipation and fulfilment. How can the latter feature in experience at all—surely, if you do not anticipate p and p does not occur, there is nothing to experience? As Husserl notes, we do not experience possibilities in isolation from each other. There is a dynamic system of largely harmonious possibilities, which are actualized in structured ways, thus pointing to further possibilities. Even if one no longer anticipates p, the anticipation of anticipating p can remain, and be disappointed when one does not anticipate p. So there is a sense that something is missing from experience. It is also possible to miss the unexpected, insofar as experience is ordinarily shaped by the sense that at least some things will transpire in ways that are unanticipated. We anticipate novelty, and a world bereft of the possibility of novelty is experienced as somehow anomalous, not quite right.

What I have outlined in this section might be regarded as a contentious account of perceptual content. By 'perceptual content', I mean simply 'whatever it is that we are able to perceive', in contrast to what we infer from perception, impose on perceptual experience or access in ways that have little or no relation to perception. There is much debate in philosophy of mind over where the limits of perceptual content lie: do we *perceive* entities, types

---

[14] There is no simple correspondence between experiences of absence, lack, or disappointment and propositional negation of the form 'it is not the case that p', given that there are several variants of the former. Saury (2009, p.254) distinguishes 'experiences of absence, lack, separation, disappearance, distance, alienation, withdrawal, rejection, end, interruption, hinder, limitation, prohibition, and obstacle' and suggests that these fall under the three broader categories of 'lack', 'otherness', and 'obstruction'. As will become clear, depression experiences encompass all three.

of entity, causes, and so on?[15] I have indicated that we perceive entities such as cups, chairs, and the like, but I do not want to be too prescriptive about what *kinds* of thing we can and cannot perceive. In addition, I have suggested that perception has a degree of intermodal structure: what is actually perceived through one sensory modality includes a sense of potential perceptions involving other modalities. I have also proposed that we perceive a range of different kinds of possibility, some of which are integral to a further perceptual achievement: the sense of something as 'here, now' or, alternatively, 'absent', 'missing', or in some way 'lacking'.[16] Nevertheless, the principal claims I make in this book do not hinge on a specific account of 'perceptual content'. I am concerned with what *experience* consists of, and not all accounts of perceptual content are driven solely or even primarily by phenomenological concerns. And, when I refer to 'perceptual experience', I am just thinking of whatever is integral to our appreciation of the 'here and now' (as opposed to what we experience as, say, 'imagined' or 'remembered'), and does not depend on conscious inference from a prior experience. So, if one chooses to think of the 'perceptual' in a different way and assert that my subject matter includes more than just what we 'perceive', the difference is a terminological one. I am interested in something else, whatever we decide to call it.

Even so, my approach is not immune to challenges that appeal to the nature of perceptual content, as there remains the possibility of conflict between my various claims and how perceptual experience is actually structured (independent of terminological disputes over what we do and do not label as 'perceptual'). However, the account of experience and possibility sketched here is not something that I will simply take for granted and then proceed to apply. My account will be refined and clarified through engagement with the phenomenology of depression. And it will also be corroborated in the process, to the extent that it allows us to understand forms of experience that would

---

[15] See, for instance, MacPherson ed. (2011) for some classic and more recent discussions of the nature of perception and the individuation of sensory modalities. See Hawley and MacPherson eds (2011) for several different conceptions of perceptual content.

[16] Increased interaction between phenomenology and work in the philosophy of mind on perceptual content offers the potential for mutual illumination. There is a degree of convergence between Husserl's view and at least some recent discussions of perceptual content. For instance, O'Callaghan (2011; 2012) maintains that perception has a rich inter-modal structure and that perception through one sense involves an appreciation of what else *could* be perceived through that and other senses: 'You hear a sound *as* the sound of something that could be seen or brought into view, and that has visible features' (2011, p.157). See also Noë (2004) and Madary (2013) for accounts of perceptual content that complement Husserl's approach in several respects.

otherwise prove intractable. Given that not much rests on the term 'perception', I tend to refer to 'experience' instead, a term that I use in two ways. In the looser sense, I mean 'any aspect of our phenomenology', but I also use 'experience' to refer to our encountering things as 'here, now', in a way that is to be contrasted with imagining, remembering and, more generally, thinking. When I use the plural, 'experiences', I am not committed to the view that experiences, in either of these two senses, can be tidily individuated and distinguished from each other. All I want to do is indicate that more than one experiential content or more than one experiencer is involved, as in 'an experience of *p*' rather than an 'experience of *q*', or 'A's experience' rather than 'B's experience'. In all instances, I hope that context will make usage clear.

Another difference between debates over perceptual content and what I am trying to do here is that I am primarily concerned with an aspect of experience that is almost entirely absent from accounts of phenomenal content, even from more inclusive conceptions of it that acknowledge 'cognitive phenomenology' alongside sensory perceptual experience. Defences of cognitive phenomenology tend to argue for one or more of the following: (a) sensory perceptual experience has cognitive content; (b) sensory phenomenology is involved in cognition as well as perception; (c) cognition has a non-sensory phenomenology of its own.[17] In so doing, they overlook something. All perceptual experiences and all thoughts are shaped by something that both presuppose; we are already *there* when we experience something or think about it. So human experience cannot be exhaustively described by addressing what experiences of perceiving, believing, thinking, imagining, remembering, and so forth consist of. The account of horizons that I have sketched so far does not itself amount to an analysis of this presupposed layer of experience. However, as I will now show, it does give us what we need in order to formulate such an analysis.

The World as a Possibility Space

Depression, I have suggested, involves a change in one's sense of belonging to the world. So it is not a localized shift in the experienced possibilities associated with however many entities or situations. However, both Husserl and Merleau-Ponty also acknowledge that we encounter entities only within the context of a pre-given experiential world, something that equally implicates

---

[17] See the essays collected in Bayne and Montagu eds (2011) for several different positions regarding the existence and nature of cognitive phenomenology. See Ratcliffe (2013f) for a broadly 'Husserlian' alternative.

a sense of the possible. Husserl claims that conflict between systems of anticipation is ordinarily experienced against a harmonious backdrop of certainty: 'without a certain measure of unity maintaining itself in the progression of perceptions, the unity of intentional lived-experience would crumble' (2001, p.64). Experiences of doubt and problematic uncertainty involve a sense of something's being potentially discrepant, anomalous. And one can only detect discrepancy if there is something harmonious to depart from. The same applies to disappointment; it is something we experience against a backdrop of cohesive, confident expectation, without which experience would lack the structure required for something to show up as anomalous. The 'world', according to Husserl, is not something we take to be the case in the way we 'perceive that a coffee cup is here, now', or 'believe that the Eiffel Tower is in Paris'. An appreciation of the world's existence, which is at the same time a sense of being rooted in the world, consists of habitual, practical, non-conceptual anticipation in the mode of certainty:

> It belongs to what is taken for granted, prior to all scientific thought and all philosophical questioning, that the world is—always is in advance—and that every correction of an opinion, whether an experiential or other opinion, presupposes the already existing world, namely, as a horizon of what in the given case is indubitably valid as existing, and presupposes within this horizon something familiar and doubtlessly certain with which that which is perhaps canceled out as invalid came into conflict. (Husserl, 1954/1970a, p.110)

As Merleau-Ponty puts it, the world amounts to a 'style' that shapes all our experiences and thoughts; 'the universal style of all possible perceptions' (1964, p.16). This 'style' corresponds to what I call 'existential feeling'. To better understand and distinguish the various forms it takes, we can draw a distinction between *instances* of possibility, such as 'this cup can be touched' or 'this cup has the potential to be seen by others', and *kinds* of possibility, such as 'being tangible' or 'being perceivable by others'. In order to encounter anything as 'tangible', 'perceptually or practically accessible to others', 'relevant to a project', 'enticing' or 'fascinating', we must first have access to the relevant *kinds* of possibility. If we were incapable of experiencing anything as tangible, we could not experience a cup as tangible. Our access to kinds of possibility is itself integral to our experience (rather than being a non-phenomenological disposition to have certain kinds of experience). To find oneself in a world is to have a sense of the various *ways* in which things might be encountered—as perceptually or practically accessible, as somehow significant, as available to others. And changes in the overall style of experience, in existential feeling, are shifts in the kinds of possibility one is receptive to.

What exactly is a 'kind of possibility'? When a hammer is encountered as 'useful in the context of a project', it might be when one is building a shed and needs to hammer in some nails. But my focus is on the kind of significance it has, not the specific projects and properties that render it significant in that way. One can only experience a hammer, a car, and a computer as practically significant in virtue of properties p, q, and r, and in the context of projects x, y, and z, so long as one is able to experience things as 'practically significant in the context of a project'. Any number of different things can be experienced as significant in the same general way—as relevant to some project, immediately enticing, or significant for someone else. This is the level of description I am concerned with. And I conceive of 'project' in a fairly loose way. It need not involve progressive pursuit of an overarching goal. Caring for one's child is importantly different from writing a book, and I want to accommodate all of the various cares, concerns, and commitments in relation to which things matter to us in the ways they do. Even at this level of description, human experience includes many different kinds of possibility, which can be characterized by drawing on distinctions made in the previous section:

Perceptual modality: Experienced possibilities can be—but need not be—specific to one or more perceptual modalities. For example, 'when I do this, I will feel this texture' is modality-specific, whereas 'something inchoate but threatening is coming' is not.

Content: What one takes to be possible—or, more specifically, what one anticipates—can have varying degrees of determinacy. 'Something is coming to get me' is less determinate than 'a tiger is coming to get me'. To this we can add some appreciation of temporal distance: 'a tiger is coming to get me now'; 'something is coming to get me, but it's not clear when'.

Mode of anticipation: When something is anticipated, its occurrence can be experienced as certain, or with varying degrees of doubt or problematic uncertainty.

Relationship to agency: A possibility can be experienced as something that one will or might bring about oneself, something that others will or might act upon, or something that will or might happen independent of any human agency. Combined with 'mode', this constitutes a sense of varying degrees and kinds of difficulty.

Significance: There are different kinds of significance or ways of mattering, such as 'practical utility', 'safety', and 'danger'. The kind of significance something has is inextricable from its 'relationship to agency'. For instance, to experience something as 'enticing' is at the same time to experience its practical pull.

Interpersonal accessibility: A possibility can relate in various ways to self and others: 'it will happen to me'; 'it might happen to us'; 'it is there for them but not for me'.

These variables combine to yield many different kinds of possibility. For instance, something could appear 'enticing but difficult to achieve', 'practically significant and yet impossible to achieve', or 'threatening, imminent, and inchoate'. Further distinctions are to be drawn on the basis of interpersonal structure. Something could be 'threatening to me and only me', 'threatening to all of us', 'threatening to them but not to us', 'practically significant for us', or 'practically significant only to me'. I will argue that this level of description is phenomenologically real: disturbances of existential feeling are changes in the kinds of possibility we are open to, kinds that can be characterized in terms of the distinctions I have drawn. At least some of these kinds of possibility are integral to the sense of reality and belonging. For instance, what would it be like to inhabit a world where nothing offered the possibility of *tangibility*? Of course, something can be experienced as real and, more specifically, as 'here, now' without its being experienced as tangible. Take clouds, for example. However, there is a difference between a cloud's lacking tangibility and an absence of tangibility from experience as a whole. If everything ceased to offer the possibility of being touched or manipulated, if that *kind of possibility* were altogether gone, then experience would no longer include a contrast between the intangibility of a cloud and the tangibility of a cup of coffee. Without that contrast, everything would look strangely distant, cut off, somehow not quite *there*, at least if one retained a *feeling* of loss (and one would, if kinds of possibility are integrated into complicated systems of anticipation, in relation to which their absence is noticeable).

The point applies equally to interpersonal possibilities. An entity can appear 'currently perceptually and practically accessible only to me' and still be experienced as 'here'. However, if nothing appeared 'practically and/or perceptually accessible to others', our sense of belonging to the world would be radically altered. According to Husserl, the ability to experience something as 'here' rather than, say, 'imagined' is tied up with an appreciation of potential interpersonal access.[18] To encounter something as an enduring entity distinct from oneself *is* to experience it as available to others, as not exhausted by one's own actual and potential perspectives upon it: 'The "true thing" is then the Object that maintains its identity within the manifolds of appearances belonging to a multiplicity of subjects' (Husserl, 1989, p.87). The point concerns our ability to experience entities as 'present' and also our more general grasp of what it is to be 'real'. There is more to the real than what is present; we can take something to be real without experiencing it as present at the time. Nevertheless, if we lacked all sense of what it is for something to be present, our broader sense of what it is to be real would be substantially eroded as well, given that the 'real' cannot be cleanly extricated from the 'potentially present'.

---

[18] See Gallagher (2008) for a discussion of Husserl on the role of interpersonal possibilities in constituting our sense of belonging to an 'objective' world.

As for the various kinds of 'significance' that things have for us, it is tempting to think of them as evaluative overcoats that cover an already established sense of reality and belonging. However, I will argue that, although changes in the kinds of significance we are able to experience need not add up to a complete loss of the sense of reality, they can affect it in a number of different and often quite profound ways.

Once we allow that experience incorporates these various kinds of possibility, we can understand how everything might look exactly the same as it did before and yet somehow different. There is a shift in the kinds of possibility that one is receptive to, as illustrated by many first-person accounts of extreme alterations in the structure of experience. Consider the following passage from *Autobiography of a Schizophrenic Girl*, where the author, 'Renee', describes a short-lived return to reality:

> ...when we were outside I realized that my perception of things had completely changed. Instead of infinite space, unreal, where everything was cut off, naked and isolated, I saw Reality, marvelous Reality, for the first time. The people whom we encountered were no longer automatons, phantoms, revolving around, gesticulating without meaning; they were men and women with their own individual characteristics, their own individuality. It was the same with things. They were useful things, having sense, capable of giving pleasure. Here was an automobile to take me to the hospital, cushions I could rest on. [...] for the first time I dared to handle the chairs, to change the arrangement of the furniture. What an unknown joy, to have an influence on things; to do with them what I liked and especially to have the pleasure of wanting the change. (Sechehaye, 1970, pp.105–6)

For Renee, everything had lost its usual practical significance. With the return of practical possibilities, a sense of reality is also recovered. As this happens, there is a pronounced awareness of what was previously lacking, of the contrast between two ways of finding herself in the world. Loss of a kind of possibility from experience need not involve a feeling of absence. Perhaps, before possibilities began to return, Renee was largely oblivious to what she had lost. However, loss of possibility often does involve a conspicuous sense of loss. This applies to many depression experiences, where the absence of hope, practical significance, and interpersonal connection is painfully felt. By appealing to an account along these lines, we can distinguish quite different experiences that would otherwise be described in much the same way. For instance, suppose two people both report that 'nothing matters anymore'. It could turn out that one finds however many previously significant states of affairs inconsequential while the other inhabits a world from which the possibility of anything mattering is gone. It is easy to misinterpret an experience of being unable to engage in any kind of meaningful project as the collapse of one or more projects that are central to a life. As we will see, this point applies more generally, to experiences of despair, guilt, agency, and interpersonal connection, amongst others.

For convenience, I will refer throughout to the *loss* of kinds of possibility. However, it is important not to construe this too literally. Alterations in the sense of reality and belonging do not involve the simple addition or subtraction of kinds of possibility. Possibility types are not separate experiential *components* that can be tweaked in isolation from each other; they are interdependent. In some cases, the dependence may be causal but, in others, it is one of intelligibility. For instance, if something appears in the guise of an imminent threat to be avoided, it cannot at the same time entice action in the way an ice cream would on a hot day; that combination does not make sense. Sometimes, the relationship is one of identity: loss of p is also describable as addition of q. The addition of an all-enveloping sense of unavoidable, imminent threat is at the same time the loss of a hopeful orientation towards the future. Furthermore, some existential changes are attributable to structural disruption, where the anticipation-fulfilment dynamic does not unfold in the usual confident, harmonious way. This is not a case of 'subtracting' the possibility type 'habitual certainty' while adding the type 'insecurity'. An existential feeling of uncertainty and insecurity manifests itself in the interplay between anticipation and fulfilment; it has a dynamic, temporal structure. For these reasons, it is better to think of *transformations* of the possibility space, and to construe talk of loss, addition, intensification, and diminishment (which remains a very convenient way of talking) in that way.

Heidegger's Moods

I have sketched an account of existential feeling by appealing to themes in the work of Husserl: by first acknowledging that token possibilities of the form 'this entity or situation offers possibility p' are experienced, we can then come to acknowledge a presupposed receptivity to various *kinds* of possibility. However, other routes could be taken to arrive at the same view (which those with an aversion to Husserl may find more appealing). One is to start from Heidegger's account of mood [*Stimmung*] in *Being and Time*. Unlike Husserl, Heidegger emphasizes the changeability of how we find ourselves in the world, as well as ways in which things *matter* to us, and my 'existential feelings' are much like his 'moods'. He uses the term '*Befindlichkeit*' to refer to *finding oneself in a world through one or another mood*. It is a difficult term to translate. Macquarrie and Robinson, in their 1962 translation of *Being and Time*, opt for 'state of mind', but this is misleading. For Heidegger, moods are not experienced as states of mind possessed by psychological subjects, and we do not experience them as 'out there' in the world either. Moods are variants of a changeable sense of belonging to the world that is pre-subjective and pre-objective. All 'states of mind' and all perceptions and cognitions of 'external' things presuppose this background of belonging. Other translations include 'affectedness' (Dreyfus, 1991), 'attunement' (Stambaugh's 1996 translation of *Sein und Zeit*), 'disposedness' (e.g. Blattner, 2006), and 'sofindingness' (Haugeland, 2000). I will replace the term 'state of mind' with 'attunement' when quoting from the Macquarrie and Robinson translation.[19]

Moods, as modes of attunement, are presupposed by the intelligibility of intentionally directed experiences, thoughts, and activities: '*The mood has already disclosed, in every case, Being-in-the-world as a whole, and makes it possible first of all to direct oneself towards something*' (Heidegger, 1962, p.176). A 'mood', for Heidegger, constitutes our sense of being there, rooted in a situation. It is not a generalized emotion, but something presupposed by the possibility of intentionally directed emotional experiences. All such experiences involve finding something significant in one way or another, experiencing it as mattering. And moods determine the kinds of significance things can have for us, the ways in which they are able to matter:

> ...to be affected by the unserviceable, resistant, or threatening character [Bedrohlichkeit] of that which is ready-to-hand, becomes ontologically possible only in so far as Being-in as such has been determined existentially beforehand in such a manner that what it encounters within-the-world can '*matter*' to it in this way. The fact that this sort of thing can 'matter' to it is grounded in one's [attunement]; and as [an attunement] it has already disclosed the world—as something by which it can be threatened, for instance. [...] nothing like an affect would come about [...] if Being-in-the-world, with its [attunement], had not already submitted itself [sich schon angewiesen] to having entities within-the-world 'matter' to it in a way which its moods have outlined in advance. *Existentially, [an attunement] implies a disclosive submission to the world, out of which we can encounter something that matters to us.* (1962, pp.176–7)

It is only insofar as we are able to feel threatened that we can find a particular situation threatening, only insofar as we are able to pursue meaningful projects that we can find something significant in one or another way in relation to a project. Hence Heidegger distinguishes 'being afraid of something' from what he calls 'fearfulness'. By the latter, he means a sense that the world includes the possibility of danger. A mood of 'fearfulness'

---

[19] Other terms, such as 'disposedness', would serve equally well. However, no English term has quite the same connotations as *Befindlichkeit*

is thus presupposed by the intelligibility of intentional states of the kind 'fear': 'Fearing, as a slumbering possibility of Being-in-the-world in an [attunement] (we call this possibility 'fearfulness' ['Furchtsamkeit']), has already disclosed the world, in that out of it something like the fearsome may come close' (1962, p.180).

Heidegger refers more specifically to 'ground' or 'basic' moods [*Grundstimmungen*], by which he means—amongst other things—moods that determine the kinds of possibility we are open to, and in a way that does not depend upon other moods.[20] His discussion also acknowledges the possibility of profound shifts in mood. For instance, the ground mood of anxiety [*Angst*] is described as involving a radical alteration in how one finds oneself in the world, amounting to a complete loss of practical significance. It is not just that however many entities cease to be significant. Rather, the possibility of encountering anything as significant in that way is altogether gone from the world: 'entities within-the-world are not "relevant" at all'; 'the world has the character of completely lacking significance' (1962, p.231). The sense that something is missing, lacking, is itself very much part of this experience. The world is experienced *as* a realm in which one can no longer engage with things in an effortless, habitual, unreflective way; 'everyday familiarity collapses' (1962, p.233). In other words, the background confidence or certainty that Husserl describes becomes salient in its absence. Mood shifts like this can therefore be phenomenologically revealing. One cannot help but acknowledge an overarching 'style' of confident anticipation when its absence is so conspicuous. Philosophical attention is drawn to what would otherwise be overlooked, nurturing what I have called a 'phenomenological stance'.[21]

Of course, moods do not fully determine the nature of what we experience. That I am capable of finding things frightening does not dictate the kind of significance that a particular thing has for me on a particular occasion. Mood is what enables me to find anything practically significant, but the content of my projects determines what I find practically significant and how. Even so, I can find an entity *threatening* only in the context of a mood

---

[20] Somewhat confusingly, 'ground mood' status also seems to depend on a mood's ability to yield philosophical insight. However, there is no reason why profundity, couched in terms of access to possibility, should correspond to a mood's having some role to play in philosophical enquiry (Ratcliffe, 2013d).

[21] See also Strasser (1977, p.192) for an account of mood [*Stimmung*] as the presupposed backdrop to all experience and thought, as 'the dispositional horizon of our commerce with the world'.

that accommodates the possibility of my being threatened, and I can embark on a project only if I have access to the kinds of mattering that all projects presuppose. So mood is essential to what Heidegger calls our 'thrownness' [*Geworfenheit*], our sense of being situated in a significant worldly situation that is not of our own making (1962, p.174).[22]

Although my 'existential feelings' have much in common with Heidegger's 'moods', there are several reasons for adopting the former term. The English term 'mood' refers to a range of different phenomena, not all of which play the phenomenological role described by Heidegger. I can be in a bad mood *with* someone, where mood is clearly an enduring but specifically focused intentional state. Other moods are intentional states with a wider range of objects (such as feeling grumpy about several things that have happened during a really bad week). So not all 'moods' determine the kinds of possibility we are receptive to, the kinds of intentional state we are able to adopt. And, as noted earlier, many existential feelings are not referred to as moods. The German term *Stimmung* does not have quite the same connotations as 'mood'. Nevertheless, it too fails to capture *all* of the relevant phenomena and *only* those phenomena. My departure from Heidegger is not just terminological though. His analysis also has shortcomings. For instance, he restricts himself to a fairly narrow range of emotional states. In *Being and Time*, we have an emphasis on fear and anxiety. In a slightly later text (Heidegger, 1983/1995), there is also a lengthy analysis of boredom [*Langeweile*]. However, the range of existential feelings is much wider than that. And we can, by drawing on Husserl's discussion of horizons, formulate a far more nuanced account of the kinds of possibility that experience incorporates. Furthermore, there is a need to accommodate the bodily dimension of existential feeling, something Heidegger explicitly declines to comment on in *Being and Time* (Ratcliffe, 2013d). In this respect, Husserl is again more informative, in explicitly linking the background 'style' of experience to our bodily phenomenology.

---

[22] Heidegger maintains that mood is not the sole determinant of 'Being-in-the-world'. Equally important are 'understanding' [*Verstehen*] and 'discourse' [*Rede*]. These, together with the having of a mood [*Befindlichkeit*], comprise the structure of care [*Sorge*], 'care' being Heidegger's term for that in virtue of which Being-in-the-world is possible. Discourse, understanding and mood are not separable components but inextricable aspects of care. I could, if I wanted, dress up various parts of my discussion in these terms, but that would amount to needless terminological complication. Hence I do not discuss the relationship between mood, understanding, and discourse any further here, but see Ratcliffe (2013d) for a detailed discussion.

Possibilities and Bodily Dispositions

I have suggested that existential feelings play a distinctive phenomenological role, amounting to a changeable sense of reality and belonging that can be conceived of as a possibility space. But *what* could play such a role—what exactly are existential feelings? In short, they are bodily feelings—a bodily feeling can at the same time *be* a sense of the salient possibilities offered by a situation. In this section, I will indicate how the body is implicated in *existential feeling*. In Chapter 3, I will make a more general case for the inextricability of bodily feelings and experiences of things that are external to the body.

According to Husserl, in addition to experiencing our bodily dispositions, we experience other things *through* them. A sense of the possibilities offered by our surroundings is inseparable from a sense of what we could do, where the latter is comprised of various bodily dispositions. Consider an experience of something as 'enticing'. This involves *feeling* ourselves being drawn towards a course of action; there is an 'affective pull of enticing possibilities' (Husserl, 2001, p.98). Hence our experience of the possible is at least partly constituted by kinaesthetic dispositions; we experience the world *through* them, and the body operates more as a 'medium' or 'organ' of perception than as an object of perception (Husserl, 1989, p.61).[23] Feelings need not be experienced as having specific bodily locations. Some involve a 'general bodily sensitivity to the world' rather than a localized bodily experience (Slaby, 2008, p.434). Existential feelings, I suggest, consist in a diffuse, background sense of bodily dispositions. I use the term 'background' to emphasize that they are presupposed by our experiences of situations *within* a world. It should not be taken to imply that existential feelings are always inconspicuous or tacit, a point that also applies more specifically to their bodily aspects. Some existential feelings are inseparable from feelings of heightened bodily awareness. Consider an experience of anxiety where the world as a whole offers only threat. One *finds oneself* in a realm that is inescapably threatening, rather than finding something threatening within a pre-given world. At the same time, it is a conspicuous, disturbing and very much bodily experience.

Hence the body provides a kind of orientation through which the world is ordinarily encountered in the style of confidence or certainty. This style

---

[23] See also Thompson (2007, p.378) for a development of the idea that fluctuating frameworks of felt dispositions shape our experience of the world. Thompson recognises that these feelings do not simply have a 'positive' or 'negative' valence; they constitute a more nuanced and multi-faceted sense of how one's surroundings are significant. See also Colombetti (2005) for a helpful discussion of the complexity of emotional valence.

wavers in various ways and to differing degrees. Binswanger (1975, pp.222–3) compares losing a confident sense of rootedness in the world to losing our balance and falling:

> When we are in a state of deeply felt hope or expectation and what we have hoped for proves illusory, then the world—in one stroke—becomes radically 'different'. We are completely uprooted, and we lose our footing in the world. [...] our whole existence moves within the meaning matrix of stumbling, sinking, and falling.

There is a sense in which talk of 'sinking' or 'falling' is to be taken literally. A type of existential predicament and an experience of losing one's balance or falling involve much the same configuration of possibility. When we begin to fall, certain kinds of possibility become salient. There is a sense of passively facing some threat, which may take on the guise of certainty: 'I *will* fall'; 'I *will* hit the ground'. At the same time, things that one more usually engages with in a habitual, confident way, such as a bicycle, a chair, or a staircase, are experienced as not offering what was anticipated. So there is a sense of disappointed expectation or surprise. Falling is thus characterized largely by a felt lack of control, by an 'I can't' in relation to imminent danger. The same configuration of possibility, Binswanger suggests, can be something that the overall structure of experience takes on. Rather than 'x no longer offers support' and 'y appears in the guise of a threat that is imminent and certain', we have 'the world as a whole no longer accommodates the possibility of anything offering support' and 'things can only appear in the guise of threat'. The existential feeling has the same structure as an experience of falling, the difference being that the world offers nothing else. Bodily experience and world experience are inseparable, just as they are when one loses balance.

In fact, first-person accounts of depression sometimes describe the experience in terms of losing one's balance, falling, or having already fallen. For instance, Solomon (2001, p.50) states that depression is akin to 'when you feel the earth rushing up at you'. However, instead of being short-lived and offering the prospect of eventual relief, it is constant and inescapable: 'I felt that way hour after hour after hour'. There is a change in the overall style of world-experience, involving erosion of the framework of confident, active anticipation described by Husserl. Just as a specific situation can involve loss of habitual, practical confidence, in a way that implicates our bodily dispositions and capacities, so too can experience as a whole. In place of the world's allure and the habitual, harmonious fulfilment of meaningful possibilities, there is passivity and helplessness: 'Someone once asked me how it felt. I lost my balance, I said. It felt as if I lost my balance. I fell flat on my face and I couldn't get up again' (Brampton, 2008, p.42).

The relationship between existential feelings and bodily dispositions is not a simple one, and possibility p is not always constituted by a bodily disposition to realize p. We have different behavioural dispositions in different situations, even though the same feeling can be said to persist across these situations. Our dispositions are not simply 'frozen in place' by an existential feeling; they are sensitive to changes in our surroundings (although I will suggest that depression is characterized in part by an experience of stasis). So the relevant bodily feelings should not be tied too closely to immediate dispositions to act. It is more accurate to say that existential feelings dispose one towards having certain kinds of behavioural disposition in certain situations. By weakening the link between existential feeling and bodily activity, we allow for the potential involvement of many different kinds of bodily feeling. Indeed, I think existential feelings are likely to have various different ingredients, which interact in all sorts of ways. Some of these will be more closely tied to specific behavioural dispositions than others. It is important not to place too much emphasis on dispositions to *act*. The world is not just something we act upon; it is also a realm in which things happen over which we have little or no control, things that matter to us in a range of ways. Bodily dispositions are equally implicated in feeling unable to act upon something. Passivity in the face of threat may involve inclinations to withdraw, to retreat, along with the absence of any other salient possibilities. And a sense of not being solicited to act is sometimes salient, in the guise of a *feeling* that something is missing from a situation. So there is no simple correspondence between 'situation x includes possibility p' and 'I could do p'.[24] Furthermore, some possibilities take the form 'available to others but not to me'. As we will see, depression often involves the feeling that 'I cannot do this' rather than 'nobody can do this'. It should be added that a given existential feeling does not depend on having specific bodily capacities. Bodily differences between people do not imply different repertoires of existential feeling. One's bodily capacities will partly determine whether and how one finds a flight of stairs, a tennis racquet or a pair of reading glasses significant, but they do not determine whether or not one is able to find anything significant in that kind of way. I am concerned not with whether or not someone

---

[24] For this reason, the term 'affordance' (Gibson, 1979), which is very much in vogue at the time of writing, cannot do the required work. Things do not simply 'afford' activities; they appear significant to us in all sorts of different ways. It is not helpful to say that a bull affords running away from, while a cream cake affords eating. What is needed for current purposes are distinctions between the many ways in which things appear significant to us and, in some cases, solicit activity. Furthermore, the significance something has for us is not just a matter of how we might act. Some significant possibilities present themselves as certain, and thus as impervious to our influence.

has the physical capacity or disposition to find *p* significant in context *c*, but with whether she can find anything significant in that way in any context.

As indicated by the theme of 'balance', existential feeling incorporates proprioceptive and kinaesthetic experience. Gallagher (2005) offers a detailed and largely complementary account of the various contributions made by the body to experience, central to which is a distinction between 'body image' and 'body schema'. The former involves the body as an object of perception or thought, while the latter involves its tacitly shaping experience and thought: 'the body *actively organizes* its sense experience and its movement in relation to pragmatic concerns' (2005, p.142). There is some degree of correspondence between my 'existential feeling' and Gallagher's 'body schema'. However, Gallagher maintains that the schema plays a pre-noetic role, meaning that it structures experience but is not itself something we are aware of; 'it helps to structure consciousness, but does not explicitly show itself in the contents of consciousness' (2005, p.32). The difference may, though, be one of emphasis. Existential feeling is something that we are frequently oblivious of; it structures experience without featuring as an object of experience. Even then, it remains accessible to disciplined phenomenological reflection (of a kind that can be cultured by reflecting on first-person descriptions of existential changes). But Gallagher does not go so far as to say that the pre-noetic body is *irrevocably* out of phenomenological reach. And, more generally, it is not clear to me that there is a clear-cut distinction between what can and cannot be accessed phenomenologically, given that phenomenological research is a skilful practice. So Gallagher's account of the body schema—which draws on a substantial body of empirical evidence for the inseparability of bodily orientation, bodily capacities and perceptual experience—can be construed as complementing and supporting my claim that a structured framework of bodily dispositions is inseparable from a sense of what the world has to offer.[25]

The admission that existential feeling does not have a singular bodily basis might be taken to suggest that it is not a unitary phenomenon but a cluster of

---

[25] My account of existential feeling is based solely on phenomenological considerations. Hence it does not imply any commitment regarding the neural correlates of existential feeling or more specific types of existential feeling. Nevertheless, Gerrans and Scherer (2013) have proposed that my conception of existential feeling is compatible with 'multicomponential appraisal theories' of emotion, and that dispositions to appraise in certain *ways* (where appraisal is understood in affective, non-propositional terms) are the non-phenomenological correlates of existential feelings. If that is right, then a phenomenological-level account of existential feeling complements a substantial, interdisciplinary literature on the neurobiological bases of affective appraisal, pointing to the possibility of fruitful interaction between the phenomenology and the science.

interconnected experiences, all of which somehow involve the body and its actual or potential movements. However, the unity of existential feeling consists in an overarching style of anticipation and fulfilment. A temporal structure unites aspects of experience that might seem separate or at least not as well integrated when construed statically. So it is important to emphasize the dynamics of feeling, as authors such as Sheets-Johnstone (2009) and Stern (2010) have done, rather than to treat feelings as synchronic episodes that occur in isolation from our activities. Feelings emerge and develop in the context of ongoing interaction with the environment. Consider the feeling of strangeness that sometimes arises as one explores a place, even a familiar place, while sick, tired, or jet-lagged. It is as one interacts with the environment that various things are anticipated and do not then appear quite as expected. This sometimes culminates in an all-enveloping sense of one's relationship with the world being somehow 'not quite right', 'out of kilter'. The overall feeling is inextricable from one's ongoing activities, from a general style of anticipation and fulfilment.[26]

Given that existential feelings are both 'bodily experiences' and 'ways of finding oneself in the world', the same existential feeling can be described in different ways. Someone with a pervasive feeling of strangeness, of being dislodged from everyone and everything, might say 'my body feels strange', the world seems strange', 'everyone looks strange', or just 'it feels strange'. When the bodily aspect is emphasized, she might say 'I feel strange' or 'my body feels strange'. 'I feel strange' can also refer to something slightly different—an altered experience *of self*. But changes in what we might call 'self-experience' are equally tied up with what I have described, at least if it is accepted that a 'core' or 'minimal' sense of self involves having a coherent set of bodily capacities and dispositions, which are also reflected in the experienced world (e.g. Slaby, 2012; Svenaeus, 2013). As the same existential feeling can be described in different ways, in terms of the body or self, the self-world relation, the impersonal world, or the social world, it is important not to double- or triple-count them.[27]

---

[26] See also Colombetti (2011) for discussion of the relationship between diffuse feelings and action-readiness. Our more diffuse feelings, she says, 'involve primarily kinaesthetic sensations or action urges' (2011, p.296). Feelings, for Colombetti, are dynamic and kinetic; they are not synchronic 'qualia'.

[27] Here, I part company with Slaby and Stephan (2008, p.510), who sketch a taxonomy of existential feeling that appeals to different 'levels of growing situational specificity and increasing conceptual impregnation'. There is the most basic level, which includes feelings such as that of being alive. Then we have feelings such as unfamiliarity, followed by vulnerability, power and control. At the most specific level, there are feelings of being watched, overwhelmed and the like. In my view, categorisations like this reflect, to some extent, different descriptions of existential feelings rather than different feelings.

How, then, should existential feelings be distinguished and categorized? I suggest that we focus on possibilities. To offer a comprehensive account, we need (1) an analysis of the kinds of possibility that are integrated into human experience and then (2) a further analysis of changes that the possibility space is susceptible to. Even (1) alone is a substantial undertaking, which would involve addressing questions about the criteria and methods employed to distinguish different kinds of possibility, how we are to distinguish a good account of the possibility space from a bad one, and whether there is a single, uniquely appropriate account of it. However, we do not need to refrain from studying changes in existential feeling until all the issues have been resolved and the work of (1) has been completed. Instead, we can address (1) by making a start on (2). By exploring altered existential feeling, in psychiatric illness and elsewhere, we can come to better understand the kinds of possibility that experience incorporates, an understanding that then feeds back into ongoing phenomenological enquiry. This is one of the things I seek to accomplish by engaging with experiences of depression. I will emphasize various different *aspects* of existential feelings in depression. The aim is to arrive at a better understanding of these feelings by approaching them from a number of directions, in a way that is analogous to looking at the contents of a room through several different windows. The same existential changes can be conveyed in terms of the body, the world, other people, one's own abilities, and one's sense of the possible, as well as types of emotion such as guilt, despair, and anxiety. The more windows we look through, the clearer the existential structure of depression experiences becomes. In the process, we come to recognize the underlying unity of what might otherwise look like several discrete symptoms. The resulting account also serves to illuminate the structure of existential feeling more generally, by telling us something about the kinds of transformation that the possibility space is susceptible to.

Eternal Incarceration

Having sketched a general framework for understanding changes in existential feeling, I will now begin applying it to the 'world of depression'. Experiences of depression are often described as being somehow akin to imprisonment without hope of reprieve. Wherever one goes, whatever one does, one remains trapped in the same unchanging, solitary realm. Perhaps the most famous statement of this is Sylvia Plath's, in her semi-autobiographical novel *The Bell Jar*:

> I knew I should be grateful to Mrs Guineau, only I couldn't feel a thing. If Mrs Guineau had given me a ticket to Europe, or a round-the-world cruise, it wouldn't

have made one scrap of difference to me, because wherever I sat—on the deck of a ship or at a street café in Paris or Bangkok—I would be sitting under the same glass bell jar, stewing in my own sour air. (1966, p.178)

Others similarly describe depression in terms of being cut-off from an inter-personal world and stranded or incarcerated for all eternity in a different *kind* of world or reality:

It is the glass wall that separates us from life, from ourselves, that is so truly frightening in depression. It is a terrible sense of our own overwhelming real-ity, a reality that we know has nothing to do with the reality that we once knew. And from which we think we will never escape. It is like living in a parallel uni-verse but a universe so devoid of familiar signs of life that we are adrift, lost. (Brampton, 2008, p.171)

Indeed, the general theme of incarceration features in one or another guise in almost every detailed first-person account of depression (Rowe, 1978, p.30). According to some authors, the experience is somehow touch-like; one is 'immersed' or 'wrapped up' in something. Others emphasize an inability to act; there is an impenetrable barrier that prevents one from engaging with the world. And others couch the experience in visual terms; the world is dark, drained of colour. Many accounts appeal to a combination of vision and agency: one can *see out* but one cannot *get out*. Despite superficial differences in how the 'world' of depression is described, consistent themes are easily discerned. The enclosure is always oppressive, suffocating. Styron (2001, p.49) compares it to 'the diabolical discomfort of being imprisoned in a fiercely over-heated room', whereas Alvarez (2002, p.293) found himself in a 'closed, concentrated world, airless and without exits'. It is also solitary and inescap-able; one is irrevocably alone, cut off from the rest of humanity. Another theme is that of stasis; the world of depression is bereft of even the *possibility* of change. One watches the dynamic lives of other people from inside a soli-tary, unchanging bubble. Alvarez (2002, p.103) thus describes a severe depres-sion as 'a kind of spiritual winter, frozen, sterile, unmoving'. This emphasis on lack of movement suggests that the sense of incarceration is temporal more so than spatial in character. It involves a feeling that things will not and cannot change. If nothing can change, then one cannot escape.

Such experiences can be understood in terms of a loss of possibility. One of the first symptoms often reported is an inability to find happiness in any-thing. It is not just that specific things cease to make the person happy in the way they once did. Instead, 'happiness' is no longer part of her emotional repertoire. For example, Solomon (2001, p.19) writes that 'the first thing that goes is happiness. You cannot gain pleasure from anything. [...] But soon other emotions follow happiness into oblivion'. It is kinds of emotion that fall into 'oblivion' rather than their instances. It is not that the person stops feeling happy about p, q, and r. She gradually loses the sense that anything in the world could offer happiness; she ceases to experience its possibility. What Solomon describes is both an inability to anticipate feeling happy and an inability to actually feel happy. However, this does not suffice to account for the sense of incarceration. If we conceive of 'happiness' as 'hedonic pleasure', our account will be overly restrictive. Granted, the person may well experience a loss of hedonic pleasure, but this alone does not add up to a sense of endless, solitary confinement. If we understand happiness in a more vague and permissive way, we might well accommodate the relevant experience, but at the expense of clarity. What is lacking from the world of depression is not simply the anticipation and/or experience of pleasure, but a sense that there could be *meaningful* change, change of a kind that matters. This is different from anticipated or actual pleasure; meaningful change might bring pleasure but it is not meaningful in virtue of its relationship to pleasure (a point to which I will return in Chapter 6).

I have indicated that there are many different kinds of significant possibility. But we can begin to understand the experience of incarceration if we start by thinking in very general terms about the possibility of 'something happening that matters in a good way'. The depressed person remains aware that change occurs and will continue to occur. What is gone from her experience is more specific than this: a sense that anything could ever change for the better. More usually, one's current situation is experienced as contingent in at least some respects, as susceptible to certain kinds of meaningful change, and this is because one's sense of the present includes an anticipatory structure. In depression, the sense of contingency is lost due to a shift in the overall style of anticipation. In extreme cases, a certain kind of change is neither anticipated nor experienced; nothing good is anticipated and nothing good is experienced as occurring. However, several qualitatively different forms of experience are accommodated by the general category 'loss of openness to the possibility of things changing in a good way'. For instance, the person might inhabit a world where things still matter, but where nothing entices or draws her in. She therefore feels unable to effect meaningful change, but is not impervious to its possibility. (Chapters 4 to 8 will describe this and other variants in detail.) Furthermore, depression can involve what might be described as the 'diminution' or 'erosion' of access to a kind of possibility, rather than its complete absence from experience. Even when an existential change does not involve total loss, it is to be distinguished from a non-existential change in experience where certain things cease to offer what they previously did. While the latter concerns what one experiences as p and to what extent, the former concerns the kinds of experience one is capable of having. Regardless of whether a loss is complete or incomplete, one is no longer able to experience things in certain ways. For instance, the *extent* to which anything *could* appear significant, and thus the extent to which anything could stand out relative to anything else, might be reduced. In the most extreme case, nothing would appear any more salient than what previously appeared as inconsequential, irrelevant; nothing would matter. As will become clear, different kinds of possibility are susceptible to different kinds of erosion, and the same kind of possibility can be eroded in different ways.

An appreciation that 'entity x is significant in way p' can take the form of an explicit judgement, sometimes arrived at through deliberation. However, significance is also something we experience as belonging to the world; the possibilities are 'there'. With the prospect of meaningful transition gone from experience, everything looks somehow different; nothing stands out from anything else anymore. As Shaw (1997, p.58) writes, 'I was looking at the world through a piece of gauze. Everything out there seemed indistinct and unimportant'. One DQ respondent similarly remarks, 'my senses are altered in that everything seems far away and strangely out of focus [. . .] I simply cannot see the wood for the trees' (#228). Whether or not we concede that an appreciation of significant possibilities is part of 'perception', it is surely integral to how we experience the world, by which I mean that it does not always require a judgment made on the basis of a prior experience. Hence we can begin to understand the 'prison' of depression by construing it in terms of a loss of possibility from experience and an associated sense of impossibility. In fact, many sufferers describe their experiences in exactly these terms. The world is bereft of possibilities with which it was once imbued and therefore seems somehow different, in a way that presents itself as inescapable. Consider the following DQ responses:

> #130. I remember a time when I was very young—6 or less years old. The world seemed so large and full of possibilities. It seemed brighter and prettier. Now I feel that the world is small. That I could go anywhere and do anything and nothing for me would change.

> #189. It is impossible to feel that things will ever be different (even though I know I have been depressed before and come out of it). This feeling means I don't care about anything. I feel like nothing is worth anything.

> #277. The world holds no possibilities for me when I'm depressed. Every avenue I consider exploring seems shut off.

> #280. When I'm not depressed, other possibilities exist. Maybe I won't fail, maybe life isn't completely pointless, maybe they do care about me, maybe I do have some good qualities. When depressed, these possibilities simply do not exist.

These and many other first-person accounts of depression explicitly implicate a sense of the possible. What is eroded or lost is the habitual, confident anticipation and actualisation of significant possibilities, something so fundamental to an experience of comfortably belonging in the world that it is often overlooked as a phenomenological achievement. Lott (1996, pp.246–7) describes it as follows:

> I have absolutely no faith, in fact, in anything. In a muddy way, I see that depression manifests itself as a crisis of faith. Not religious faith, but the almost born instinct that things are fluid, that they unfold and change, that new kinds of moment are eventually possible, that the future will arrive. I am in a time-locked place, where the moment I am in will stretch on, agonizingly, for ever. There is no possibility of redemption or hope. It is a final giving up on everything. It is death.

Of course, it might be objected that what I am offering here is a contestable interpretation of ambiguous first-person testimonies. However, the many superficially different first-person descriptions of depression all gravitate toward this same theme. So it does not take an elaborate hermeneutic exercise, involving precarious inferences, tenuous interpretations, or the postulation of hidden meanings to reach the conclusion that depression experiences involve a loss of possibility. Although any one testimony might be contested, the sheer weight of consistent testimony is—in my view—quite compelling, even when we take into account the various methodological concerns raised in Chapter 1. Furthermore, once it is acknowledged that depression involves an alteration in one's sense of the possible, everything else fits into place. As we will see, all sorts of seemingly disparate phenomenon can then be recognized as symptomatic of a unitary shift in existential feeling.

Take, for instance, the belief that recovery from depression is impossible, something that features in many first-person accounts. This could be construed as the depressed person's belief that *not p*, where *p* is the proposition 'I will recover from depression'. However, people do not state that they believed *not p* rather than *p*. What they almost always say is that they could not even *conceive* of the possibility of *p*. By implication, they could not entertain the possibility of a choice between *p* and *not p*. *Not p* struck them as the only available option; it presented itself to them as absolutely certain. When we acknowledge that depression involves loss of any sense that things could change in a good way, it becomes clear why this is so. That kind of possibility is absent from the experienced world and, importantly, from thought too. The depressed person finds herself in a place where the possibility is lacking, and she cannot somehow 'leave' that place in order to think; her thoughts are as constrained by the world's possibilities as her experiences are. Insofar as recovery from depression amounts to things changing in a good way, it is something she cannot entertain; the possibility is not there: 'When I'm depressed life never seems worth living. I can never think about how my life is different from when I'm not depressed. I think that my life will never change and that I will always be depressed' (#75). What might otherwise be interpreted as a localized belief with a specific propositional content, 'I will not recover', is actually an expression of something much more pervasive. Once this is recognized, we can better understand numerous remarks, all of which convey—in slightly different ways—the impossibility of recovery. Here are just a few examples from recent depression memoirs:

> There was and could be no other life than the bleak shadowland I now inhabited. (Shaw, 1997, p.25)

> A human being can survive almost anything, as long as she sees the end in sight. But depression is so insidious, and it compounds daily, that it's impossible to ever see the end. The fog is like a cage without a key. (Wurtzel, 1996, p.168)

> It was inconceivable to me that I should ever recover. The idea that I might be well enough to work again was unimaginable and I cancelled commitments months ahead. (Wolpert, 1999, p.154)

> In the middle of a depressive episode, it is impossible to believe it will pass. It is, oddly, a problem of believing that one is seeing the world 'as it really is' and unable or unwilling to put a gloss on that perception. (Burnard, 2006, p.244)

The conviction that one cannot recover is closely associated with something else that might otherwise be construed in terms of a belief with a specific content: the sense that 'depression reveals the world as it truly is'. Solomon (2001, p.55) describes this as the feeling of 'deep knowledge' that you are 'in touch with the real terribleness of your life'. The world of depression is imbued with certainty because it is bereft of other possibilities. The feeling of conviction, of revelation, arises from privation. Yet there is usually some recognition that things remain meaningful to others. The world is not 'gone'. Instead, one is irrevocably cut-off from a realm that others continue to inhabit. Some compare this to having died or ceased to exist: 'I was certain, quite certain, that I was already dead. The actual dying part, the withering away of my physical body, was a mere formality' (Wurtzel, 1996, p.19); 'I didn't exist, so I could take no pleasure in the material world' (Steinke, 2001, p.64). Remarks like these need not be interpreted as expressing the apparently self-contradictory or, at the very least, counter-intuitive negation of the belief 'p exists' where p is oneself. They concern a level of experience that is presupposed by judgements about what is and is not the case. When we assert that p exists or p does not exist, we do so in the context of already belonging to a world, a space of possibilities where we are able to encounter things as 'the case' or 'not the case'. This sense of being part of the world is eroded in depression, and utterances to the effect that one has died express existential changes rather than circum-scribed experience or belief contents.[28]

Although depression involves loss of the sense that things could change in a good way, the depressed person may still be open to other kinds of significant possibility, such as 'something bad is possibly or certainly going to happen, imminently or in the longer term'. In the absence of the potential for positive change, there is often an all-enveloping feeling of helplessness in the face of some inchoate threat. One is not anxious about something specific, which one might or might not be able to prevent. Instead, experience as a whole is shaped by a *feeling* of one's surroundings as globally oppressive, or takes on the form of waiting for something horrible and inevitable to happen:

> ... ordinary objects—chairs, tables and the like—possessed a frightening, menacing quality which is very hard to describe vividly in the way that I was then affected. It was as though I lived in some kind of hell, containing nothing from which I could obtain relief or comfort. (Testimony quoted by Rowe, 1978, pp.269–70)

> There is something in the future which is coming... I am afraid it will suck out my core and I will be completely empty and anguished. (Thompson, 1995, p.47)

First-person accounts consistently emphasize several further themes, which—I will suggest—concern inseparable aspects of unitary existential changes. For instance, a feeling of being disconnected from other people features in almost every account. The experience is not one of contingent isolation or loneliness, of a kind that could be remedied by a change in social circumstances. Rather, the depressed person feels irrevocably estranged from the rest of humanity. As Thompson (1995, pp.199–200) writes, 'I wanted a connection I couldn't have. [...] The blankness might not even be obvious to others. But on our side of that severed connection, it was hell, a life lived behind glass'. Interpersonal experience in depression comes in a number of different forms. Others might appear threatening or distant, or feelings of worthlessness and guilt might take centre stage. I will address the interpersonal aspects of depression in the chapters that follow, along with several other themes, in order to further clarify the phenomenology

---

[28] The most extreme form of this is the so-called 'Cotard delusion', which is said to involve the belief that one is dead or non-existent. One might attempt to distinguish this from expressions of deadness and non-existence associated with depression on the basis that the depressed person only takes it to be *as if* she is dead; she does not really believe it. However, the difference is not so clear-cut. Many people with severe depression do say that they really believed they were dead, at least in some sense of the word 'dead'. See Ratcliffe (2008, Chapter 6) for an interpretation of the Cotard delusion in terms of existential feeling, and for the view that there is a continuum here, rather than a clear-cut distinction between believing that *p* and merely feeling as if *p*.

of depression and tease out subtle differences between qualitatively different types of depression experience. Despite the heterogeneity that I will emphasize, it should be added that there is also a degree of phenomenological unity to 'depression'. The majority of predicaments associated with diagnoses such as 'major depression' involve existential changes, all of which can be understood in terms of the loss, diminution, or increased salience of certain kinds of possibility. At a very general level of description, the phenomenology of (existential) depression can be characterized as follows:

The practical significance of things is somehow diminished; they no longer offer up the usual possibilities for activity. Associated with this, there may be a sense of impossibility; possibilities appear as 'there but impossible to actualize'. There can also be a sense of estrangement, as possibilities that are inaccessible to the self appear as 'accessible to others with little effort'. Other people might continue to offer possibilities for communion, but these possibilities appear at the same time as 'impossible for me to take up'. Together, these alterations in the possibility space constitute a feeling of isolation, which is experienced as irrevocable because depression does not include a sense of its own contingency. The resultant estrangement from the world amounts to a change in the sense of reality and belonging—things no longer appear available; they are strangely distant, not quite 'there' anymore. Certain kinds of possibility may also be heightened. A world that no longer offers up invitations to act can at the same time take the form of an all-enveloping threat, before which one is passive, helpless and alone. Hope, practical significance and interpersonal connection are not just gone. Their loss is very much part of the experience; it is *felt*.

The Existential Basis of Cognitive Style

The view I have sketched in this chapter parts company with cognitive approaches to depression, which focus on a depressive 'cognitive style' involving characteristic reasoning biases. According to my account, biases towards the adoption of certain kinds of belief are symptomatic of existential feeling; cognitive style arises out of how we find ourselves in the world. Take beliefs such as 'I will not recover', 'things will not get better' and 'I have no future'. It would be a mistake to construe these as convictions that the person is merely *disposed* to adopt. She 'adopts' them because her world is bereft of other possibilities; she cannot even contemplate alternatives. My approach thus differs from cognitive theories such as that of Beck (e.g. 1967), which emphasize reasoning biases. And it differs equally from 'depressive realism', the view that depression involves a *loss* of reasoning biases or a shift from one kind of bias to another (e.g. Alloy ed. 1988). These conflicting positions place a common emphasis on 'cognitive styles' or 'cognitive schemata' and associated 'attributional biases' (see Alloy and Abramson, 1988). Depression, on both accounts, involves distinctive kinds of schemata. That view is closely associated with work on helplessness and depression, particularly the 'reformulated learned helplessness' hypothesis. According to this hypothesis, the depressed person not only finds himself in a seemingly helpless predicament but also asks *why*. Depression is associated with a tendency to answer the question in terms of internal, stable, global factors, such as 'the kind of person I am', and therefore arises due to the combination of bad outcomes with a distinctive attributional style (Abramson et al, 1978; Seligman et al, 1979).

What are cognitive 'schemata'? Alloy and Abramson (1988, p.249) describe one of them, the 'self-schema', as comprising 'an individual's generalized beliefs, attitudes, and assumptions about the self and its relation to the environment as well as specific self-relevant thoughts and behaviors'. So the main difference between my view and cognitive approaches to depression is that they focus on belief contents. A cognitive schema is an entrenched system of (often very general) belief contents, which is employed to evaluate situations and make inferences. However, I have suggested that depression implicates an aspect of experience that is presupposed by any such schema. It is not just a matter of believing that *p*, however many beliefs one might appeal to, and even if we add to the mix the various emotions and feelings associated with those beliefs. Taking something to be the case or otherwise, in the form of a perceptual experience or a non-perceptual belief, presupposes existential feeling. And a change in existential feeling is a change in the *form* of experience and thought. It is not just that one's belief contents change; the *way in which one believes* changes too.

Of course, I do not deny that people with depression diagnoses have systems of beliefs and are disposed towards certain belief contents. But cognitive schemata, conceived of in terms of belief contents, are symptomatic of changes in experiential form. In the case of the belief that recovery is impossible or that depression reveals things as they really are, the 'belief content' is an expression of something much more general, a loss of access to kinds of possibility. For many other belief contents, the link is not so direct and depression does not render them inevitable. Even so, stopping at cognitive schemata leaves us with a comparatively superficial appreciation of what depression experiences consist of. Biases are symptomatic of changes in the possibility space, something that is not itself a belief system.[29] My account is compatible with the view that depression often involves a sense of 'helplessness'. However, as I will show in Chapter 6, this does not consist in an appraisal of one's situation *plus* a set of beliefs about the self. The sense of being constitutionally incapable of acting in a meaningful way is a unitary experience, a way of experiencing the possible.

I concede that *some* instances of diagnosed depression will most likely conform to cognitive approaches, that they will involve systems of intentional states rather than existential feelings. However, this is just to say that labels such as 'major depression' are not sufficiently discriminating to tease apart the majority of 'depressions', which are existential in nature, from superficially similar-sounding predicaments that are actually very different. In these latter cases, the world remains undisturbed—the person can contemplate recovery and meaningful change more generally, as well as hope for things and feel connected to other people. But she lacks certain hopes, she thinks things might not get better, and she feels detached from however many people. I also acknowledge that existential feelings can be affected, in various ways, by changes in belief. Even if a 'cognitive schema' arises out of existential feeling, it may be possible to manipulate a backdrop of feeling by addressing certain beliefs (a point I will return to in Chapter 5). So my position is compatible with the efficacy of cognitive therapies.

Can an account of existential feeling also accommodate the findings of cognitive approaches? It is fairly clear how certain 'beliefs' arise due to a loss of possibility. Haaga and Beck (1995, p.46) observe that 'a salient feature of depressive biases appears to be the underappreciation of potential for improvement in current negative circumstances'. What looks like a circumscribed appraisal is in fact attributable to a shift in the kinds of possibility that the person is open to. It is not a matter of how likely x or y is taken to be; her future offers only more of the same. What about the bias of attributing failures to 'internal, stable, and global causes' (Seligman et al., 1979)? This can also be accounted for in terms of existential feeling. The person lacks any sense that things could be different in ways that matter and thus that she could ever be any different; there is a loss of contingency from her world. So she is inevitably biased towards construing her failures as non-contingent and inescapable. The existential change *explains* the bias, by revealing it to be an inevitable symptom of experiences that people with depression consistently describe. However, a person can also have some of these biases without being depressed. Hence we have the 'cognitive vulnerability hypothesis', which treats cognitive style

---

[29] See also Varga (2014) for a critique of cognitive approaches to depression that emphasizes the rootedness of cognitive schemata in background feeling.

as something that renders one susceptible to depression under certain circumstances, rather than something that makes it inevitable (e.g. Alloy et al., 2006). There are various scenarios to consider here. It could be that an existential feeling gradually becomes more pronounced or that one such feeling disposes a person towards cognitive styles, which in turn provoke existential changes, which precipitate further changes in cognitive style, and so on. But, whatever the case, unless people who are currently severely depressed reason in *exactly the same way* as those who are vulnerable to depression, despite their living in different 'worlds', there is no threat to the view that reasoning biases and existential feelings in depression are inseparable.

Another bias sometimes documented is the tendency to attribute good things to external, contingent causes (Abramson et al., 1978; Seligman et al., 1979). This can be accounted for by acknowledging that loss of possibility in depression often applies to memory and imagination, as well as to what is anticipated:

> I cannot understand what is happening to me. I have felt this way for so long now, it seems hard to imagine that I ever felt any other way, that I was once a different person, with life and heart and libido. (Lott, 1996, p.229)

The ability to appreciate anything that happens as 'good' is lessened, considerably so in some cases. Even so, there is a difference between anticipating the good and recognising something as good when it actually happens. Although anticipation of good things will be substantially diminished, the person may remain able to reliably identify things as good when they do happen. However, insofar as anything is still recognized as good, it is only registered as such in a transient way. Soon it is gone, not part of a world that fails to incorporate the anticipation or memory of anything having that kind of significance. Its contingency is symptomatic of a fleeting appreciation of its import. As for externality, if something good arises due to one's own agency, it will not have been anticipated as an outcome of one's agency and is therefore less likely to be credited to one's agency. Depression therefore goes a lot 'deeper' than cognitive style. An existential approach can accommodate and—to some extent also explain—much that is emphasized by cognitive theories. Up to this point, I have offered only a preliminary sketch of that approach. In order to clarify and elaborate it, I will now turn to more specific aspects of depression's existential structure, beginning with bodily experience.

Chapter 3

Depression and the Body

Depression is generally regarded as a psychological rather than somatic/bodily condition, but is also acknowledged to have a range of bodily symptoms. In this chapter, I challenge the distinction between psychological and somatic illness on phenomenological grounds. In so doing, I introduce a theme that runs throughout the remainder of the book: diagnostic categories such as 'major depression' are insufficiently discriminating and accommodate a variety of predicaments. I begin by drawing on first-person testimonies in order to emphasize the extent to which depression is a *bodily* experience. Although it is not exclusively bodily, I suggest that the same applies to experiences of somatic illness; 'bodily feelings'—in illness and more generally—are seldom, if ever, experiences of *just* the body. Then I turn to some recent empirical work on the relationship between depression and inflammation, which indicates that depression and bodily infection are associated with similar neurobiological changes. It could be maintained that, even if depression has much in common with some experiences of somatic illness, it has additional characteristics that render it distinctive. However, symptoms that are largely or wholly attributable to inflammation could, I argue, meet current DSM criteria for a major depressive episode. Hence some cases of diagnosed 'depression' may well be phenomenologically and neurobiologically indistinguishable from some cases of 'somatic' illness. In other cases, differences may be attributable to greater duration of symptoms in depression and/or changes in self-interpretation and social relations that are associated with depression diagnoses. However, different symptoms, of a kind not associated with inflammation, could equally meet the same diagnostic criteria. It is doubtful that this diverse phenomenology is united by a common aetiology. I thus conclude that, if the label 'major depression' is supposed to identify a unitary category of illness, it is too broad.

The Bodily Phenomenology of Depression

It is often claimed that the expression or even the experience of depression is cross-culturally variable. For instance, some non-Western depression narratives are said to include a 'predominance of somatic symptoms' (Kleinman, 1988, p.41). However, it is important not to understate the place of bodily symptoms in contemporary Western accounts of depression.[1] Bodily experience is a conspicuous theme in all of the depression memoirs I have come across. For example:

> Why do they call it a 'mental' illness? The pain isn't just in my head; it's everywhere, but mainly at my throat and in my heart. Perhaps my heart is broken. Is this what this is? My whole chest feels like it's being crushed. It's hard to breathe. (Brampton, 2008, p.34)

DQ respondents similarly indicated that depression is very much a 'bodily' experience. Of 136 people who answered the question 'how does your body feel when you're depressed?', only two reported no bodily ailments, while two others were unsure. One or more of the words 'tired', 'heavy', 'lethargic' and 'exhausted' appeared in 96 of the other responses. Most of the remainder included closely related terms. There were complaints of lacking energy, feeling drained or fatigued, and having a sluggish or leaden body. Along with experiences of heaviness, exhaustion, and lack of vitality, a range of other bodily symptoms were mentioned, including general aches and pains, headache, feelings of illness, sickness or nausea, joint pain, pressure or pain in the chest, numbness, and loss of appetite. Some also reported a sore throat and blocked nose. Responses varied in detail, with some consisting of only brief remarks:

> #8. Very tired and uncomfortable.

> #26. As heavy as lead. I can't drag it out of bed most of the time.

> #41. Tired, aching.

> #66. Tired and painful. I feel like gravity is pushing me down.

> #129. My body seems very heavy and it's an effort to move.

> #133. Exhausted, drained, no energy.

> #180. Tired but not sleepy. Tight neck and shoulders giving headaches.

> #228. It aches. I can feel fluish. My stomach and throat can ache and I feel anxious.

> #266. Exhausted, heavy limbs, aching, headaches, tired, spaced out.

> #312. Heavy, arched and with hot and cold sweats. Vulnerable and hollow.

> #357. No energy. Just totally run down.

Other responses were more elaborate:

> #14. Slow, heavy, lethargic and painful. Every morning I wake with a sore throat, headache and blocked nose. Everything feels 1000 times harder to do. To get out of bed, hold a cup of tea, it's all such an effort. My entire body aches and feels like it is going to break.

---

[1] Kirmayer (2001) observes that 'somatization of depression and anxiety is ubiquitous and not characteristic of some specific ethnocultural group' (p.24). He adds that we should, in any case, be wary of the 'colonialist dichotomy' between 'Western' and 'non-Western', which is simplistic and anachronistic when applied to an era of 'mass migration and globalization' (p.27). See also Fuchs (2013a) for the point that depression is often described in bodily, rather than affective or cognitive terms, and that this applies cross-culturally.

#22. Lethargic, like it's full of lead. My legs felt heavy all the time and I felt ridicu-lously tired. It was a horrible cycle—the more I felt tired, the more I stayed in bed, so that when I did get up I'd feel even more lethargic. Sometimes I would feel so numb I felt like I couldn't eat anything, or I'd feel 'too sad' to eat. I think a lot of people have this impression that depression is a purely mental illness, and I can't explain it but it totally affects you physically as well and your body just goes into meltdown mode.

#166. It would feel like I had a large nautical rope threaded through my stomach, with a knot bigger than both my fists together at the front pushing on me under the weight of an anvil behind me (1.5–2 meters) on the other end of the rope.

Several respondents added negative evaluations of their bodies or of some bodily characteristic. These were mostly self-evaluations, but a few also referred to how others 'saw' them. The most frequent complaint was that of being 'big', 'fat' or 'ugly', the more general theme being disgust at one's body and sometimes at oneself too. Some wrote that their bodies were 'pointless' or 'useless', where the theme of having a useless body was closely related to that of being a useless person or self:

#110. It feels fat and useless...

#200. Fat, ugly and pointless, fatigued.

#224 Huge, an appendage. Grotesque.

#311. Heavy, tired, useless.

#326. Heavy, slow, big, hideous, painful, pain in my hands and my neck.

#370. Like a useless blob of inconvenient fat.

Only around 10% of responses included such remarks, and some of these also mentioned accompanying diagnoses such as anorexia nervosa (#370) and psychotic episodes (#224).[2] In what follows, I will restrict myself to the core bodily symptoms that feature in almost every account, and will exclude the theme of bodily- and self-evaluation, my aim being to provide an account that is more generally applicable.[3] Many of the bodily experiences

---

[2] All of these respondents were female, raising the issue of whether and to what extent bodily experiences of depression are gendered (in ways that may be historically and/or culturally variable).

[3] It is debatable whether and to what extent an attitude of disgust or shame directed at the body can be extricated from a more immediate bodily experience. It is arguable that a sense of how others perceive one's body is inseparable from how it is experienced (Sartre, 1989, Part 3; Ratcliffe and Broome, 2012). Perhaps one *feels* fat, ugly or disgust-ing in the eyes of others. On the other hand, it could be that one's body is judged to appear disgusting or ugly on the basis of prior experiences and beliefs. It is difficult to arbitrate between these two interpretations in any given case.

described by DQ respondents do not seem so different from experiences associated with acute somatic illnesses such as influenza, but perhaps they only *seem* similar because an exclusive emphasis on bodily experience gives us a very partial picture of the phenomenology of depression. There is a lot more to depression than a way of experiencing one's body and, as discussed in Chapters 1 and 2, much of it is embedded within a more pervasive 'existential change'. This, rather than an associated 'bodily' experience, is surely what distinguishes an experience of depression from one of somatic illness. However, I will now suggest that somatic illnesses can likewise involve disturbances of 'world'.

The World of Illness

On the basis of first-person testimonies, it might seem that many illnesses have an exclusively 'bodily' phenomenology. It is easy enough to find reports of experiences of influenza and other acute illnesses. For example, one website on 'cold and flu' includes (at the time of writing) 153 first-person accounts.[4] They refer to a number of symptoms, including headache, sore throat, stomach ache, congested nose, throat, lungs and/or sinuses, soreness, stiffness, aches, joint pain, feeling hot or cold, sweating, diarrhoea, watery and/or itchy eyes, weakness, and exhaustion. A few posts also mention crying all the time and wondering when it will end. One person remarks, 'I just want to die', and goes on to say 'this one makes me feel like absolute crap and I am just whinging and complaining and I just want to cry all the time'. Aside from that though, the emphasis is almost entirely on unpleasant bodily experiences.

However, those who have explored the phenomenology of somatic illness in any detail tend to describe wider-ranging and more profound phenomenological changes. To quote Merleau-Ponty (1962, p.107), illness can amount to a 'complete form of existence'. Consider some remarks by Virginia Woolf, in her essay *On Being Ill*. First of all, Woolf emphasizes both the difficulty of describing bodily experience and its neglect in literature: 'English, which can express the thoughts of Hamlet and the tragedy of Lear, has no words for the shiver and the headache' (1930/2002, p.6).[5] She adds that experience of illness is not restricted to the body; it transforms one's relationship with the world and with other people. Reflecting on being

---

[4] <http://coldflu.about.com/u/ua/flu/flusymptomsstories.htm>. Originally accessed 11 December 2011. By 20 May 2014, the number of accounts had risen to 667.

[5] Scarry (1985) makes similar points about experiences of pain, claiming that they are indescribable.

in bed with influenza, Woolf notes how 'the world has changed its shape'; 'the whole landscape of life lies remote and fair, like the shore seen from a ship far out at sea' (2002, p.8). This is not unlike the feeling of detachment that many depressed people describe. We find similar themes in J. H. van den Berg's essay on the phenomenology of illness, *The Psychology of the Sickbed*. He focuses on experiences of serious, chronic illness, but much of his discussion is also intended to apply to more mundane cases of acute illness.[6] Again, a shift in how one finds oneself in the world is described. Along with altered bodily experience, the world looks different—familiar things seem somehow strange, distant. There is a feeling of being dislodged from the realm of everyday activity: 'I have ceased to belong; I have no part in it'; the world has 'shrunk to the size of my bedroom, or rather my bed' (van den Berg, 1966, pp.26–7). This shrinkage is attributable in part to one's no longer being practically, purposively immersed in projects that more usually determine whether and how worldly entities appear significant and solicit activity. Things can also become salient in new ways. Their appearance is no longer constrained by what is practically salient in relation to a backdrop of habitual concerns, and so all sorts of ordinarily overlooked details begin to show up:

> The blankets of my bed, articles so much devoted to utility that they used to disappear behind the goal they served, so that in my normal condition I could not possibly have said what color they are, become jungles of colored threads in which my eye laboriously finds its way. (Van den Berg, 1966, p.29)

As van den Berg says elsewhere, to be ill 'means first and foremost that the surroundings have changed' (1972, p.45). And of course, the body is experienced differently as well. What was taken for granted becomes conspicuous: 'The healthy person is allowed to *be* his body and he makes use of this right eagerly; he *is* his body. Illness disturbs this assimilation. Man's body becomes foreign to him' (1966, p.66).[7] Van den Berg also stresses the extent to which experiences of body and world in illness are regulated by interpersonal relations. How the patient 'experiences his sickbed depends to a great extent on the behavior of the visitor: the way he enters, the way he finds a seat and the way he talks', especially where more serious, chronic illnesses are concerned (1966, p.18). An experience of somatic illness can involve, amongst other things, a pervasive feeling of estrangement from others, who either refuse or are unable to engage with the world of illness.

---

[6] See also Carel (2008) for a detailed first-person account of serious, chronic illness, which conveys the extent to which illness changes one's world.

[7] See also Toombs (2001) for a discussion along similar lines.

Bodily Feeling and World Experience

Why are experiences of body and world so intimately connected? I suggested in Chapter 2 that they are sometimes one and the same: a way of experiencing one's body is at the same time a way of experiencing the world and one's relationship with it. But the point does not apply solely to existential feelings, and I will now make a more general case for the inextricability of bodily feeling and world experience. The phenomenology of the body is not exhausted by its featuring as an *object* of experience, as something we perceive and think about. The body is also *that through which* we experience other things. This is a consistent theme in the phenomenological tradition. As Husserl (1989, p.61) puts it, 'the Body [*Leib*] is, in the first place, *the medium of all perception*', something that is '*necessarily* involved in all perception'. It is, he says elsewhere, 'constantly there, functioning as an organ of perception' (2001, p.50).[8] Consider Sartre's (1989, p.332) example of reading when you have tired, sore eyes:

> ...this pain can itself be indicated by objects of the world; i.e., by the book which I read. It is with more difficulty that the words are detached from the undifferentiated ground which they constitute; they may tremble, quiver; their meaning can be derived only with effort...

Before you reflect on the pain, the sore eyes are not an object of perception; the pain manifests itself as how the words on the page appear. And, when the painful eyes do become an object of perception, the experience is quite different.[9] Terms such as 'bodily feeling' and 'bodily experience' are therefore equivocal. There is a distinction to be drawn between the *feeling* body, which is a medium through which something else is experienced, and the *felt* body, which is an object of experience (Ratcliffe, 2008). It is thus a mistake to think of bodily experience as something that occurs in isolation from experience more generally; the two are often inseparable. To illustrate the relational phenomenology of bodily feeling, we can appeal to experiences of touch. When I run my hand along the surface of a desk, what I perceive is not a feeling *in my hand* but the texture of the desk. My hand is not wholly absent from the experience, but neither is it an

---

[8] Merleau-Ponty (1962, p.146) similarly maintains that the active body and its habitual dispositions comprise 'our general medium for having a world'.

[9] We also find something along these lines in Heidegger. Although he neglects the body in *Being and Time*, he does address it at length in his *Zollikon Seminars* (held at the home of Medard Boss between 1959 and 1969). For instance, he says that 'precisely when I am absorbed in something "body and soul", the body is not present. Yet, this "absence" of the body is not nothing, but one of the most mysterious phenomena of privation' (Heidegger, 2001, p.85).

additional *object* of experience, one that is eclipsed by the texture. The hand features as something *through which* I experience something else. The difference is illustrated by the example of two hands touching, used several times by Merleau-Ponty (e.g. 1968, p.9). When you actively touch one hand with the other, only the touched hand is experienced as an object of perception. When you try to bring the other hand into focus, there is a kind of 'gestalt switch', as the perceiving hand becomes the perceived. This does not simply involve a previously recessive *object* of perception becoming dominant; the experience of a perceived hand is qualitatively different from that of a perceiving hand.

One might accept that tactual feeling can involve experiencing the body as perceiver, but insist that touch differs from other kinds of bodily feeling, given that it relies on physical contact between perceiver and perceived. So, what applies to tactual feeling need not apply to feelings that are internal to the body. However, experiences of distance touch count against this. If you write on a rough surface with a pencil, you perceive the surface through the pencil, rather than the boundary between pencil and hand. And when you cut through a steak with a knife, it seems that you perceive the texture of the steak through touch, regardless of whether or not you also perceive the steak knife. Indeed, distance touch is ubiquitous in the context of tool use. One could respond that it does indeed *seem* as though you perceive the surface or the steak, but appearances are deceptive. But, even if we disregard the possibility of distance touch, it is unclear why the scope of 'feelings that reach out beyond the body' should be restricted to those feelings generated by physical contact between an entity and one's skin. More generally, that an experience is caused by physical contact with entity x does not make it an experience of x. In vision and audition, we do not see the proximal stimuli that make contact with the retina or hear the vibrations detected by the inner ear. Similarly, it should not simply be *assumed* that a bodily feeling caused by physical contact with x can have only x and/ or the body as its object. Once it is conceded that some bodily feelings have world-directed intentionality, the default position should be that other kinds of bodily feeling, which equally seem to have world-directed intentionality, have it too. Hence I suggest that we generalize from the case of touch and grant that many other 'bodily feelings' are not just experiences of the body.[10]

Some philosophers of emotion have adopted similar views. For instance, Goldie (2000) distinguishes 'bodily feelings' from 'feelings towards', where the

---

[10] We can also appeal to neurobiological evidence in support of the view that many feelings are relational in structure, rather than being perceptions of bodily states that are contingently associated with externally directed perceptions (Northoff, 2008). Some authors specifically associate bodily feeling, bodily disposition and experience of the environment. For instance, Panskepp (e.g. 1999, p.113) proposes that feeling is bound up with the 'neural

latter are feelings that have intentional objects other than the body. Stocker and Hegeman (1996) draw much the same distinction in terms of 'bodily' and 'psychic' feelings. Although I agree that not all feelings have the body or part of it as their primary object, I reject the proposed distinction between two types of feeling. Instead, I suggest that most, if not all, bodily feelings are relational. They are seldom, if ever, experiences of *just* the body.[11] Even paradigmatically *bodily* experiences such as pains have a relational phenomenology, at least in some instances.[12] The painful body is at the forefront of awareness, but the feeling of pain is not exhausted by its bodily phenomenology. Pains also shape how we experience and relate to our surroundings. To quote the phenomenologist and psychiatrist Eugene Minkowski (1958, p.134):

> ...pain evidently opposes the expansive tendency of our personal impetus; we can no longer turn ourselves outward, nor do we try to leave our personal stamp on the external world. Instead we let the world, in all its impetuousness, come to us, making us suffer. Thus, pain is also an attitude toward the environment.

There may also be more specifically 'existential' experiences of pain, which involve changes in the *kinds* of possibility offered by the world. When we experience intense and enduring pain, the world can cease to be a realm of significant possibilities that draws us in and become something before which we are passive, vulnerable and threatened. Scarry (1985, p.35) goes so far as to say that pain can be 'world-destroying'; it 'destroys a person's self and world, a destruction that is experienced spatially as either the contraction of the universe down to the immediate vicinity of the body or as the body swelling to fill the entire universe'.[13] It is difficult to make confident generalizations about experiences of pain, as it is unclear what 'pain' actually is. There is arguably no single, simple

---

schema of bodily action plans'. In fact, it would be odd, to say the least, for an organism that spends almost every moment of its waking life interacting in some way with its environment to perceive its body and its environment in complete isolation from each other, and only afterwards somehow match the two together in a behaviourally relevant way.

[11] In some of his later writings, Goldie (e.g. 2009) moved in a similar direction, acknowledging that many bodily feelings are also feelings towards. If there was a disagreement between us, it concerned which feelings are exclusively bodily. He maintained that some of them clearly are, but I am not sure we should concede even that much.

[12] Merleau-Ponty (1964, p.5) writes that 'even our most secret affective movements, those most deeply tied to the humoral infrastructure, help to shape our perception of things'. I think this is right.

[13] Cole (2004, p.8) makes the same point in his first-person account of participating in an experiment where intense pain was induced. In his words, 'my immersion in the pain was so consuming that the world, as an external place to calibrate myself in, and from, no longer presented itself to me'.

'feeling of pain', to be extricated from memories, emotions, self-interpretations, and expectations. At the very least, pain has both sensory and affective aspects, which can occur in isolation from one another (Grahek, 2007; Radden, 2009, Chapter 7). Hence I restrict the scope of my claim about pain's relational structure to 'at least some of those experiences that are uncontroversial instances of bodily pain'. It is also worth noting that first-person accounts of depression often remark on its inseparability from pain or something pain-like: 'the gray drizzle of horror induced by depression takes on the quality of physical pain' (Styron, 2001, p.49). Interestingly, there is neurobiological evidence of 'common substrates' for pain and emotional attachment (Kirmayer, 2008, p.322). So the 'painful' estrangement from other people that is central to many depression experiences may be painful in a literal sense.

We can distinguish three broad categories of feeling, all of which are affected in depression. There are 'noematic feelings', which involve the body as a central or peripheral *object* of experience. And there are also 'noetic feelings', where the body is that *through which* something else is experienced (Colombetti and Ratcliffe, 2012). Both of these are experienced against a backdrop of existential feeling.[14] One might worry that the distinction between having a noetic feeling and having no feeling at all is a tenuous one. On one interpretation, when we experience something *through* our bodies, the body disappears altogether from experience. Sartre (1989, p.322), leans towards that view, in maintaining that, when we are unproblematically immersed in projects, our bodily phenomenology consists of nothing more than an organized system of practical possibilities integrated into the experienced world.[15] However, there is a difference between the feeling body and the phenomenologically absent body, as illustrated by cases where a bodily feeling is an object of experience and, at the same time, a way of experiencing something else (Ratcliffe, 2012c).

Let us return to the phenomenology of touch. When holding a pen and effortlessly writing, how one perceives the pen is inextricable from how one's hand is perceived. Consider what happens when the hand starts to ache and tire. When it is no longer a medium of effortless activity, the pen is experienced differently too. One could not experience a pen in the same way with a tired, uncomfortable hand as one does when comfortably absorbed in writing. The aching hand is also a way of perceiving the pen; it is both an object and a medium of perception. A single, unitary feeling is at the same time 'noematic' and 'noetic'. So it

---

[14] There is a further distinction to be drawn between reflective and pre-reflective noematic feelings; something can be an object of experience without our reflecting on what we experience.

[15] See also Leder (1990) for an account of the 'absent body'.

would be more accurate to speak of the noematic and noetic *aspects* of feelings than of two different types of feeling. But in many cases the noetic or noematic aspect is considerably more salient, thus allowing us to distinguish two ends of a spectrum. An experience where one's hand is absorbed in the activity of comfortably writing is at the noetic end. Even then, it does not disappear completely from experience, as illustrated by the phenomenological difference between a hand that 'disappears' into one's activities and one that is completely numb.

Our phenomenological access to noetic feeling could be construed in either of two ways: (1) some feelings are purely noetic but at the same time phenomenologically accessible; (2) a recessive noematic aspect remains, facilitating phenomenological access to a feeling that is primarily noetic. I am not sure which of these is right. In fact, they may well amount to different ways of saying the same thing. On one view, *x* cannot be studied phenomenologically at all without its being the *object* of a certain kind of reflective experience, and the possibility of *x*'s becoming an object of experience implies its having a noematic aspect. Cases of (1) can thus be construed as cases of (2) that fall at the extreme noetic end of the spectrum. And, where *x* is not phenomenologically accessible at all, the body is indeed *absent* from experience rather than noetic. However, even if we accept that there are phenomenologically accessible *purely* noetic feelings, cases such as the uncomfortable hand complicate a simple either/or account of bodily awareness, where the feeling body is contrasted with the felt body. Contrary to Merleau-Ponty's account of two hands touching, a hand need not completely lose its role as perceiver when it becomes an object of perception. A more accurate way of putting things is to say that whether and how the hand is experienced as an object of perception is inseparable from the way in which one perceives through it. The same feeling has two inseparable aspects; we experience it and we experience something else through it.[16]

The view that bodily feeling and world experience are inextricable is consistent with first-person accounts of depression. The body is not experienced in isolation from the world; there is a unitary experience involving both. This unity is something that people often struggle to communicate, perhaps due to well-established distinctions between how the body feels and how we experience and think about our surroundings. For example, Thompson (1995,

---

[16] This account of the touching hands is closer to that of Husserl, who suggests in *Ideas II* that both hands are experienced noetically and noematically at the same time. In his words, 'the sensation is *doubled* in the two parts of the Body [*Leib*], since each is precisely for the other an external thing that is touching and acting upon it, and each is at the same time Body' (Husserl, 1989, p.153). Merleau-Ponty's discussion of touch was influenced by Husserl's.

p.246) remarks on how 'the mental pain was physical, as if the marrow of my bones were being ground into dust'. Some DQ responses similarly draw attention to the inextricability of depression's 'bodily' and 'mental' aspects:

#17. Often the emotional and mental pain during depression was so severe it was very nearly a physical pain. It often felt as though I literally had a broken heart and my chest was tight. I also suffered symptoms of anxiety with depression, which tightened my stomach.

#22. I think a lot of people have this impression that depression is a purely mental illness, and I can't explain it but it totally affects you physically as well and your body just goes into meltdown mode.

Although my emphasis in this book is on existential feeling, depression experiences also involve changes in noetic and noematic feeling. Existential feeling is a phenomenological context within which these feelings occur, a general style of experiencing that determines the *kinds* of more localized feeling a person is able to experience, as well as the overall *balance* between noetic and noematic aspects of experience.[17] A world bereft of any practically significant or enticing activities is one from which certain kinds of noetic feeling, those associated with effortless immersion in activity, are absent. And the lethargic, uncomfortable body that depressed people describe involves a shift towards the noematic. One DQ respondent answered the question about bodily experience as follows: 'Tired—really, really tired—the stairs in my house seem like a mountain' (#147). The stairs are perceived as mountain-like *through* the body. Indeed, everything is experienced through a lethargic, heavy, aching body, and therefore appears uninviting, difficult, daunting.

Fuchs (2003, 2005) suggests that the body ordinarily operates as a medium *through* which the world is experienced but becomes uncomfortably obtrusive and object-like in depression. There is thus a change in one's relationship with the world as a whole, along with a 'reification' or 'corporealization' of the body. I think this is along the right lines, but it is important not to over-emphasize the contrast between a conspicuous, alienated body and one that is harmoniously entwined with its surroundings, as though that difference consisted of having *only* noematic feelings in one case and *only* noetic in the other. According to Fuchs (2003, p.225), 'primordial or lived bodiliness is a constant outward movement, directed to the environment from a hidden center, and participating in the

---

[17] My claims about the phenomenological inextricability of body and world in psychiatric illness are not specific to depression. It is just as plausible to maintain that other psychiatric conditions involve changes in bodily feeling that also amount to alterations in 'how one finds oneself in the world' (Ratcliffe, 2008). For instance, Sass (2004) suggests that a loss of bodily affect in schizophrenia is bound up with what he calls 'unworlding', where the world is stripped of practical potentialities.

world'. Experienced corporeality is a matter of this being 'paralysed or stopped'.[18] However, everyday experience seldom involves effortless participation in the world. We routinely meet with impediments to activity, which take the form of dangers, obstructions, uncertainties, things that require effort, interpersonal confrontations, and so on. In all these circumstances, the body or parts of it become conspicuous to varying degrees and in different ways. Furthermore, not all bodily conspicuousness is a matter of unpleasant alienation. Take the experience of being massaged or caressed, or the feeling of stepping into a hot shower after a long day working outside in cold weather. It can be added that, in the case of the massage or the caress, conspicuousness does not interfere with the body's role as perceiver. If anything, perception of what comes into contact with the body is heightened. Even forms of conspicuousness that are enduring and pervasive need not be estranging. For instance, Young (2005, p.47) describes changes in bodily experience that can occur during pregnancy, where the 'transparent unity of self dissolves and the body attends positively to itself at the same time that it enacts its projects'.[19] Here, and in many other circumstances, bodily awareness does not amount to alienation from one's surroundings.

Experiences of bodily conspicuousness and inconspicuousness are in flux throughout the course of everyday life, and there are many different kinds of conspicuousness. So changes in existential feeling do not just involve the body becoming more or less conspicuous, but changes in *when* and also *how* it is conspicuous. If the approach sketched in Chapter 2 is broadly right, existential feelings are inextricable from felt bodily dispositions, and any existential disturbance will be associated with some sort of change in bodily experience, however subtle. Hence different kinds of depression experience, involving different configurations of the possibility space, will also implicate the body in slightly different ways. A world that fails to entice, to draw one in, corresponds to a sluggish body, one that is not primed for action. A heavy, aching body is a world full of difficulties, where tasks appear daunting, insurmountable. And a world that threatens, overwhelms or suffocates in some inchoate way is at the same time an experience of bodily tension, tightness and pressure. So, although altered bodily experience in depression is ubiquitous and common themes can be discerned, there is also variation. When two people complain of a lethargic, heavy, painful body, one but not the other may have additional feelings of tension and restless. Or one may feel vulnerable or awkward in social situations, while another feels a need to be with others that cannot be satiated.

---

[18] See Stanghellini (2004) for a similar view.

[19] See also Legrand and Ravn (2009) for the view that the body can be phenomenologically conspicuous in various ways while remaining a medium of experience.

Depression, Somatic Illness, and Inflammation

I want to suggest that some—but not all—depression experiences are indistinguishable from types of experience that are attributed to somatic illness. Experiences of bodily lethargy, heaviness and pain characterize somatic illnesses in general. In the context of health, different parts of the body are conspicuous at different times, to varying degrees and in various ways. The body as a whole becomes more salient in illness, in a way that is not so responsive to changes in one's activities or surroundings. This applies equally to the phenomenology of depression. More generally, it is arguable that there is no principled distinction to be drawn between experiences of 'somatic' and 'psychiatric' illness. As Kendell (2001, p.491) remarks:

> That most characteristic of all psychiatric disorders, depressive illness, illustrates the impossibility of distinguishing between physical and mental illnesses. [...] The fact is, it is not possible to identify any characteristic features of either the symptomatology or the aetiology of so-called mental illnesses that consistently distinguish them from physical illnesses.

Even if this is accepted, it can be maintained that depression has distinctive symptoms which set it apart from other types of illness or—at the very least—from non-psychiatric illnesses. All one need concede is that depression is not to be distinguished on the basis of its having a 'psychological' phenomenology in contrast to a 'bodily' one. I doubt, though, that even this much is defensible. Of course, experiences of serious, chronic illness are routinely distinguished from depression, as exemplified by the observation that depression is sometimes but not always co-morbid with them (National Collaborative Centre for Mental Health, 2010). It is also possible to have a general sense of well-being during illness, something that is incompatible with a depression diagnosis.[20] But I want to focus on the more specific question of what distinguishes the phenomenology of depression from a certain kind of all-over bodily experience that is commonly associated with a wide range of illnesses. This general 'feeling of being unwell' arises during acute infections such as influenza, and in chronic illness as well, although it need not be a *constant* accompaniment to the latter.

Nothing I have said so far rules out the possibility that illnesses such as influenza involve an experience of the body, pure and simple. That many (or

---

[20] The possibility of well-being in illness shows that there is no simple correlation between the presence of disease, conceived of biologically, and a certain kind of experience. I am using the term 'illness experience' to refer to kinds of experience that consistently arise due to the presence of some disease, kinds of experience that may well turn out to be quite heterogeneous. When it comes to 'psychiatric illness', however, matters are more complicated, as it is often unclear what—if anything—the relevant disease process consists of.

even most) bodily experiences are inseparable from world experience does not rule out the possibility that others are principally or even exclusively of the body. Perhaps what Woolf, van den Berg and other phenomenologically inclined writers describe are exceptions to the rule. However, as Woolf points out, the phenomenology of somatic illness has been neglected to the extent that we lack the language required to convey it adequately. That may account for the paucity of testimony. But surely influenza symptoms are routinely and unproblematically described, as illustrated by the 153 accounts mentioned earlier? In fact, people seldom offer anything approximating a *description*. Instead, they *name* various phenomena and emphasize how unpleasant they are. Furthermore, a diagnosis of influenza gives one a disease entity and aetiology to refer to, along with an established canon of *bodily* complaints to list. In the case of depression, no disease process has been identified and there is greater emphasis on phenomenological changes that many sufferers find hard to describe. It is therefore likely that a diagnosis of depression disposes one to (attempt to) convey symptoms that are more easily ignored when reporting an experience of influenza.

It is interesting to note that people who have suffered from depression sometimes report confusing its return with the onset of an infection. One DQ respondent comments, 'It [the body] aches. I can feel fluish. My stomach and throat can ache and I feel anxious' (#228). And someone I spoke to while writing this chapter told me how he thought he was becoming depressed, but was subsequently relieved when he developed a cough and a runny nose. Such experiences are by no means unusual. Healy (1993, p.29) reports on a study of depression where the three symptoms most commonly reported were lethargy, followed by a sense of detachment (especially from other people) and then 'physical changes that were described in terms of feeling that the subject was coming down with a viral illness, either influenza or glandular fever'. So we cannot rule out the possibility that differences between narratives of somatic illness and depression are largely attributable to established styles of report, rather than marked phenomenological differences. At this point, one might be tempted to concede that the necessary phenomenological work has not been done yet, that we do not know how to draw the distinction even though we know that there is a distinction to be drawn. However, I will now turn to some neurobiological findings, which support the view that certain experiences of 'depression' are indeed indistinguishable from experiences that would, in other circumstances, be regarded as symptoms of somatic illness.

Distinguishing influenza from depression is usually easy enough, given that influenza involves more than just a vague feeling of being unwell. There are more specific symptoms too, and the same applies to other illnesses. In fact, one might think that the 'feeling of being unwell' to which I refer is an abstraction from experience, rather than something that can be experienced in isolation and legitimately compared to depression. However, I reject that view, on the basis of both phenomenology and immunobiology. What I have in mind is something we often experience before the arrival of more specific symptoms, something that can also linger on for a time after those symptoms have passed. It is not pathogen-specific, and many acute and chronic illnesses involve much the same kind of experience. There is a lack of vitality, inability to concentrate, diminished inclination to act and a feeling of being disconnected from things. This is largely attributable to an immune response common to many illnesses, involving increased release of protein molecules called pro-inflammatory cytokines by white blood cells (particularly monocytes). These cytokines play a regulative role, serving to increase the body's inflammatory response to infection.

It has long been recognized that inflammation in illness is correlated with behavioural changes (which have also been observed in animal studies) and low mood. Correlation does not add up to cause, but the view that pro-inflammatory cytokines play a causal role in feelings of lethargy and low mood is supported by experimental studies where inflammation is induced in healthy subjects (by injecting them with a vaccine, for instance) and mood changes are monitored. Participants report or display symptoms such as 'fatigue, psychomotor slowing, mild cognitive confusion, memory impairment, anxiety, and deterioration in mood', which are strikingly similar to depression (Harrison et al., 2009, p.407). According to Capuron and Miller (2011, p.226), effects of increased pro-inflammatory cytokine activity include 'depression, anxiety, fatigue, psychomotor slowing, anorexia, cognitive dysfunction and sleep impairment; symptoms that overlap with those which characterize neuropsychiatric disorders, especially depression'. Longer term inflammatory responses in patients treated with interferon (an artificial inflammatory cytokine) are associated with diagnoses of major depressive episodes in approximately 50% of cases. There is also a characteristic time course: lethargy is more salient in the first two weeks, while anxiety and depressed mood become more pronounced after one to three months of treatment (Harrison et al., 2009, pp.407–8). So the effect may be attributable to duration more so than degree of inflammation, with lower grade but longer term inflammation having more significant effects (Krishnadas and Cavanagh, 2012, p.495). The mechanism whereby pro-inflammatory cytokines induce sickness behaviour is not well understood. However, it is accepted that they are somehow able to act across the blood-brain barrier, and it seems that sickness-associated experiential changes owe much to their influence on activity in specific areas of the brain, including some of those implicated in the regulation of mood.[21]

Depression is often associated with high levels of inflammatory cytokines. Several markers of inflammation have been found in depressed patients, regardless of age of onset, severity, and more specific diagnosis (Raison et al. 2006; Miller et al. 2009). This is perhaps unsurprising, as acute/chronic psychological stress causes the increased release of inflammatory cytokines, and episodes of depression are frequently preceded by stressors (Raison et al., 2006; Miller et al., 2009). Hence it has been proposed that depression is wholly or partly attributable to over-activation of the immune system: 'depressive disorders might be best characterized as conditions of immune activation, especially hyperactivity of innate immune inflammatory responses' (Raison et al. 2006, p.24). In support of this hypothesis, there are studies reporting that anti-depressants used in conjunction with anti-inflammatory drugs are more effective in treating depression than anti-depressants alone (e.g. Müller et al., 2006). And, as Raison et al. (2006) observe, the inflammation hypothesis of depression also accounts for the increased prevalence of depression in medical illness (which they claim to be five- to ten-fold), given the near ubiquity of inflammation in illness. Furthermore, depression is especially prevalent in illnesses involving higher levels of inflammation. In auto-immune diseases such as multiple sclerosis, lifetime rates of major depressive disorder are reportedly as high as 50% (Krishnadas and Cavanagh, 2012, p.497). That said, we should tread cautiously here, as it is difficult to isolate the effects of inflammation from other factors, including level of distress caused by illness.

Phenomenological research need not (and, in my view, should not) proceed in isolation from relevant science. When it comes to determining whether and to what extent the phenomenology of depression is akin to that of a general 'feeling of being unwell', the neurobiology can help to arbitrate. Changes in brain activation associated with inflammation-induced mood changes were investigated by Harrison et al. (2009), who conducted an fMRI study monitoring brain activation in subjects injected with typhoid vaccine (which causes inflammation). They found that areas showing increased activation corresponded to those identified by Helen Mayberg and colleagues as centrally involved in depression, principally the subgenual cingulate (e.g. Mayberg, 2003; Mayberg et al, 1999, 2005). These changes in brain activation were correlated with first-person reports of fatigue, low mood, anxiety and other symptoms. Harrison et al. (2009, p.407) therefore propose that there is

---

[21] See Capuron and Miller (2011) and Krishnadas and Cavanagh (2012) for further discussion of mechanisms.

a 'common pathophysiological basis for major depressive disorder and sickness-associated mood change and depression'[22] I do not want to put too much weight on neurobiological data. Nevertheless, I think the following methodological principle is generally sound: where there seems to be no phenomenological difference between experiences of type p and type q, an absence of associated neurobiological difference supports the view that there is indeed no phenomenological difference.

Where does this leave us? The most radical conclusion to draw would be that depression and a feeling of being ill are one and the same: depression is a form of experience associated with chronic inflammation. In line with this, many DQ respondents reported experiences that appear indistinguishable from those involved in a wide range of illnesses (at least in the absence of further qualification):

#155. Tired, achy, unwell.

#334. When I first started to suffer from depression I always used to say that it felt as though something 'wasn't quite right' in that I generally felt under the weather. It felt as though I was always coming down with a cold in that I felt 'below par'. My swings in mood are generally accompanied by headaches, sometimes quite bad, and I will always wake up with them. If that is the case I know that my mood is changing and that my headache will not go until I go to sleep that night.

#352. I notice small aches and pains more and also feel nauseous and have an indefinable feeling of being unwell.

Such a conclusion would cast doubt on the legitimacy of 'depression' as an illness category. Given that forms of experience associated with influenza, tonsillitis and a range of other infections are not categorized as 'depression' but as symptoms of infection by some pathogen, it would be dubious to insist that all those other inflammation experiences where the aetiology is unknown constitute a single 'disorder'. Of course, one could maintain that depression is not to be identified with its symptoms; it is what causes them.

---

[22] It is also interesting to note that the same inflammatory cytokines (e.g. IL-6) have been implicated in alcohol hangovers. Verster (2008) suggests that a hangover involves two largely independent factors: dehydration symptoms and the effects of increased concentrations of pro-inflammatory cytokines, although he adds that matters are complicated by additional factors such as tiredness, food, smoking and congeners (colourings and flavourings in drinks). Depression is sometimes compared to a bad hangover. One DQ respondent describes it as a 'permanent hangover', in order to 'illustrate the sense of everything closing in and the feeling of hopelessness' (#60). Another says that it is 'like when you have just had a load to drink the night before and just woken up with a desire to stay put and sleep' (#242). Furthermore, depression is often associated with heavy drinking, and it is generally accepted that the two can feed off each other.

Radden (2009, pp.79–80) makes the helpful distinction between an aetiological/causal conception of depression and an 'ontological descriptivism' that identifies depression with a cluster of symptoms. But to appeal to aetiology here would be to mortgage the integrity of the construct 'depression' on the future discovery of a common cause of all those phenomena currently falling under the category 'symptoms of inflammation not currently attributed to known pathogens'. And that would surely be wishful thinking. Depression is often associated with stressors. However, there is a need to distinguish between proportionate and disproportionate reactions to stressors, and there are different kinds of causal story to be told about stressors, probably many different kinds. There is also appropriateness to consider, which differs from proportionality. A kind of reaction could be entirely inappropriate or, alternatively, appropriate in kind but excessive in its intensity and thus disproportionate. In other cases, 'depression' might arise due to undiagnosed or as yet unidentified pathogens, or some other trigger of inflammation. Hence, even if all cases were largely attributable to inflammation, we would expect the origins of depression to be causally diverse. It is already well established that the relevant immune system responses have a variety of causes and there are no grounds for thinking that cases of 'inflammation: cause currently unidentified' are exceptions to the rule. So, if the radical view is correct, 'depression' is best regarded as a temporary placeholder, to be discarded once we have a more refined understanding of the different phenomena it encompasses.

An obvious objection to the radical conclusion is that symptoms such as low mood are not constant accompaniments to all cases of inflammation, and so the phenomenology associated with inflammation does not add up to that of depression. Indeed, van den Berg (1966, p.73) points out that an experience of illness can give things a new significance; the sick person can make 'his room, his window sill, his window and his view a world full of significant and breathtaking events'. He goes so far as to say that bodily illness gives one a 'soundness of mind' that is often lacking in health. This is in stark contrast to depression, which drains the world of its significance and enticement. We can respond by making clear that the relevant phenomenology is a *common* symptom of inflammation, rather than a *universal* symptom. In those cases where that phenomenology is causally attributable to infection by some pathogen, it is generally regarded as a symptom of somatic illness rather than depression. Hence the claim is that depression is indistinguishable from the kinds of experience associated with *some* inflammatory responses to infection, rather than *all* such responses. To insist that something be present in all cases of x in order to qualify as a symptom of *x* would be too strict a criterion. (In fact, it is not at all clear how the line should be drawn between (a) a 'symptom' of an illness and (b) something caused, however indirectly, by the illness that does not qualify as one of its symptoms.)

A more promising objection is that not all of those illnesses that do involve a general feeling of being unwell (which the radical view takes to be indistinguishable from depression) are co-morbid with depression. Therefore, depression is different from the experience of inflammation. However, in cases where a somatic illness has already been diagnosed, the fact that symptoms *p*, *q*, and *r* can be attributed to that illness rather than depression does not imply a phenomenological difference between the two. In the absence of a diagnosed somatic illness, exactly the same symptoms would be attributed to depression instead, as exemplified by the DSM-IV instruction to disregard what would otherwise be depression symptoms when they can be blamed on another medical condition:

> The evaluation of the symptoms of a Major Depressive Episode is especially difficult when they occur in an individual who also has a general medical condition (e.g. cancer, stroke, myocardial infarction, diabetes). Some of the criterion items of a Major Depressive Episode are identical to the characteristic signs and symptoms of general medical conditions (e.g., weight loss with untreated diabetes, fatigue with cancer). Such symptoms should count toward a Major Depressive Episode except when they are clearly and fully accounted for by a general medical condition. (DSM-IV-TR, p.351)[23]

Nevertheless, the very possibility of co-morbidity implies that at least some cases of depression involve something more. Otherwise, depression could not be diagnosed in conjunction with *any* of those inflammatory conditions that themselves involve an alteration in how one 'finds oneself in the world', and it often is. One might further argue that, contrary to the radical view, depression *always* involves something more, that a general feeling of sickness is common to depression and somatic illness but never sufficient for depression. However, where there are phenomenological differences between a case of depression and a general feeling of being ill, it is arguable that at least some of these are attributable to duration of symptoms. As noted earlier, it has been suggested that symptoms of inflammation follow a temporal course, with mood changes becoming more prominent in the longer term. So perhaps the initial sickness feeling is not sufficient for

---

[23] The DSM-5 update consists of a few changes in wording, but the only substantive alteration in content is the addition of 'pregnancy' as an example of a 'general medical condition' (2013, p.164). I assume we would not want to label all pregnancies 'pathological', and so this addition makes it unclear what a 'general medical condition' actually is.

depression but predisposes one towards other phenomenological changes that are. A comparison could be drawn here with Sass's (e.g. 2003) account of negative symptoms in schizophrenia, according to which initial symptoms such as affective changes and a loss of practical significance constitute a shift in the sense of reality and belonging, of a kind that is presupposed by the intelligibility of later psychotic symptoms. Perhaps the experiences of inertia and despair associated with depression are to be interpreted as arising in the context of already having a body that is drained of its vitality and having a world that is no longer alive with the potential for bodily activity. Alternatively, there could be a simple causal relation here. It is surely plausible to maintain that living with chronic illness *makes* some people feel depressed. Another possibility is that some illnesses cause physiological changes, which then lead to depression. Whatever the case, there is a process involved, rather than a static experiential state that can be compared to another such state.

Even so, there is often more to an experience of depression than an overall feeling of being unwell, regardless of how long the person might have been inflamed for. Depression symptoms such as despair do not relate in a systematic way to experiences of inflammation. As we will see in Chapters 4 and 10, despair takes several different forms. Some of these are plausibly associated with inflammation. In short, bodily fatigue can add up to a feeling of being unable to do various things. So various tasks 'look' difficult or impossible and hope in one's ability to achieve anything is progressively eroded. But not all experiences of despair take that form. For instance, a kind of 'existential despair' that I will describe in Chapter 10 is quite different (which is not to imply that it bears no relationship to bodily feeling). To this, we can add that there is a need for caution regarding the inflammation data. Raison et al. concede that some studies have failed to find a correlation between inflammation and major depression. They acknowledge that 'strong pronouncements about the role of the immune system in depression might be premature', and suggest that 'inflammation contributes to some, but not all, cases of depression' (2006, p.25). In fact, Krishnadas and Cavanagh (2012, p.495) maintain that only about a third of those with major depression diagnoses have raised levels of inflammatory biomarkers.

The Heterogeneity of Depression

How can we arbitrate between different accounts of the relationship between an experience of depression and the kinds of experience associated with inflammation? The problem we eventually have to face is that current conceptions of depression, as well as subcategories such as 'major depression', are too permissive to facilitate the required distinctions. They accommodate and fail to distinguish a range of different predicaments, which are likely to differ from the phenomenology of somatic illness in different ways and to differing degrees. Ehrenberg (2010) remarks on the 'incredible heterogeneity' of the 'depressive phenomenon' (xv), adding that 'depression, far from being a problem of distinguishing the normal from the pathological, brings together such a diversity of symptoms that the difficulty of defining and diagnosing it is a constant fact of psychiatry' (xxix). This is just what we find when we try to compare depression experiences with something as seemingly different as an experience of influenza. Consider the DSM diagnostic criteria for a major depressive episode, which I summarized in the Introduction. The majority are implicitly or explicitly phenomenological, and all are under-described. 'Depressed mood' can surely refer to a range of experiences. And consider feelings of guilt and worthlessness. As we will see in Chapter 5, there are importantly different kinds of guilt, all of which can feature in depression narratives. Thus, as with 'despair', 'guilt' in depression can refer to any of several different predicaments. Given how phenomenologically permissive the DSM criteria are, a pronounced feeling of being unwell, of the kind associated with illnesses such as influenza, could indeed meet the criteria for a major depressive episode, at least when no other illness has been identified. It might well involve depressed mood and loss of interest in activity for at least two weeks, along with other symptoms such as decreased energy, difficulty thinking and changes in sleep patterns. And a common neurobiology corroborates the view that there is no principled way of distinguishing the two phenomenologically. That they share neural correlates suggests they are indeed what they seem to be: much the same.

However, a predicament that did not involve this general sickness feeling could equally meet the same criteria. One might lose interest in activity without having a flu-like bodily experience, and—depending on the circumstances—this could be associated with weight change, guilt, lack of concentration, or even thoughts of suicide. So certain experiences of 'major depression' may be only superficially similar. In the absence of a common phenomenology or aetiology that unites them and sets them apart from other forms of illness, it is not clear what does unite them, other than established diagnostic practice. This is not a new problem. Freud (1917/2005, p.203) made much the same point regarding the category 'melancholia':

> Melancholia, the definition of which fluctuates even in descriptive psychiatry, appears in various different clinical forms; these do not seem amenable to being

grouped together into a single entity, and some of them suggest somatic rather than psychogenetic diseases.

To further complicate matters, diagnosis can itself shape how a person experiences, interprets, and responds to her condition. Although people with influenza sometimes ask 'when will this end?', the time scale is fairly predictable. The appreciation that one's situation is longer-term and of unpredictable duration may influence how it is experienced. A diagnosis of depression implies greater uncertainty, and the sense that 'this might never end' or 'this will never end' could surely precipitate or further fuel feelings of despair.[24] More generally, how one responds to a depressed mood will affect the mood. Not knowing what is happening to you and feeling cut off from others could provoke negative emotions that exacerbate or change the existential feeling that disposed one towards those emotions in the first place. As Healy (1993, p.25) puts it, 'the more people become emotional about being depressed, the deeper the pit they dig for themselves'.

Depression is often interpreted by the sufferer in a way that differs from how somatic illnesses are generally conceived of. Influenza is a foreign invader that inflicts symptoms on the person from the outside, whereas many depression narratives construe depression as integral to the self. As Radden (2009, p.16) puts it, accounts of depression often have a 'symptom-integrating structure', as opposed to one that sets the illness apart from the self.

This interpretative tendency may partly account for the prevalence of feelings of worthlessness and guilt in depression. Whereas influenza temporarily stops one from doing things that one is capable of doing, or prevents one from acting in ways that are consistent with who one takes oneself to be, depression is often construed by sufferers as inextricable from who they are and what they are capable of. Much the same point applies to social relations. I might feel socially uncomfortable or estranged from others due to an external constraint that gets in the way of my normal social dispositions, or I might construe myself as cut off from them due to an enduring attribute of myself. It is arguable that certain depression symptoms are attributable to how the person interprets her predicament, and that self-interpretation is partly responsible for setting some depression experiences apart from some somatic illness experiences. So there is a story to be told about the relationship between existential feelings and the narratives through which we interpret and regulate them, one that I will turn to

---

[24] With this in mind, and also the earlier observation that more severe depression symptoms may be associated with longer term inflammation, it would be interesting to explore the comparative phenomenology of longer term infections such as glandular fever (mononucleosis), as well as that of chronic fatigue syndrome (myalgic encephalopathy).

in Chapter 5. There are also social and interpersonal norms associated with diagnoses of depression and with psychiatric illness more generally, which regulate the behaviour of friends, family and clinicians, and thus play a role in shaping the depressed person's experience and behaviour.

So, what we have is a dynamic and potentially diverse phenomenology, which is associated with a range of causes and embedded in systems of meaning that involve various norms of self-interpretation and performance. The radical conclusion that there is no difference between the phenomenology of depression and a chronic, pronounced feeling of sickness should therefore be rejected, not because depression is something else but because the category is so untidy. The literature on depression and inflammation tends to assume the legitimacy of the diagnostic category 'major depression'. Raison et al. (2006) even engage in some speculative evolutionary theorizing about how depression might involve an adapted immune response that becomes maladaptive in modern social environments. Harrison et al. (2009, p.413) similarly accept the category 'major depression' and speculate over what the mechanisms underlying it might be: 'neurobiological circuits supporting adaptive motivational reorientation during sickness might be 'hijacked' maladaptively during clinical depression'. However, the findings of their studies, when combined with the kind of phenomenological investigation pursued here, render the category highly problematic. It is based largely on phenomenological considerations but encompasses a range of different kinds of experience, while offering us no reason to think that they are aetiologically united. And it fails to distinguish these from other kinds of experience that it does not encompass.[25]

In the absence of phenomenological clarification, the category 'depression' risks being a 'catch-all' term. This raises issues for the treatment of depression. If the diagnosis accommodates different experiences with different causes, there is every reason to suspect that an effective treatment for one of them will not be an effective treatment for some or all of the others. This is consistent with recent literature reporting the limited, variable and/or unpredictable efficacy of current antidepressant treatments. Ghaemi (2008, p.965) summarizes the situation as follows: 'since nosology precedes pharmacology, if we get the diagnosis wrong, the treatment will be ineffective'. In the case of major depression, he argues, we have a category that is 'excessively broad', and the efficacy of pharmaceutical intervention is limited by this.

---

[25] Krishnadas and Cavanagh (2012) also point out that inflammation is present in a range of other psychiatric conditions too, including schizophrenia and post-traumatic stress disorder. Hence, they maintain, it is neither necessary nor sufficient for 'major depression'.

More discriminating methods are needed in order to identify the distinctive sub-group of patients who benefit from SSRIs and other drugs more than they would from placebos, as well as other groups of patients who are likely to be harmed.[26]

I have already suggested that there is an important distinction to be drawn between existential changes and other experiences that might be described in similar ways, and that the category 'major depression' is permissive enough to accommodate both. Most first-person descriptions of depression suggest the former (at least where more severe cases are concerned). However, there are also qualitative distinctions to be drawn between kinds of existential change associated with depression, distinctions that may prove relevant to research, nosology, and treatment. It cannot be determined whether any of the existential variants are more closely associated with inflammation than others until some of the phenomenological work has been done, thus facilitating a more discriminating approach to depression experiences. I will continue that work in Chapter 4, where I turn to the varieties of hopelessness and despair.

---

[26] See also Kirsch (2009) and Undurraga and Baldessarini (2012). Kirsch goes so far as to claim that antidepressants are no more than 'active placebos' (placebos that have a noticeable effect on the person, by making him feel sick, for example). However, if sub-types of what we currently call 'major depression' are better distinguished, we may find that they are effective (that is, more effective than active placebos) for some types but not others. Hence reports of their limited effectiveness or even ineffectiveness could be partly attributable to an inadequate nosology, as argued by Ghaemi (2008).

Chapter 4

Loss of Hope

What is it to lose hope, in the way that many depressed people describe? One might think of hope as a type of intentional state, of the form 'A hopes that p'. That being the case, it would seem that loss of hope is not specific to depression or in any way unusual; people give up on hopes all the time. Perhaps, one might add, depression involves loss of more hopes or of hopes that the person has invested more in. However, in this chapter, I draw a distinction between our 'intentional' hopes and a different kind of hope: 'pre-intentional' or 'existential' hope. I argue that the experiences of hopelessness associated with depression diagnoses are generally of this latter kind. Intentional and existential experiences of hopelessness can be described in similar ways, and are therefore easily confused. As a result, loss of hope in depression is often misconstrued in intentional terms, and the profundity of the experience is not acknowledged. I go on to distinguish several different subtypes of existential hopelessness that feature in depression, thus showing that there are qualitatively different kinds of existential depression experience. Experiences of profound hopelessness or despair are closely associated with suicidal thoughts, feelings and behaviours: 'I see life as meaningless and long to exit so I don't have to deal with it any more' (#66). I suggest that a better understanding of the different forms that loss of existential hope can take (and how they relate to different experiences of agency, time, guilt, and other people) can feed into the task of identifying and responding to kinds of depression experience associated with an especially high risk of suicide.

Hope as an Intentional State

What kinds of predicament are expressed by statements such as 'I've lost hope', 'there is no hope', 'it's hopeless', 'I despair over this', and 'I am in despair'? We could explore whether different kinds of experience are associated with different terms—perhaps an experience of 'hopelessness' differs in some way from one of 'despair'. I doubt that this would be very informative though, as terms like 'despair' and 'hopelessness' are used interchangeably to refer to a range of subtly different experiences. In this chapter, I will describe and distinguish some of these. One way of approaching the loss of hope is to first offer an account of what it is to hope and then treat loss of hope as the subtraction of a state or states of that kind. Hope, one might suggest, is an intentional state of the form 'I hope that p'. And the task of understanding it involves distinguishing hope from other kinds of intentional state, such as belief, desire, and expectation. Hope is sometimes construed as a desire for something, accompanied by an assessment of its likelihood or at least an appreciation of its uncertainty. Bovens (1999, p.674) proposes that hope further involves the investment of 'mental energy' or 'mental imagining'. It has been argued in response that imaginings and the like are expressive rather than constitutive of hope, and that endorsed desire (in contrast to a desire that the person wishes not to have) plus recognition of uncertainty is sufficient (Martin, 2010). However, Meirav (2009) argues that the 'desire plus uncertainty' approach remains unsatisfactory, as two people can have the same level of desire for p and assign much the same probability to p, while one of them hopes for p and the other does not. For example, A and B might buy lottery tickets, find the prospect of winning equally desirable, and know the likelihood of its happening, while A hopes and B does not. Meirav adds that a mental energy criterion does not help matters, given that it is just as compatible with ruminating despair as it is with passionate hope. This objection applies equally to the view that hope is analogous to precaution, insofar as hope involves investing in a prospect and acting as though it will occur while acknowledging that it might not (Pettit, 2004). It is possible to continue investing in a scenario while feeling a deep sense of despair or futility over what will actually happen. Of course, it could be objected that the despairing person does not act as though something will occur, as despair implies otherwise. But then there is a risk of circularity: hope is to be understood as a kind of investment, one that is distinguishable from other kinds of investment on the basis that it involves hope.

Meirav instead proposes that hoping for p involves desire, uncertainty, and also recognition that p's occurrence depends—to some extent—on something outside of one's control. What distinguishes hope from lack of hope or even despair is *trust* in this external factor, a sense that it is ultimately good or on one's side. This emphasis on externality is questionable though. One could hope in the face of adversity, where there is confidence in the justness of one's own stance and actions, along with a kind of trust or faith in one's own ability to perform, despite a sense that 'the world is against me'. It is also unclear what kind of dependence is required. When hoping that a good decision will be reached, one might place trust in an organization, where the emphasis is on reliability and efficiency more so than moral goodness. In other circumstances, one might trust that things will somehow turn out for the best, in a way that rests on the attribution of moral goodness. If the kind of dependence and trust needed for hope comes in several different guises, it is doubtful that all of them will be specific to hope. For instance, similar points can be made about belief: to believe anything with any confidence, we must assume that our cognitive abilities are to some extent 'trustworthy' and that our interactions with the environment can be depended upon to nurture an appreciation of what is actually the case.

So the nature of intentional hope is not so easy to pin down. However, without endorsing a specific analysis, let us assume—for now—that something along these general lines is right, that hope is a distinctive kind of intentional state with some or all of the characteristics mentioned above. That still leaves us with the task of distinguishing and characterizing the various subtypes of intentional hope. For example, McGeer (2004) observes that hope has a normative dimension; one can hope well or badly. 'Wishful hope' involves insufficient reliance on one's own agency, whereas 'wilful hope' is active but involves excessive fixation upon the hope content. Both are ways of hoping badly, in contrast to what McGeer calls 'responsive hope', something that involves neither extreme. And Steinbock (2007, p.438) treats 'desperation' as a distinctive style of hoping, where there is recognition of one's helplessness along with an enduring sense that one has to do something, anything; one attempts to 'force the issue' rather than waiting for it to resolve itself. There is a further distinction to be drawn between hoping for the actualization of x and hoping to avoid it. Consider the kind of hopeful anticipation that can accompany dread, where one clings to the possibility that the dreaded event will not happen. One could 'force the issue' when hoping for x or when hoping for anything but x. We can also draw a more general distinction between passive hope, where one waits for something to happen or for someone else to do something, and active forms of hope, which involve hoping that one's actions will achieve some outcome. These do not map neatly onto the normative categories 'wishful' and 'wilful'. When we hope for something, our ability to influence the outcome varies considerably, and the level of influence we actually have over a situation is what determines whether a hope is appropriately or inappropriately active or passive.

Setting aside the nuances, all of these ways of hoping have the same general structure: 'I hope (in some way and to some extent) that/for p'. So it seems reasonable to assume that 'I've lost all hope of p' communicates the fact that one no longer has an intentional state of the kind 'hope' with content p. However, not all loss of hope is so content-specific. What about complaints such as 'I have lost all hope' or 'all I feel is utter despair'? We could simply extend the same account by maintaining that more hopes are lost, perhaps even all hopes. It should also be acknowledged that loss of hope is not just the absence of something. People often complain of a painful awareness of loss. So it can be added that intentional states of the kind 'hope' have been replaced by other kinds of intentional state, such as disappointment, sadness, or regret.

I am not sure whether anyone explicitly endorses such a view, but something like it is implicit in various contexts of enquiry and practice. Consider the Beck hopelessness scale, a device used in clinical psychology to quantify a person's level of hopelessness (Beck et al., 1974). It is premised on the view that hopelessness is not just an inchoate feeling, but something that consists—at least in part—of evaluative judgments. The data used to measure a person's degree of hopelessness consist of yes/no responses to twenty propositions, most of which explicitly concern the future. They include, for instance, 'my future seems dark to me' and 'I don't expect to get what I really want'. Loss of hope thus appears to involve a switch in attitude towards various propositions. The scale does not make clear what it is that renders one experience of hopelessness more profound than another. Perhaps greater profundity involves loss of more hope contents or, alternatively, loss of hope contents that are more encompassing in scope and have a more significant effect on a person's life. For example, loss of the hope that 'my life will have some kind of purpose' will inevitably affect a person more than loss of the hope that 'I will do something today that has some kind of purpose', as the former implies the latter but not vice versa. Another possibility is that of fading: a more profound loss of hope could involve a greater drop in the level of hope for various things. But, regardless of which account is adopted, losing hope is construed as a loss or weakening of however many attitudes of a given type.

Even if the Beck scale does not actually entail this view, it is at least insensitive to the distinction between hopelessness as a loss of intentional states and the 'existential' forms of hopelessness that I will focus on here. This criticism applies more generally. Take, for example, a hypothesized subtype of depression called 'hopelessness depression', for which hopelessness is taken to be a sufficient cause (Abramson, Metalsky and Alloy, 1989). How is 'hopelessness' to be understood? We will not be able to reliably identify a type of depression unless we are at least clear on that much. Here is the proposal:

> According to the hopelessness theory, a proximal sufficient cause of the symptoms of hopelessness depression is an expectation that highly desired outcomes will not occur or that highly aversive outcomes will occur coupled with an expectation that no response in one's repertoire will change the likelihood of occurrence of these outcomes. (Abramson, Metalsky and Alloy, 1989, p.359)

There is no mention of feeling. What we have instead is an emphasis on reasoning biases and life events, which together lead to a preponderance of beliefs of the form 'horrible event x will occur; nice event y will not occur; and nothing I can do will change things'. The resultant predicament is referred to as 'generalized hopelessness'. Again, it is not clear what this consists of. It could involve piecemeal loss of many intentional hopes, loss of intentional hopes that are fundamental to life projects and thus serve as the basis for lots of other hopes, or a global 'diminution' of intentional hopes. Much of the recent philosophical literature on emotion is equally insensitive to the difference between intentional and existential forms of hope and hopelessness. As discussed in Chapter 2, there is a tendency to construe emotional experiences as intentional states (such as judgments, appraisals, or perceptions), feelings, or a combination of the two.[1] I also noted in Chapter 3 that some philosophers question the feeling/intentionality distinction, maintaining that certain feelings have world-directed intentionality. However, the assumption remains that emotions and their constituents can fall into one or the other of only two categories: 'intentional' and 'non-intentional'. This obscures an important aspect of emotional experience. Certain established emotion categories include forms of experience that are not intentional or non-intentional but, rather, 'pre-intentional'.

I accept that some of the experiences we describe in terms of losing hope involve loss of intentional states of a given kind. And this no doubt applies to at least some statements by people with depression diagnoses to the effect that they have 'lost hope'. But there is another kind of hope, the loss of which is central to many depression experiences. It is not an attitude with a specific content, however vague or general that content might be. Instead, it is a phenomenological backdrop against which states of the kind 'I hope that p' are possible. It can—in principle—survive the loss of all intentional hopes: one can lose 'all hopes' without losing 'all hope'. And when this 'pre-intentional' or 'existential' hope is itself lost, what is gone from experience is not however many hopes but the possibility of adopting an attitude of the kind 'I hope that p', something that can be experienced *as* a loss.

It could be maintained that 'existential hope' is just a disposition towards experiences of hope and has no phenomenology of its own. However, I reject that view. That existential hope is part of our experience becomes clear when we turn to depression. Many depression experiences involve disturbances of existential hope and thus serve to make its phenomenology salient. Existential

---

[1] See, for example, Solomon ed. (2004) for a representative selection of recent approaches to emotion, where this assumption is in evidence throughout.

hope, I will argue, is not simply 'lost' or 'retained'. It is susceptible to various kinds of change, which affect a person's capacity for intentional hope in different ways. Any of these could be described in terms of 'despair' or 'hopelessness'. Hence, when it comes to the experiences of hope and its loss, we miss something philosophically important, something essential to an understanding of certain kinds of human suffering, if we restrict our thinking to intentional states of a given type.

Existential Hope

The difference between 'losing hopes' and 'losing existential hope' can be illustrated by addressing a particular *way* in which hopes sometimes become unsustainable. 'Lost hopes', in the relevant sense, differ from disappointed hopes. Disappointment involves recognition that 'it is not the case that p', whereas loss of hope over p is a matter of 'it will not be the case that p' or, alternatively, 'p is not the case, even though I don't have confirmation of this yet'. Losing the hope that p sometimes involves adopting a different attitude towards p, such as 'I am resigned to the fact that *not p*'. In this case, the proposition p (or *not p*) continues to feature as the content of some attitude. However, another way of losing hope, which I will focus on here, is when the attitude becomes unsustainable because its content loses meaning. Suppose someone hopes to score a goal in a cricket match, but comes to realize that he was confused about the rules of cricket. Here, hope is not replaced by a different attitude with that same content, such as 'it is sad that I will not score a goal in cricket'. Perhaps some hopes are like this—confused from the start. (The hope of surviving one's death as a disembodied soul strikes me as a plausible candidate.) But more common are cases where once meaningful possibilities are lost due to social or cultural changes. For instance, in a country where the monarchy has been overthrown, it no longer makes sense to hope that one will meet the Royal Family.

Is it possible for all of one's hopes to lose their intelligibility in this way? Jonathan Lear (2006) thinks so. He considers the testimony of Plenty Coups, the last chief of the Native American Crow tribe, and suggests that the Crow may well have endured the collapse of a system of meanings that all their hopes and activities depended upon. Various practices around which the Crow structured their lives lost their intelligibility due to historical change. Take the example of planting a 'coup-stick' in the ground, which served as a commitment to not abandoning the stick or retreating in battle. When anticipating a battle, everyone accepted the proposition 'either our warriors will be able to plant their coup-sticks or they will fail' (Lear, 2006, p.25). There were no other possibilities to consider. A warrior might hope to place a coup stick in the ground or, alternatively, consider the situation hopeless and resign himself to failure. But both attitudes presuppose placing a Coup stick in the ground as an intelligible possibility. Once the Crow were moved to a reservation and the US government enforced a ban on tribal warfare, such actions were no longer possible; their meaning was lost. How wide-ranging was this meaning loss? One might think that many other activities, like cooking, would have remained unaffected. But Lear maintains that such activities were embedded within a 'larger scheme of purposefulness'. The meaning of cooking was not restricted to preparing food in order to feed hungry mouths; 'every meal was in effect the cooking-of-a-meal-so-that-those-who-ate-it-would-be-healthy-to-hunt-and-fight' (2006, pp.39–40). Although the Crow could still cook and eat, the richer meanings of these practices were gone and a way of life was lost.

Is what Lear describes something that can happen to a person or group, regardless of whether or not it actually happened to the Crow? It is plausible to suggest that major cultural changes can involve a significant *degree* of meaning loss, but what about a complete loss of the practical meanings upon which hopes rest? Whether or not such a fate can befall an entire culture, something along these lines can and often does happen to individuals. Take experiences of profound grief. Suppose a person has spent the last thirty years in a loving relationship with a partner. It could well be that all or almost all of her activities and projects (other than mechanical routines that would not ordinarily be associated with attitudes such as 'hope') make explicit or implicit reference to the partner in some way, take on the significance they do because of the relationship, and are regulated by the relationship. Every Saturday, it is 'we' who get up and head to the café for breakfast, 'we' who take it in turns to make lunch, and 'we' who enjoy drinking wine together in the evening. When options such as 'a bottle of wine tonight or no bottle of wine tonight' are considered, the partner's participation in both scenarios is taken for granted. Even activities that the partner is not directly involved in somehow implicate him. For instance, money is earned in order to sustain 'our' life together. The contents of all the person's hopes, all her aspirations, thus involve the partner in one way or another. For someone with that kind of life, the partner's death could, I think, impact on all hopes. It is not that she would cease to hope for various states of affairs, but that these states of affairs would no longer make sense. Consider Auden's poem *Funeral Blues*, which ends with the words 'nothing now can ever come to any good'. This is reminiscent of Lear's interpretation of Plenty Coups' assertion that 'after this, nothing happened' (2006, p.2). There comes a time when the meaningful possibilities presupposed by all one's hopes cease to be. After that, nothing of any consequence *could* happen.

Auden's poem also emphasizes how all the meanings of a life can depend on another individual: 'He was my North, my South, my East and West, My working week and my Sunday rest'. Grief is experienced as a catastrophe that befalls one's entire world.[2] C. S. Lewis (1966, p.12) describes the experience as follows: 'The act of living is different all through. Her absence is like the sky, spread over everything'. There is a pervasive feeling of dislocation, implicating all of the meaningful practices that one previously took as given.

Various other life events can be construed in a similar way. Consider, for example, a dedicated employee who loses a job she has performed with pride for many years. What she hopes to achieve, hopes to be, hopes to experience and hopes to avoid all implicate that professional role. In its absence, very little survives intact. So it is arguable that meaning catastrophes of the kind Lear describes are not so uncommon at the level of the individual. A collapse is surely no less severe *for an individual* when it affects only her own idiosyncratic system of meanings. Granted, she still has access to the broader meanings of a culture, but these alone are not enough to constitute the meaningfulness of *her* life. She must also be able to make some of these meanings significant in ways that are specific to her. It is not enough that one's culture offers the possibilities of being a chef, a police officer, or an academic. The contents of a person's hopes depend more specifically on which of these possibilities she has made her own. In fact, when meaning loss is specific to the individual, rather than shared, it is perhaps more troubling, given that she feels estranged from everyone else, different from them in a way they may not understand.

Let us accept that it is possible to lose all or most of one's hopes due to a breakdown of content-intelligibility: one recognizes that the content no longer makes sense and is consequently unable to adopt an attitude with that content. Does this amount to a 'loss of hope'? Lear's answer is no—a kind of hope can remain. He calls this 'radical hope', because it is directed at a good that one currently lacks the conceptual resources to understand (Lear, 2006, p.103). Somehow, the Crow found the ability to carry on, rather than giving up completely. Lear suggests that their ability to do so may have rested on how they interpreted a dream vision experienced by Plenty Coups in 1855 or 1856. The dream pointed to something that could not be fully understood, while at the same time offering the reassurance that it could somehow be endured. So the kind of hope they retained was devoid of specific content; it included only the 'bare idea *that something good will emerge*'. All Crow possibilities might be gone, but what remained was 'the possibility of new Crow possibilities' (2006, pp. 94–8).

---

[2] This kind of meaning loss does not exhaust an experience of grief. My claim is only that it can be an aspect of grief.

The point applies equally to bereavement and other life events. Reflecting on his own experience of grief, Whybrow (1997, p.2) offers this description:

> When it strikes, the raw intensity of the feeling comes as a surprise. Life is rolled on its head, and we find ourselves off balance. Routine patterns and familiar assumptions are called into question. Social attachments of love and friendship that gave life meaning and purpose are fundamentally changed. Inevitably we are confronted with the challenge of finding for ourselves a new fit with the world, for that which was once a stable and accustomed part of life's routine has been irretrievably lost. The external world has changed and with it the inner world of personal meaning.

What he describes is similar in some respects to first-person accounts of depression, but Whybrow distinguishes the two, suggesting that severe or 'melancholic' depression is an 'emotional pole we glimpse while in the throes of grief' (1997, p.15). What is the difference? In both cases, we might say that the world 'looks' different—it is no longer imbued with the possibilities it once was; things are no longer significant in the ways they were. However, Whybrow also refers to the 'challenge' of finding a 'new fit' with the world, that of immersing oneself in new systems of meaning. What is lost, it seems, is a system of meanings and an associated system of hopes, rather than a capacity to hope and find meaning. I do not want to make generalizations about what *the* experience of grief amounts to, any more than I do in the case of depression. Grief can be thought of as a process that takes various forms, rather than as a singular state of varying intensity. As Goldie (2011a, p.125) observes, a grieving process involves 'characteristic thoughts, judgments, feelings, imaginings, actions, expressive actions, habitual actions, and much else besides, unfolding over time, but none of which is essential at any particular time'. We can distinguish existential forms of depression from many experiences of grief on the basis that this dynamism is lacking in depression. In Chapter 2, I emphasized how the world of depression seems inescapable; there is a feeling that one's predicament will not and cannot change in a good way. Grief, in contrast, can include openness to the possibility of positive change, and thus the ability to engage in a process. There are grief experiences that lack this dynamic process shape, which I will further discuss in Chapter 7. And I also acknowledge that a loss of habitual meanings, hopes and aspirations can itself take the form of an existential change (of a kind that I will describe later in this chapter as a 'loss of trust in the world'). So the distinction between existential and non-existential grief is difficult to draw, as is that between some experiences of grief and some experiences of depression. For now, though, suffice it to say that certain grief experiences can be understood as involving the complete or near-complete loss of a system of intentional hopes, along with the retention of what Lear calls 'radical hope'.

Radical hope might be interpreted as an intentional state of the form 'I/ we hope that p', with a vague or very general content, such as 'good will ultimately come of this'. However, although it is easy enough to describe it in such terms, that interpretation is implausible. First of all, it is not at all clear what p is. The same 'hope' can be expressed in all sorts of ways, such as 'possibilities will return', 'we can continue', 'things will eventually work out', 'we must have courage', 'nobody knows what the future might bring', 'we will survive or prevail', 'the world is ultimately good', and 'life will go on'. Not all are synonymous and it is doubtful that they all express a single, core propositional content. Second, it is only given very general possibilities of the kind 'things may turn out for the good' that one can adopt attitudes with the more specific content 'this particular state of affairs may turn out for the good' and, by implication, the more specific attitude of hoping for something. That there are possibilities of that *kind* is something all intentional experiences of 'hoping' presuppose. Radical hope is not an intentional state with some specifiable content but, rather, a sense of the kinds of possibility that the world contains. It is a context in which intentional states of the kind 'I hope that p' are possible. By analogy, having a sense that 'there is a future' might be described as the belief that p, where p is 'there is a future'. As in the case of 'the hope that p', it is trivially easy to offer such linguistic constructions but also misleading. A sense of there being a future is presupposed by the possibility of intentional states of various kinds, such as desire, hope and anticipation. Without it, those states would not be intelligible. It is also doubtful that one could have beliefs without any sense of the future. The concept of belief surely implicates possibilities such as checking, confirming and repudiating, all of which presuppose some sense of future possibility. The difference is that radical hope is more specific than 'there is a future'. It is also a sense that the future offers kinds of significant possibility that attitudes of intentional hope depend upon.[3] It is not the bare appreciation that 'something is coming', but a more specific kind of anticipatory structure that includes possibilities such as 'things could change for the better' and 'bad things might not happen'.

An implication of my interpretation, which parts company with Lear's account, is that what he calls 'radical hope' is not something people only occasionally have, at times when other hopes have lost their meaning. It is

---

[3] An alternative approach is to construe radical hope as 'meta-hope', the intentional state of hoping for the return of hope. However, as I will show in the remainder of this chapter, loss of radical hope can amount to a sense that intentional hope (including the hope that hope will return) is impossible. 'Loss of meta-hope' might account for an absence of hopes but it cannot account for a sense of impossibility.

something most of us have most of the time, a backdrop against which our various hopes are formed, nurtured and lost. What Lear succeeds in doing is distinguishing two very different types of hope by showing how a type of 'hope' can remain even when all 'hopes' are lost.[4] What is notable about Plenty Coups is not that he summoned up radical hope in such circumstances but that he managed to retain it. He might not have done, and the same goes for those suffering from profound grief—loss of a system of hopes can erode the capacity for hope. One can lose the 'will to go on'. The fact that some people do and others don't, even though both may have suffered a comparable erosion of hopes, makes the contrast between 'loss of hopes' and 'loss of hope' all the more salient.

A less extreme erosion of past meanings and openness to new meanings characterizes human life more generally. And the background orientation through which change and uncertainty are met varies in structure from person to person and time to time. The degree to which we 'have hope' is affected by life events, health, mood, and other factors. On some mornings, one gets out of bed to find the world thoroughly enticing, filled with possibilities for good things. On other days, the world can seem dull, threatening, bereft of the possibility of positive change. But, for most of us, most of the time, there is at least some degree of hope, a general sense that things might turn out for the good. It is in the context of this that more specific hopes are formed and projects take shape.[5]

A loss of radical hope is therefore a deeper or more profound kind of experience than a loss of all hopes, as one not only loses however many actual hopes but also an orientation that is presupposed by the possibility of hoping for anything. Steinbock (2007) aptly describes this as a loss of the 'ground of hope'. Like Meirav (2009), he proposes that the capacity to hope for p presupposes trust in something external, something that also amounts to a sense

---

[4] Existential hope is thus akin to faith in some respects, but they also differ. Faith can have a determinate content, whereas existential hope can survive the loss of all such contents. And faith can involve unwavering *certainty* whereas radical hope is a sense of there being certain kinds of *possibility*.

[5] Webb (2007, p.68) makes a similar distinction in terms of 'goal-directed' and 'open-ended' hope (along with several further distinctions), where the latter is much like my 'existential hope'. However, a hope can be open-ended without amounting to a way of finding oneself in the world. In the context of already inhabiting a world that includes the possibility of hope, one can have intentional hopes with indeterminate and wide-ranging contents. McGeer (2004) also describes something along the lines of existential hope. Rather than assuming that hope is a kind of intentional state, she construes it as a drive towards the future that is integral to human life and inseparable from the capacity for action.

of the kinds of possibility the future has to offer. Its loss, he says, is the most profound challenge to hope one could ever face. Steinbock (2007, p.449) calls this 'despair': 'when I despair, I experience the future as closed of meaning-ful possibilities that should otherwise be there'. This does not capture all or perhaps even most everyday uses of the word 'despair'. If despair were a com-plete loss of the intelligibility of hope, people could not—as they sometimes do—talk about 'depths of despair'; one would either despair or one wouldn't. And the term 'despair' can also be used to communicate an intentional state with a specific content, such as 'I despair over the increasingly managerial culture of British universities'. Such talk conveys a painful sense of resigna-tion regarding a specific state of affairs that one finds undesirable. But the fact that Steinbock's use of the term 'despair' is either a technical or revisionary one does not detract from his distinction between loss of intentional hope and loss of what it depends upon: 'even if I experienced hopelessness in every particular instance, the sum of these experiences would not equal despair because the ground of hope can still function guidingly' (Steinbock, 2007, p.448). His 'ground of hope', which I identify with Lear's 'radical hope', is not a system of hopes embedded in a pre-given world. It is a sense of the kinds of possibility the world incorporates, an aspect of existential feeling. Many experiences of depression, I will now suggest, involve loss of existential hope, rather than of however many intentional hopes. I will also describe some of the different forms this loss can take.

The Impossibility of Hope

First-person accounts of hopelessness in depression often indicate that it involves more than a lack of however many specific hopes, regardless of how wide-ranging their content might be. A capacity for hope presupposes a sense of the future as a dimension in which significant possibilities can be actual-ized. Those possibilities need to have a certain kind of significance; they have to be 'good' in some way, rather than—say—threatening. In more severe cases of depression, an orientation towards the future that intentional hope presup-poses is transformed in such a way as to prohibit the possibility of hoping. Karp (1996, p.27) describes this as follows:

> Although depression alters perceptions in multiple ways, the social world seems to lose its normal temporal dimension for most sufferers. Their present bad feelings so thoroughly capture them that the sense of hope and security normally framing images of a future is destroyed.

Where Karp writes of a sense of hope and security 'framing' the future, he is not referring to a specific hope content but to a more general sense of the future that shapes all experience and thought. A style of anticipation is absent; nothing is practically significant anymore, nothing beckons activities, and so nothing offers the possibility of meaningful change. Without a sense of the future as a dimension of meaningful change, one cannot hope—it is 'hope' itself that is gone, and experienced *as* gone. Many other accounts convey much the same thing. For instance, Styron (2001, p.58) describes reaching a stage where 'all sense of hope had vanished'. What is lost is something so fundamental to our experience of the world that we are more usually oblivious to it. Its loss is therefore unfamiliar, difficult to understand and express. As Brampton (2008, p.18) writes, 'There were no words to explain the depths of my despair. I didn't understand it myself'. As mentioned in Chapter 2, such a predicament underlies seemingly more localized expressions of hopelessness, such as having no hope of recovery from depression. When hope itself has lost its intelligibility, recovery inevitably strikes one as impossible:

> My father would assure me, sunnily, that I would be able to do it all again, soon. He could as well have told me that I would soon be able to build myself a helicopter out of cookie dough and fly on it to Neptune, so clear did it seem to me that my real life, the one I had lived before, was now definitively over. (Solomon, 2001, p.54)

What is missing is openness to kinds of possibility that hoping depends upon. The perceived world is devoid of the potential for certain kinds of significant change, and so it looks somehow different, diminished:

> #23. The world looks very different when I am depressed, because everything looks dark/black and bleak. To me it looks like the colour and joy has been sucked out of the world and that the world looks completely dull.

The loss is not specific to perceptual experience. Certain kinds of possibility can no longer be imagined either and are inaccessible to thought more generally, gone from the world *within* which one's experiences and thoughts reside:

> #22. Life seems completely pointless when depressed. Depression is the worst feeling in the world and when you're absorbed in its depths you just don't even want to be there, anything to stop the numbness and pain. You can't see far into the future so you can't see aspirations or dreams. Everything I ever wanted to do with my life before seemed impossible now. I also would think that I would never get out, that I'd be depressed forever. It brings quite irrational thinking because it's not a rational illness. It makes you think all sorts of things about life and yourself that aren't true. I thought I'd never escape from the depths of depression and never achieve anything with my life.
>
> #343. See no future or a hopeless future.

The nature of the existential shift can vary in subtle ways. Sometimes the emphasis is on one's own life. It is 'I' who lack access to the kinds of possibility upon which hopes rest. So the prospect of any improvement in 'my' life is absent: 'When depressed I feel I have no future and lose any hope in things improving in my life. I feel generally hopeless' (#158). This need not imply that the depressed person still recognizes others as having access to hope. It could be that she emphasizes her own life because her sense that other people matter has also been eroded. However, the feelings of estrangement and isolation that are often described indicate that some degree of recognition remains. Others are seen to go about their business in a place where hope is possible; it is only 'my' world that is bereft of hope. This contrast is partly constitutive of the glass wall between self and others, the division between a solitary, static realm and a public world where others continue to reside. But the sense of impossibility is circumscribed to varying degrees: one might find the possibility of hope unintelligible in the context of one's own life or in a more enveloping way that applies to all human life, any conceivable human life, or even any conceivable kind of life: 'I can't see any future for myself or the rest of the human race' (#26). Regardless of whether or not the loss of hope is experienced as self-specific, what makes the predicament distinctive is the associated sense of impossibility. With this, it is not just that the depressed person ceases to hope, but that she *experiences herself as unable to*, even though she may continue to recognize that others possess something she lacks.

Within the general category 'loss of existential hope', there is a distinction to be drawn between losses of active and passive hope. A person might experience herself as incapable of actualizing meaningful possibilities: 'I feel hopeless, as though there is nothing I can do that will ever truly improve my life. I often feel like I'm in a rut, like I'm stuck' (#171). Loss of active hope (something that is inextricable from changes in a person's experience of agency, which I will turn to in Chapter 6) is compatible with retention of passive hope and thus with reliance upon others. However, the sense of loss often envelops both: 'I have a feeling of pointlessness and inevitability of outcome so feel powerless to make changes' (#352). Insofar as something is pointless and also inevitable, passive hope is equally unsustainable. Where something is inevitable, nobody can act so as to avoid it; alternative possibilities are absent.

In many cases of existential hopelessness, the world is not simply 'dead'. In place of a structured system of significant possibilities, of the kind required for the intelligibility of projects, goals and hopes, sufferers often report that things are anticipated in the guise of fear, dread or horror. Purposive action is stifled because the world offers only danger. Passive hope is usually unsustainable too, given that other people appear as a source of threat and often the primary source (a point I will return to in Chapter 8). So the experience frequently includes a sense of one's own impotence and, with it, an inability to depend on others:

#14. [The world] seems to be full of more hatred, evil and fear. When I am depressed, the world is a truly awful place to be.

#34. The problem with depression is you lose hope and then you get very self-destructive. I also find that the world becomes a dark and dangerous place and I become unable to find any joy or happiness in it.

#324. The world seems pointless because when I am depressed I can't see the world in a positive way. All I see is a place full of suffering which I often feel I would be better off escaping from.

#347. When depressed I see life as pointless and sometimes cruel. I cannot see any possibilities for change or improvement.

#367. Whilst depressed, I feel an impending sense of doom. I feel hopeless and use-less, and my self-confidence drops so low that sometimes I cannot even leave the house to buy food as I don't feel worthy to be taking up any space and time.

The future is there, but it offers nothing of the kind that would allow one to form hopes. Openness to the possibility of something good happening is replaced by the certainty of something bad happening. The experience does not just con-sist of however many intentional states. It is a shift in the kinds of possibility one's world incorporates, which constrains the kinds of intentional state one can adopt. Now, one might object that even the most severely depressed person does not lack 'all hope', as he can and often does hope for death. For example:

#14. When I am depressed I want to die. I want to go to sleep and never ever wake up. When I am depressed the world seems such an awful place I no longer wish to be part of it.

#23. When I am not depressed my feelings/emotions are totally different, because I can think clearly. I can see a future for myself. I can feel happiness. I can see the joys in life. I can socialize. I can be loving and friendly. When I am depressed, I am unable to think clearly. I feel sorrow, anger, frustration, sadness, lonely, worthless, despair and mainly I feel like my life is not worth living and I would rather be dead!

However, we should not read too much into the fact that the word 'hope' can be used to describe a 'wish' or 'want' for death that arises against the back-drop of a more general loss of hope. Ordinarily, we form our hopes within a world where the future can differ from the present in all manner of significant ways, where a situation we hope to realize or hope to avoid may or may not come to pass. In depression, as one DQ respondent remarks, 'there is the feel-ing that your life "contracts"—you stop seeing it as an expansive project and it all zeroes in on feelings of despair and wanting to escape' (#61). What we might call a 'desire', 'wish', or 'hope' for death does not resemble 'hope' in the more familiar sense, as an attitude of hope presupposes an open future. The kinds of possibility that hope depends on are absent, and the only meaningful distinction left is that between inhabiting a world bereft of the potential for positive change and ceasing to be. This contrast, at least, continues to make sense; the depressed person still finds himself in a world that offers suffering, something that can be distinguished from 'nothing whatsoever' (which is not to insist that death is always conceived of by the person simply in terms of 'nothing'). Hence he does not hope for death in the way one might hope for some future event within the world—it is a different *kind* of attitude.

Although passively hoping for death is to be distinguished from actively seeking death, the point applies equally to suicide. Drawing on my work on existential feeling, along with a substantial body of first-person testimony, Benson, Gibson and Brand (2013) identify what they call a 'feeling of being suicidal', an existential feeling of a kind that drives the person towards suicide. Suicidal feeling, they maintain, does not consist in a system of beliefs, emotions, or intentions, at least not in any familiar sense. The very form of motivation has been altered. Sometimes, the depressed person no longer experiences or thinks of herself as an agent in a way that most of us take for granted. A process occurs whereby her world is sapped of the possibilities that experiences of agency and choice presuppose. So much is already gone from it that she experiences herself as no longer fully alive. Suicide presents itself as the final stage in a process that is already close to completion: 'You feel tempted to end the suffering—however this is not a calculated decision (to end the suffering); it is feeling as though it's a natural next step to take (just like animals seek solitude to die)' (#117). The experience thus involves a way of 'wishing' that is quite alien to many of us.

I do not want to suggest that there is a single 'experience of being suicidal'. Another kind of experience to consider is that of existential guilt (which will be addressed in Chapter 5). Fuchs (2003, p.239) proposes that 'suicide for the melancholic does not mean anticipated relief (as it often does for the neurotic patient), but rather adequate punishment, the execution of a death sentence'. The sense of hope, of an open future, is gone. This adds up to a feeling of inescapable guilt, which nurtures the conviction that one should be punished. And where some sense of agency remains, this is something one may act upon. I say 'where some sense of agency remains' because I also want to acknowledge that there can be a sense of inescapability and incapacity so profound that even death, through suicide or any other cause, does not present itself as an alternative. The predicament seems eternal, irrevocable, and no possibility for efficacious action remains. In such a case, the risk of suicide would be higher were the person to recover some sense of her capacity to effect change, while continuing to inhabit a world that is devoid of hope and offers only suffering.[6]

---

[6] This is consistent with the view that risk of suicide is heightened as a person starts to recover from depression. That view is not uncontroversial though. See, for example, Mittal, Brown and Shorter (2009). However, what I have suggested only applies to a certain kind of depression experience, one where—at some point—the loss of hope is so profound that even death does not present itself as offering an alternative.

The ability to distinguish existential hopelessness and its variants thus has a potential role to play in identifying those depression experiences associated with especially high risks of suicide, improving our understanding of them and perhaps—in the process—informing our response to them.[7] There are also more general implications for psychiatric classification and diagnosis. Current diagnostic practices are not guided by an explicit distinction between losing existential hope and losing intentional hopes. Consequently, it is likely that both are associated with diagnoses of major depression. Carl Elliott raises similar concerns in relation to the use of antidepressants. These, he says, are often used to treat something that is 'not so much depression as a peculiar sense of feeling lost in the world, the sense that all the old structures that once gave life sense have disappeared, that we have been abandoned and lost at sea, castaways on a lonely island' (1999, p.53). This is much like the kind of experience Lear describes, where the meanings of a life are eroded and the intentional hopes that presuppose those meanings are consequently lost.

In most of those cases where existential hope is lost, it is not altogether *absent* from experience, analogous to someone who quietly leaves a party without saying goodbye. Its absence is unpleasantly salient, very much *there*. How do we account for that? A person might remember that things used to be different, but this does not suffice for a feeling of absence or loss. That I remember *p* does not imply that the current absence of *p* is itself experienced. However, there are all sorts of circumstances where things change and we *do* have a sense of loss or absence. When a piece of furniture is moved from its usual place in your home, you might enter a room and be immediately struck by a feeling that something is missing, somehow wrong. What is disappointed is not an explicit propositional attitude of the form 'I expect that *p*', but a kind of habitual, bodily expectation. When I enter my office in the morning, I do not at that moment have propositionally structured expectations concerning the precise locations of hundreds of different artefacts (although I do for some of them). Nevertheless, any number of different alterations could give rise to a feeling that something is not quite right. Of course, one might claim that I possess all of these expectations implicitly. But that would be to insist on an implausible proliferation of propositional attitudes. Furthermore, disappointment of

---

[7] A research team associated with the mental health charity SANE employed the concept of existential feeling to interpret experiences of suicidal feeling, experiences that cannot be understood against the backdrop of an intact possibility space, their intention being to facilitate more effective ways of identifying and responding to those who are at high risk of suicide. See Benson, Gibson and Brand (2013).

a propositional attitude does not always involve experience of something being absent from a scene or not quite right (as exemplified by the difference between Pierre's and Darth Vader's absence from Sartre's café, mentioned in Chapter 2). The two therefore need to be distinguished.

What is more likely, as I indicated in Chapter 2, is that a certain kind of anticipation is absent from experience, along with its fulfilment, but that the relevant anticipation-fulfilment dynamic continues to be anticipated and is therefore experienced as missing. It is still anticipated that certain things will look as they would have looked if the world included hope. In Husserl's sense, the world 'disappoints'—things appear different from how they did before, somehow lacking. By analogy, one can return to a place in which one once lived and find that it looks strange and unfamiliar, in a way that is difficult to pin down in terms of specific discrepancies between perceived and remembered physical properties. The place is no longer significant in the way it once was, but one still expects it to 'look' how it did when it embodied that significance. Now think of world-experience as a whole in this way—nothing offers what it once did; everything looks different. It can be added that, when hopelessness is partly attributable to impotence before a world that offers only threat, things are not merely lacking. They also take on a new and unfamiliar kind of significance, which conflicts with how they were previously encountered.

Steinbock (2007, pp.448–50) makes the complementary point that even despair somehow depends on hope: it is experienced as a loss of the ground of hope and therefore presupposes some lingering sense of what it is to hope. Despair is not just the absence of hope, as hope is 'experienced as impossible'. However, there is no reason to rule out forms of despair so profound that the person no longer experiences a lack; the absence of hope ceases to be conspicuous. I have suggested that depression often involves something akin to a pervasive feeling of unfulfilled anticipation, but suppose one endures this for a prolonged period. Might the sense of anticipation itself fade, along with the feeling of loss? Might one forget—in a habitual, practical way—what it was like not to be depressed? Many remarks suggest that depression can involve forgetting how things were before one was depressed. For example:

> You can't…even remember what it's like to go and do something and feel pleasure from it. You look at the world, the array of things that you could do, and they're completely meaningless to you. (31-year-old woman quoted by Karp, 1996, p.32)

It is not clear from this passage whether the author is saying that she could no longer rekindle the relevant feelings or that she could not even remember *that* she used to feel pleasure. I suspect it is only the former. Even so, if this were the case for hope as well, a sense of its absence would not be part of one's current experience. By analogy, my memory that I used to experience the world differently when I was a five-year-old does not shape how I experience the world at this moment. So it is not clear that loss of hope has to involve retaining a sense of what it is to hope. The deepest or most profound loss of hope would be one involving no awareness of what had been lost. And we can admit that the difference between the two experiences is a matter of degree; a person could come to miss hope less and less, as the anticipatory structure of experience adjusts to a world without it.

Loss of Aspiration and Demoralization

I will now distinguish two other forms that a loss of existential hope can take, which are qualitatively different from and less profound than the kinds of experience so far described. The first is what we might call a lack of *aspiring hope*. On one account, an unknowing absence of aspiring hope is quite widespread. It need not involve 'losing' something either, as some may not have had it to begin with. Consider someone bereft of any aspiration to be better, any hope of improving her situation, or any sense of there being worthwhile, long-term projects to engage with. The only possibilities for hope that life offers her are tied up with transient pleasures and distractions. Although she might still hope for many things, there is still a privation of existential hope, which limits the *kinds of hope* she is capable of. In *The Sickness unto Death*, Kierkegaard refers to something like this as a form of 'despair'. Writing as Anti-Climacus (and explicitly acknowledging a discrepancy between his own view and that of his pseudonym), he distinguishes several different kinds of despair. All involve impoverishments of self that we are usually unaware of, rather than phenomenologically conspicuous absences. Most people, he claims, are in unknowing despair most of the time, and their obliviousness to it renders their despair all the more profound.

For Anti-Climacus, despair is a failure to recognize potentialities that are integral to one's being, with only Christianity offering the possibility of salvation from it. So despair is ubiquitous amongst non-Christians. His conception of despair therefore departs substantially from more familiar uses of the term, and it departs equally from my own subject matter, given that it is not first and foremost a matter of 'lacking hope'. Nevertheless, Kierkegaard's discussion remains relevant to a consideration of what it is to lose existential hope. He characterizes certain forms of despair in terms of lacking any appreciation that there are non-trivial possibilities. A person might only do what is safe, what is laid out by the norms of his society, to such an extent that he forgets there are any other options; he 'finds being himself too risky, finds it much easier and safer to be like the others, to become a copy, a number, along with the crowd'. Kierkegaard describes this as a retreat from 'venturing' into the world (1849/1989, p.64).[8] 'Despair' of this kind is a limit on the kinds of aspiration a person is capable of having, and Kierkegaard explicitly construes it in terms of the absence of possibility (1989, p.70). What is missing is a sense of certain *kinds* of self-transformative possibility. There is a distinction between hoping to obtain something and aspiring to be something—to accomplish something or to improve one's life. The sense that 'I am not all I could be', 'I am not all I should be', or 'I could/should be better' is surely integral to many lives; it is a background drive or orientation that shapes one's various activities and projects. It involves a distinctive *kind* of hope, the hope of being able to surpass one's current predicament, to improve oneself or one's situation in ways that might evade concrete linguistic description. Its lack need not manifest itself as the positive acknowledgement 'I am complete' or 'I am all I could be'. It is a failure to recognize the possibility of there being significant alternatives to one's current situation. That situation is not contrasted with anything else; it is taken as given, as the space of possibilities within which one resides. So the contrast between having and lacking aspiring hope is not just a matter of one person having various hope contents that the other does not have. Different hope contents are symptomatic of the different kinds of possibility they take the world to offer, their different senses of what the future might bring. It is an existential difference.

Now, someone who lacks aspiring hope might be untroubled by it, even completely oblivious to it. However, it can also take a salient and troubling form; one experiences oneself as having lost something, and the world as no longer offering any basis for a certain kind of hope. One feels that life is lacking, that one is not all one could or should be and that one cannot be. Some people describe depression as removing the possibility of aspiring to be something; it 'prevents you from seeing who you might someday be' (quoted by Karp, 1996, p.24). The difference is that the depressed person is aware—to some extent, and for a time at least—that something has gone from her world; it is permeated by the impossibility of aspiration. She is still able to immerse herself in trivial pastimes, hope for various outcomes in relation to those pastimes, and interact with other people in meaningful ways. Even so, she is resigned to the fact that any aspiration towards self-betterment is senseless. The world still offers the possibility of changes that matter, insofar

---

[8] This is similar to what Heidegger (1962) calls 'das Man' and Sartre (1989) 'bad faith'.

as they are preferable to current situations or to other potential changes, but a more radical sense of contingency is absent from it. It is difficult to pin down exactly what is missing here. After all, the person feels that the world offers nothing more than transient pastimes and superficial distractions, and that it never did. So what does she take to be lacking; how else might things have been? The experience could be construed in terms of the recognition that a once taken-for-granted style of hoping is in fact incoherent, that some forms of aspiration were senseless or futile from the outset. This presents us with the difficult question of whether certain kinds of despair are rational or appropriate responses to human life, which I will address at length in Chapter 10. But, regardless of how we answer that question, the point remains that a distinctive *way of hoping* can be experienced as irrevocably absent without one's losing all active and/or passive hope.

A slightly different privation of existential hope is what we might call 'demoralization' or 'giving up on life'. Here, one retains a sense of what it is to hope; what is missing is any hope regarding one's own future. This differs from loss of aspiring hope because one becomes demoralized in relation to trivial pastimes as well. It is not just self-transformative possibilities that cease to nurture hope; one's future is altogether bereft of hope. It also differs from the more profound losses of hope described in the previous section, as the person continues to appreciate the counterfactual 'my prospects could have been otherwise'. It is not that she cannot conceive of the possibility of a hopeful future; she just resigns herself to not having one. Furthermore, she retains a sense of what it was to hope, as well—perhaps—as the hope that others' lives will go well. But her actual future is experienced as no longer offering the possibility of intentional hopes; her life is over, even though it might not have been. One might argue that this is better construed in terms of losing a system of intentional hopes, where a very general intentional hope, that of 'my future including the possibility of good things happening', is lost along with all the hopes that rest upon it. And it is indeed a system of significant possibilities that has been lost here, rather than the sense of significance full stop. But this is inextricable from the loss of another *kind* of possibility. The world no longer 'draws one in'; its enticement is diminished or absent, in a way that will be further described in Chapters 6 and 7.

I have borrowed the term 'demoralization' from Kissane and Clarke (2001) and Clarke and Kissane (2002), who propose that two distinct psychiatric categories be recognized: 'depression' and 'demoralization syndrome'. They define demoralization syndrome as follows:

> ...a psychiatric state in which hopelessness, helplessness, meaninglessness, and existential distress are the core phenomena. Hopelessness and helplessness arise

from an experience of feeling trapped or of not knowing what to do. (Kissane and Clarke, 2001, p.13)

One reason offered for the distinction is that demoralization differs qualitatively from depression, as anhedonia (inability to experience pleasure) is characteristic of depression but not of demoralization syndrome. However, to complicate matters, they also acknowledge that the two frequently occur together and that untreated demoralization can lead to depression. Demoralization, as they describe it, is compatible with a DSM major depression diagnosis, and their proposed classification is therefore revisionary. But the above description is not very clear, accommodating losses of intentional hope as well as existential forms of hopelessness. There are also several further problems with the proposal. Clarke and Kissane suggest that we regard 'demoralization' as a medical condition, to be distinguished from that of depression. The view that all such predicaments be regarded as pathological is contentious to say the least. For one thing, it implies that anyone who requests euthanasia should be diagnosed with a psychiatric disorder (Parker, 2004). So the category fails to acknowledge a normative distinction between accurately appraising one's situation as hopeless and mistakenly seeing no future for oneself. Furthermore, the only criterion Kissane and Clarke (2001, p.16) offer for distinguishing pathological demoralization from non-pathological losses of hope is that demoralization is more intense or pronounced. They do not consider whether equally pronounced feelings could be 'normal' in some life situations, and neither do they indicate what the normal range is. The suggestion that we can draw a line between those experiences typical of depression and of 'demoralization' is similarly contentious, in the absence of more refined phenomenological distinctions.

However, if we set aside the issue of whether demoralization should be construed as a psychiatric illness, one to be distinguished from depression, we can help ourselves to a useful phenomenological distinction that Kissane and Clarke at least hint at. The 'demoralized' person, we are told, complains that 'I can't see the point anymore. There is no reason to go on' (Kissane and Clarke, 2001, p.12). This sounds like a loss of 'hope' rather than 'hopes'. It is a general orientation towards one's future that is altered or lost, rather than a number of intentional states. It differs from lack of aspiring hope because someone without aspiration can still hope for all sorts of things, look forward to them, and find various possibilities enticing. How, though, does it differ from cases where hope loses its intelligibility? Kissane and Clarke suggest that the demoralized person lacks hope (which they construe rather narrowly, in terms of 'anticipatory pleasure'), whereas the depressed person lacks 'consummatory pleasure' too.[9] Loss of pleasure thus extends further in the latter case (Kissane and Clarke, 2001, p.15). But elsewhere they also indicate that loss of hope in depression is somehow deeper:

> The demoralized feel inhibited in action by not knowing what to do, feeling helpless and incompetent; the depressed have lost motivation and drive even when the appropriate direction of action is known. (Clarke and Kissane, 2002, p.736)

Jacobsen, Maytal and Stern (2007, p.140) similarly state that demoralization involves 'distress and a sense of incompetence that results from an uncertainty about which direction to take. Individuals with depression and those with anhedonia cannot act (even if they know the proper direction to take)'. The demoralized person does not lack the capacity for motivation, or indeed for hope, but she does experience her future as devoid of meaningful possibilities for action. And, unlike Plenty Coups, she gives up; nothing draws here in anymore, propels her forward. So demoralization can be described as a resignation of radical hope. The person retains a sense of what it would be to have a hopeful orientation towards her future but does not have one.[10] This differs from a loss of active hope, as she gives up on passive hope too— there is no hope of rescue. Hence demoralization is not an intentional state or cluster of intentional states, with the overall content 'my future is bleak' or something similar. It is a more general sense of what the future offers. Loss of however many intentional hopes is compatible with retention of a 'hopeful' orientation towards the future. Demoralization also differs from experiences of the form 'my future *could not* offer any possibilities for hope'. Because the demoralized person retains some capacity for hope, she is able to imaginatively relive past hopes; loss of hope is not backdated to include all of one's

---

[9] I am not sure that the proposed distinction differs substantially from the DSM distinction between 'major depression' and 'major depression with melancholic features', where melancholic depression involves 'loss of interest or pleasure in all, or almost all, activities or a lack of reactivity to usually pleasurable stimuli' and 'the individual's depressed mood does not improve, even temporarily, when something good happens' (DSM-IV-TR, p.419).

[10] Something slightly different from 'demoralization' may be experienced by some of those who face terminal illness or other circumstances: not all hope in one's future is lost, but one does cease to experience and think about the world in relation to longer term possibilities. To a greater extent, one 'lives in the present'. This is structurally similar to a loss of aspiring hope but is not the same—one could retain shorter term aspirations and distinguish these from more trivial pastimes. Giving up on certain possibilities or kinds of possibility may not be experienced as a bad thing. Indeed, it may even involve a sense of relief and an increase in happiness. Thanks to Havi Carel (personal communication) for these points.

life. Demoralization is also not so recalcitrant to change as more profound forms of hopelessness. A reappraisal of what the future offers, brought about by significant and unanticipated events, has the potential to re-instil hope (Jacobsen, Maytal and Stern, 2007, p.141).

I think demoralization may well be an appropriate response to certain situations, but my aim here is to describe depression experiences, rather than determine whether or why they are pathological (although I will turn to that issue in Chapter 10). Should demoralization be distinguished from depression though? The category 'depression' is currently so permissive that it makes little sense to distinguish the two, even when demoralization is understood in the more specific way I have suggested. It would be analogous to distinguishing 'primates' from 'all other mammals', a move that would be unwarranted given that other mammalian orders are no less worthy of being singled out. Hence a distinction between two syndromes is not especially informative. Demoralization is one of several qualitatively different privations of hope, the distinctive characteristics of which are obscured by their inclusion under the undifferentiated category 'experience of depression' and by undiscriminating use of the labels 'hopelessness' and 'despair'.

Loss of Trust

Various life events can ultimately lead to demoralization, loss of aspiration, or even a complete loss of hope. However, some traumatic events provoke a different kind of change in the structure of hope, where all hopes are rendered 'fragile' rather than lost. For example, Jean Améry (1999) vividly describes his experience of torture at the hands of the SS. With the first blow, he says, the prisoner loses 'trust in the world' and, more specifically, trust in other people. The kind of 'trust' in question is something that is more usually taken as given: 'In almost all situations in life where there is bodily injury there is also the expectation of help; the former is compensated by the latter' (pp. 28–29). This expectation, Améry says, was shattered by torture, leading to an enduring change in how he found himself in the world:

> Whoever has succumbed to torture can no longer feel at home in the world. The shame of destruction cannot be erased. Trust in the world, which already collapsed in part at the first blow, but in the end, under torture, fully, will not be regained. (1999, p.40)[11]

----

[11] Scarry (1985, pp.40–41) describes torture as the destruction of a person's 'world'.

Other kinds of traumatic experience can also lead to losses of trust in the world and, more specifically, in other people.[12] Reflecting on several first-person testimonies, Bernstein (2011, p.398) describes this 'trust' as follows:

> ...the existential confidence that permits the rational suppression, overlooking, forgetting, or fortunate ignorance of each individual's utter dependence on surrounding others, and hence each's categorical helplessness; with our helplessness no longer in conscious view, we can attend to the world rather than ourselves, or ourselves as fully worldly beings.

So trust—in the relevant sense—is not an explicit attitude that one adopts, of the form 'I trust A to do p', 'I trust A', or 'I trust that p will be done'. It is a habitual, confident style of anticipation, in the context of which danger and threat appear as localized anomalies or disruptions.[13] Certain experiences can lead to an erosion of this confidence, replacing it with a pervasive sense of dangerous uncertainty. Even when the person does feel, to some degree, 'at home again in a situation', there lingers a heightened sense of contingency, of vulnerability. As Stolorow (2007, p.16) puts it, emotional trauma reveals the 'inescapable contingency of existence on a universe that is random and unpredictable and in which no safety or continuity of being can be assured'. Trust and its absence are thus integral to existential feeling, to a sense of the kinds of possibility offered by the world. What we have is not a complete loss of hope but an enduring sense of its fragility; it is no longer implicitly taken for granted as a firm and unwavering basis for intentional hopes. The 'ground of hope' is not absent, but one lives with the sense that it—and everything that rests upon it—is unsafe, lacking firm foundations, perhaps even inevitably doomed to collapse. So there is a modification of the 'style' in which one hopes. All hope is shaped by a loss of confidence, something that also limits the scope of potential hope contents. One might no longer be able to hope that 'things will all turn out for the best in the end', as the existential structure that shapes one's hopes incorporates a sense that

---

[12] See, for example, Brison (2002).

[13] See also Baier (1986, p.245) for the view that there is a kind of trust that is 'automatic and unconscious', as exemplified by the 'primitive and basic trust' between infant and parent. Jones (2004) refers to it as 'basal security', an affective state that is presupposed by more specific relations of trust that take the form 'I trust A to do p'. See also McGeer (2008) for an interesting discussion of the close relationship between hope and trust. McGeer prioritizes hope as a precondition for some forms of trust, but does not address more specifically existential variants of trust and hope.

they will not. Hope contents are thus more modest, such as 'situation x will work out well'.

This fragility is not always to be contrasted with other ways of losing hope, as it can play a role in their development. Many first-person accounts of depression describe not just a loss of hope or meaning, a 'sterile promontory', but a feeling of being unsafe, of residing in a bad and inescapable place: 'the world seems like a negative and bad place to be. It looks as if nothing is going right, and everything on the news is always bad news. The world feels out of control and dangerous' (#45). An increasingly pronounced sense of the world as dangerous and unpredictable could lead to the progressive collapse of systems of hope. Furthermore, when people offer only threat, all those hopes that explicitly or implicitly depend on entering into trusting relations with others are affected. A growing sense of the world as unsafe, of people as bad or dangerous, and of hope as unfounded could develop into loss of aspiration, demoralization, or an even deeper loss of hope. The differences between these experiences can therefore be difficult to discern, at least on the basis of brief first-person descriptions. A profound loss of trust in the world or other people could be described as having no hope, even when a fragile sense of hope lingers on. This is also a reason why the distinction between depression and grief is sometimes difficult to draw. Earlier in the chapter, I suggested that grief can involve the loss of systems of hope, which cease to be intelligible in the absence of a particular person. But grief can also involve an erosion of trust in the world. One's sense of belonging to the world is different; everything seems finite, no longer dependable (Stolorow, 2011). An increasingly profound loss of trust along these lines could extinguish not just systems of hope but kinds of hope, and so there is a fine line between the existential structure of some grief and depression experiences.

Hence the kinds of hopelessness I have distinguished here are not just static forms of experience. It is also likely that they are integrated into processes, and we can better understand those processes if we are sensitive to the relevant phenomenological distinctions. The provisional taxonomy I propose, which will be further refined in Chapters 6 and 7, is as follows:

1. Absence of the capacity to hope

2. A more specific loss of aspiring hope (hope of bettering oneself or improving one's life)

3. Demoralization (loss of a sense of one's actual future as a dimension of hope)

4. Loss of trust in the world, which renders all hope 'fragile' and may restrict the scope of potential hope contents[14]

This list is complicated by further subdivisions. (1), (3), and (4) can all involve different balances of active and passive hope, whereas (2) principally involves loss of a certain kind of active hope. (1), (2), and (3) can all involve differing levels of awareness. Hope might be sorely missed or inconspicuously absent. However, a lack of trust is always 'there'; one *feels* unsafe. There are also differences in scope. What distinguishes (1) is the sense of hope as unintelligible, but this can take an egocentric focus, with some awareness of the hopeful lives of others remaining. (2) and (3) are self-specific, whereas (4) varies in a range of ways; it could be 'me' that is 'unsafe' or 'us', where the scope of 'us' is more or less encompassing. In the case of (4), the principal focus of insecurity could be other people, the world, the efficacy of one's agency, one's bodily functions, or even one's own thoughts (where the latter takes us into the domain of psychosis). Furthermore, degree of distrust varies considerably. The world might seem irrevocably different in a way that is inescapable. Alternatively, one might feel lost, in need of solid ground, and—by implication—able to conceive of there being solid ground. Any of these predicaments could be associated with a depression diagnosis. More than one could be involved during a single 'episode' of depression, and some may be more typical than others of first or later episodes, or of chronic depression.

In summary, everyday terms such as 'hopelessness', 'despair', and the like do not serve to convey the structure of existential hopelessness or the different forms it takes. But more detailed first-person descriptions can do so, at

---

[14] I have not included 'pessimism', which I take to involve a disposition to form fewer intentional hopes and/or hope to a lesser degree, rather than a loss of something that is presupposed by the intelligibility of one or another subtype of intentional hope. One might respond that there are also existential forms of pessimism. However, even if the term 'pessimism' is used to refer to certain privations of existential hope, I do not think it points to a distinctive kind of existential change that differs from those already described. 'Existential pessimism' could be conceived of in terms of 'loss of hope', 'demoralization', and/or 'loss of trust'. Even so, my list may not be comprehensive, and I do not rule out the possibility that there are other ways of losing hope, which differ from what I have described here.

least if we are sufficiently sensitive to the relevant phenomenological distinctions. For instance, there is a fine line between demoralization and intentional states that can be described in similar ways. A person might respond to questions about his life by saying 'I've given up hope'. Further questioning could reveal that the 'giving up' actually relates to a number of intentional hopes, perhaps concerning employment, a relationship with someone, or the chances of achieving a particular goal. However, if he further insists that the future offers nothing, he looks forward to nothing, and he has no hopes about anything, matters are different. A demoralization experience like this also needs to be distinguished from no longer being able to entertain the possibility of hoping, and from a loss that is restricted to certain kinds of hope, such as aspiring hope.

Many descriptions of hopelessness and despair, even those that do draw attention to different subtypes, are ambiguous. For example, Garrett (1994) distinguishes project-specific despair (despair over failing to achieve some outcome), personal despair (despair over one's whole life), and philosophical despair (despair over all life). Project-specific despair clearly involves an intentional content, but it is not clear whether or not personal and philosophical despair are to be thought of in terms of the progressive widening of that content. There are various options to consider. 'Personal despair' could be an intentional state with oneself as its object, a loss of aspiring hope, demoralization, or a deeper loss of hope. As for philosophical despair, if it is conceived of as an instance of intentional despair that involves accepting a very general proposition along the lines of 'all life is irrevocably pointless', it is not the deepest or most profound form of despair. It needs to be distinguished from a predicament that is only superficially similar, where one is no longer able to hope. (I will return to philosophical despair, construed in existential terms, in Chapter 10.)

The same concerns apply to the Beck hopelessness scale, where it is not at all clear what is being measured. Take propositions such as 'I don't expect to get what I really want' and 'It is very unlikely that I will get any real satisfaction in the future' (Beck et al., 1974, p.862). Someone might put a tick next to these because a specifically focused intentional hope or a more general hope is absent. Alternatively she might have lost all sense of hope, lost aspiring hope, or become demoralized. Or maybe she lives with an enduring feeling of fragility and distrust. A similar ambiguity is generated by an assumption that frames discussion of emotion more generally: emotions must be intentional states, non-intentional states, or a combination of the two. As an alternative to these options, I have proposed that some established emotion types, amongst which I include hope and its contraries, have intentional and pre-intentional variants.

At several points in this chapter, I have referred to emotional 'depth' or 'profundity'. There are qualitative differences between some of the existential changes I have described, such as demoralization and loss of aspiring hope, but I have also indicated that some of them are 'deeper' or more 'profound' than others. For instance, the most profound form of despair is one involving loss of the intelligibility of hope, a loss so enveloping that the person is not even aware of it. In making such claims, it is important to be clear about what 'depth' consists of. This theme will be further addressed in Chapter 5, where I turn to the depths of guilt.

Depth, Guilt, and Narrative

In the previous chapter, I described several different 'hopelessness' experiences and indicated that some of them differ in relative depth or profundity. Such differences are also hinted at by everyday language; people talk of 'the depths of despair', 'deep depression', 'a profound sense of hopelessness', and the like. One of my aims in this chapter is to clarify the notion of 'depth' that I am appealing to. I distinguish two kinds of 'depth' that feature in our discourse about emotions and feelings. One is content-based and applies to intentional states, while the other concerns the overall form of experience and applies to existential feeling. I suggest that, although existential feelings cannot themselves be compared in terms of depth, changes in existential feeling can be. To apply my account of existential depth, as well as further develop my analysis of depression experiences, I turn to another familiar emotion category that accommodates intentional and existential variants: guilt. The DSM mentions guilt as a common symptom of depression, but its nature is not made clear. Consequently, both existential and intentional types of guilt are compatible with depression diagnoses. Unlike losses of hope (whether existential or intentional in nature), guilt is not ubiquitous in depression. To be more specific, not all existential forms of depression incorporate existential guilt. I propose that this is partly because guilt involves a distinctive modification of interpersonal experience. Whether or not an existential feeling amounts to one of guilt also depends on how it is conceptualized and narrated, by the depressed person and by others. So the feeling is not simply one of guilt but one that lends itself to being interpreted and experienced as guilt. The chapter concludes with a wider-ranging discussion of the relationship between existential feeling, narrative, and self-regulation in depression.

Depths of Feeling

Talk of 'emotional depth' is fairly commonplace, but its nature is seldom addressed by philosophers.[1] The term 'depth' is often used in a comparative

---

[1] For an exception, see Cataldi (1993), who also observes that the topic of emotional depth has been neglected by philosophers.

way. A given feeling might be described as deeper than love, regret, or shame, or as deeper even than words can express. First-person accounts of depression often refer to unusually deep feelings of dread, despair, hopelessness, or guilt. For example, in describing a period of depression that followed the onset of blindness, Hull (1990, p.168) remarks that 'the deepest feelings go beyond feeling. One is numbed by the feeling; one does not experience the feeling'. I do not seek to offer a comprehensive analysis of how the term 'depth' is used in relation to emotional experience. It most likely has all sorts of different connotations, some clearer than others. Instead, I want to focus on two conceptions of depth, both of which correspond to at least some everyday talk of 'depth'. One of these applies to intentional emotions and feelings. Consider 'loss of the hope that p'. There is a sense in which loss of the hope that I will manage to write well today is not as deep or profound as loss of the hope that I will ever write well. One content is more enveloping than the other, and the effect its loss has on one's life is therefore greater. In this case, one content also includes the other, and so the difference in scope is especially clear. Pugmire (2005) offers a sophisticated account of emotional depth or 'profundity', which appeals to this kind of difference. According to his account, emotional profundity depends—amongst other things—on how significant an emotion's content is to a person, 'on how much of a person's life is affected by what evokes the emotion' (2005, p.43).

When referring to the depth or profundity of existential feelings, I am concerned with something different. An existential feeling determines which kinds of intentional emotion are amongst one's possibilities, in a way that is independent of content. In depression, there is a shift in the *kinds* of emotion one is able to experience: 'Depression is when your normal range of emotional functioning contracts so that it shrinks to just the portions where you experience negative feelings' (#61). For instance, a loss of existential hope (as described in Chapter 4) is not a matter of losing however many hope contents but of losing the capacity for intentional states of the kind 'hope', regardless of what their contents might be. In Chapter 2, I offered a phenomenological account of our receptiveness to kinds of significant possibility, an account that can be applied more specifically to our *emotional* repertoire. Different types of emotion are associated with different kinds of significance. For instance, fear is tied to danger, and grief to a form of loss. The kind of significance associated with a type of emotion is sometimes referred to as its 'formal object'. There is debate over what the relationship is between emotions and their formal objects. Perception or cognition of the relevant formal object could be construed as a causal prerequisite for an emotion or, alternatively, as integral to that emotion (see e.g. Teroni, 2007). I favour the latter view but, regardless of how exactly we conceive of the relationship between emotions and their formal objects, it is plausible to maintain that anyone incapable of experiencing things as significant in some way will also be incapable of the associated emotion type(s).[2] This is not a causal dependence but one of sense. And the point does not apply solely to what we might call 'classical emotions'. A world bereft of all kinds of practical significance would be a world in which many different kinds of experience and activity were impossible. We could not encounter things as useable, functional, useless, appropriate or inappropriate for a task, required, inadequate, and so on, and there could be no projects or goals.

A loss of existential hope is not merely a matter of having an experience that is *incompatible* with hoping for various things. It is importantly different from a case of conflicting intentional emotions, where one emotion 'I hope that p' is incompatible with another emotion 'I feel hopeless in relation to p'. A particular existential feeling, 'loss of hope', does not cancel out however many particular hopes. It cancels out a *type* of intentional state, the attitude of hope itself. For this reason, an existential change can be described as 'deeper' or more 'profound' than a change in intentional emotion, however widespread the effects of the latter might be. So, when we say that existential changes are 'deeper' than changes in intentional emotions, the relevant conception of 'depth' differs from that employed to gauge the relative depth of intentional emotions. This conception can also be used to compare different existential feelings in terms of depth. Existential feelings are configurations of a possibility space. One configuration of that space is different from another, not deeper. However, *changes* in existential feeling are comparable in terms of relative depth or profundity. This also accounts for our phenomenological access to existential depth; one often experiences the profundity of an existential change as it happens, the extent of the shift from one feeling to another. Following such a shift, one may continue to experience the gulf between one's current existential feeling p and an earlier existential feeling q. Loss of existential hope is experienced *as* a loss (a point that applies to losses of intentional hope too).

How are we to make existential depth comparisons, given that they are not to be construed in terms of more or less encompassing contents? There is no simple formula for doing so. Consideration of relative depth needs be accompanied by an appreciation of qualitative differences in existential feelings. For instance, demoralization and loss of aspiring hope involve different sub-types

---

[2] Several philosophers have argued that emotions involve *perceiving* the significance of things. See, for example, de Sousa (1990, Chapter 7), Deonna (2006), and Goldie (2007).

of hope and thus different *kinds* of existential change. Where the kinds of existential change involved in experiences p and q do not overlap substantially, differences render depth comparisons difficult. But, where there is substantial overlap, it is often clear that one change involves a more profound shift in the possibility space than another. The most clear-cut cases are those where change p is included in change q. Demoralization and loss of aspiring hope are not so deep as a complete loss of hope, given that loss of all hope affects the same kinds of intentional state that they do, and others as well. All sub-types of hope are lost, rather than just one. The point similarly applies to losses of practical significance. Its loss might be specific to one's own possibilities, in which case the sense that things are significant to others remains intact. The possibility of a type of intentional state is still gone from one's world, that of encountering things as 'practically significant to me'. However, the loss is deeper when any sense of anything being significant for anyone is gone, as it impacts on a wider repertoire of intentional state types.

We can construe such experiences in terms of a progressive departure from an existential feeling that accommodates the possibility of hope and practical significance, one that the person might previously have taken for granted as 'the world' and not even recognized as a contingent phenomenological achievement. The notion of depth is therefore contrastive in the following way: an existential feeling p is deep compared to q in virtue of its greater departure from starting point r. Existential changes are not always described in a way that is explicitly contrastive. When an experience, such as that of despair, is described simply as 'profound' or 'deep' rather than 'deeper than q', the contrast is implicit. Its departure from a non-despairing way of belonging to the world is unusually pronounced, relative to certain other kinds of shift that are similar in structure. Clear comparisons are only possible when p and q are similar in kind, but this conception of depth is still informative when it comes to depression. Although two depression experiences might involve existential changes that are qualitatively different, many of the existential changes that feature in depression are comparable in terms of relative depth or profundity.

When interpreting depression experiences, it is important to keep the distinction between existential and intentional depth in mind, as the two are easily confused. I will now illustrate this by turning to guilt in depression. I will show that, as in the case of hope and its privations, guilt has intentional and existential forms, either or both of which can arise in depression. That 'guilt' is a familiar emotion category makes our task easier in one respect, as we do not need to first identify and then describe something that lacks an established name. However, the fact that we are able to label something 'guilt' exacerbates a tendency to construe it as a type of intentional state, as something more familiar and less profound than it actually is. I will start by offering some general remarks on the nature of guilt, after which I turn to guilt in depression.

The Nature of Guilt

What is guilt? As noted in Chapters 2 and 4, a fairly standard philosophical approach to emotions is to consider the respective contributions made by bodily feelings and evaluative judgments. Hence what distinguishes one emotion type from another is the contribution of a distinctive type of feeling, judgment, or both. Feelings surely have some role to play in guilt, as a person can recognize that she has done something morally wrong and that she is deserving of punishment without feeling any guilt. But this does not imply that the emotion of guilt consists solely of feeling. Indeed, it is arguable that a kind of cognitive judgement is what distinguishes guilt from a range of similar emotions, such as shame and regret. Guilt is sometimes claimed to involve internalizing and thus accepting moral judgements concerning one's actions or omissions, judgments made by actual or imagined others (e.g. Elster, 1999, pp.152–3). Shame, in contrast, need not be associated with moral transgression. A person might feel ashamed of aspects of his appearance that are morally inconsequential and also beyond his control. Regret can likewise concern all sorts of non-moral acts and omissions.[3] Several other criteria have been proposed for distinguishing guilt from shame and other emotions. Blackburn (1998, pp.17–19) suggests that guilt is associated with 'reparation' and shame with 'concealment'. Another potential criterion is that guilt is directed towards the irrevocable effects of one's deeds. One might compensate for those effects, with varying degrees of success, but the deeds themselves cannot be undone. To quote Viktor Frankl (1973, p.90), 'guilt is responsibleness without freedom—without freedom, that is, except for the freedom to choose the right attitude to guilt'. In contrast, the causes of shame can often be removed (for example, by losing weight, staying away from people who make you feel ashamed, or getting a new job).

None of these criteria apply to every experience of guilt. Seemingly irrational guilt is commonplace, where strong feelings of guilt persist alongside the judgment that one has done nothing wrong. Take 'survivor guilt', where someone who has survived an event feels guilty for having done so when others did not.[4] In addition, people sometimes feel free-floating or 'diffuse' guilt, which is not obviously associated with a specific act or omission (Roberts, 2003, p.223).

---

[3] See, for example, Stocker and Hegeman (1996, p.285) for the claim that guilt involves attribution of responsibility whereas shame need not.

[4] There are also more mundane experiences of irrational guilt. For example, Elster (1999, p.151) says that he feels guilty when friends travel a long way to see him and it rains throughout their stay.

A person can also feel guilty about things that nobody else regards as a moral transgression. For instance, an academic might feel guilty about not finishing a book on schedule or declining a conference invitation due to lack of time. And guilt feelings are frequently associated with concealment rather than an urge towards reparation. Hiding the wine bottles from one's spouse is not inconsistent with feeling guilty about one's excessive drinking. The deeds a person feels guilty about are not always irrevocable either. One might feel guilty about a habitual behaviour or other ongoing activity that can be stopped, rather than one's role in a particular event. Furthermore, guilt and other emotions such as shame often occur together, in response to the same actions and events, making them hard to disentangle (Blackburn, 1998, pp.17–19; Stocker, 2007).

If we are to understand the nature of guilt in depression, some importantly different kinds of guilt experience need to be distinguished. Feeling guilty about an act or omission is not the same attitude as feeling that one *is* guilty. Although I might feel guilty about something, feeling that I actually *am guilty* of it requires an additional acceptance of guilt, as guilt feelings are consistent with doubt over one's guilt. However, not all guilt is *guilt about* something. Another variant of guilt is feeling that one simply *is guilty*, independent of any particular act or omission, as though there were a moral flaw in one's being. Here, the person 'reproaches himself *in general*, as if his very existence is an offense as well as any particular action' (Solomon, 1993, p.259). This kind of personal guilt is different from an experience of diffuse guilt where one feels guilty about something but does not know exactly what. There is a further distinction to be drawn between experiences of contingent and irrevocable guilt (where irrevocable guilt generally involves the feeling of 'being guilty', rather than 'feeling guilty about something'). When one feels that one has become guilty due to some deed, the recognition that things could have been otherwise remains and a sense of contingency thus attaches to the experience. Similarly, one might feel that one's existence is contingently flawed, that there is hope of redemption. Irrevocable guilt, however, involves the sense that being guilty is integral to one's essence: one could not have been otherwise and could never be otherwise (although I grant that there are in-between cases, such as feeling that one has become guilty but that this guilt is now inescapable). Hence we can make the following distinctions:

1. Feeling guilty about something specific
2. Feeling guilty about something but not knowing what
3. Feeling that one really is guilty of something specific
4. Feeling guilty
5. Feeling irrevocably guilty

In referring to a feeling as one of 'guilt', I want to emphasize certain common themes: a focus on past deeds, recognition that effects of one's deeds are unchangeable, an awareness of estrangement from others, a sense of having done wrong or of being intrinsically flawed, and an anticipation of being harmed or punished. But I do not seek rigid criteria for distinguishing every one of those emotional experiences we might call 'guilt' from those we might call 'shame', 'remorse' or 'regret'. Our phenomenology is unlikely to map neatly onto distinctions made by natural language, and the practice of offering criteria, counter-examples and then further criteria could happily go on forever.[5] So my quarrel is not principally with criteria that are invoked to distinguish kinds of emotion, and I am happy to leave the boundaries blurred. What I will challenge, though, is the assumption that guilt invariably consists of intentional states of one or more types (such as perceptions, intentional feelings, factual beliefs, and evaluative judgements) and/or non-intentional bodily feelings. Types 1, 2 and 3 (above) all involve intentional states. Their relative profundity can be understood in terms of their scope, the extent to which they impact on concerns that are central to a person's life. Another factor is the degree of conviction; feeling that one is guilty of something will have a more decisive effect on those concerns than just *feeling guilty*. However, types 4 and 5 are 'deep' or 'profound' in a different way. Both are existential forms of guilt, 5 being the deepest. They are to be characterized in terms of a change in one's sense of what is possible.

All five kinds of guilt can occur in depression. First-person accounts often report experiences of intentional guilt, which tend to focus on not being able to do what one ought to do, or causing others distress by being depressed: 'I [...] feel incredible guilt due to the fact that I can see their pain at my situation (although they try to hide it). I tend to close off more from them as I feel this is the only way to spare them from suffering because of me' (#282). However, intentional states also arise in an existential context, and some expressions of intentional guilt are symptomatic of more profound existential changes. The DQ response just quoted also includes the following, which suggests some kind of existential change: 'It is as though a black blanket smothers me and takes away all pleasure, interest or enthusiasm for anything. I just withdraw into my own very dark world'. In some cases, it may be that the person feels 'existentially guilty' and her expressions of guilt latch onto more

---

[5] See Stocker (2007) for a comprehensive discussion of the various criteria that have been proposed for distinguishing guilt from shame. He concludes that they all fail but retains the view that shame and guilt are importantly different, maintaining that the relevant criteria have yet to be identified.

specific objects, which are to some degree arbitrary: I am irrevocably guilty and I feel guilty about everything; hence I feel guilty about p, given that p is what I am currently attending to. This would be analogous to the belief that recovery is impossible, something that looks like a content-specific evaluative judgment but is symptomatic of a wider-ranging inability to register the possibility of anything good happening.

Depression experiences often involve feelings of all-enveloping, irrevocable guilt.[6] These cause considerable suffering and are sometimes singled out as the most troubling symptom. Rowe (1978) quotes several interviewees with depression diagnoses who complain of profound guilt. One states that the depression itself is 'a sign that I'm not what I should be' (p.39). Another describes the experience as follows: 'I feel I am suffering more than a murderer is suffering. In the end a murderer forgets and it all goes away from him. [...] I know I'm not the only one that suffers from depression, but it's my guilt—it's worse than the depression' (p.173). Talk of 'guilt' usually features alongside a host of related themes, including 'inadequacy', 'shame', and 'damnation'. 'Self-hatred' is very common (e.g. Rowe, 1978, p.215), as is worthlessness (e.g. Styron, 2001, p.3). Several DQ respondents similarly describe a feeling of *being guilty*, of a kind that does not attach to anything specific and permeates one's relationship with the world as a whole:

> #16. When I am depressed everything seems so bad. It seems as if there is nothing good in the world and that all the bad is because of me somehow.

> #179 [When depressed] I hate myself. The reason my life is so awful at these times is because I am a terrible, wicked, failure of a person. I'm not a proper human being, I am a failed human being. Everything that goes wrong in my life is directly my fault; I caused it by not doing things I should have done, or doing things I shouldn't have done. I am a waste of a human life. No-one knows just what a horrible useless nothing of a person I really am, because I hide it from people—if they ever found out the truth, they will all hate me and I will never have a single friend in the world ever again.

This kind of guilt is inseparable from despair. If I am irrevocably guilty, then there is no hope of reprieve, of things changing for the better, of my acting in a way that could alleviate my situation. But this is only one form that existential despair might take; irrevocable guilt implies loss of hope, whereas loss of hope does not imply something as specific as irrevocable guilt. Existential guilt can

---

6 This applies especially to 'melancholic depression', a proposed subtype that has been the primary focus of phenomenological research on depression (e.g. Tellenbach, 1980; Fuchs, 2003; Stanghellini, 2004). It corresponds roughly to the DSM category of 'major depression' with 'melancholic features'.

also underlie suicidal thoughts, and is more generally associated with feelings of worthlessness, especially with respect to interpersonal relations and commitments:

> #88. Deep despair, hate myself, feel like I can't do anything right, everyone would be better off if I wasn't here to fuck their lives up, feel useless, why was I even born, I shouldn't be here, I don't belong here, just want to go to sleep and never wake up.

> #97. Feel hopeless, like I shouldn't exist and it would be better for family and friends if I wasn't here. Just feel dark, worried, impending feeling of doom.

In some first-person accounts of depression, relations with and commitments to specific individuals constitute a reason to live. Existential guilt removes that possibility from consideration, as it includes a sense that others would be better off in one's absence. So it is implicated in the loss of reasons for living, and can also motivate a 'wish' to die, where death presents itself as a form of punishment and/or a way of relieving others of their misery. However, the term 'guilt' is arguably too specific to convey the relevant existential change. It can equally be described in terms of self-disgust, self-hate, or a feeling of utter worthlessness: 'I often feel hate and disgust towards myself—I can't see pictures of me without wanting to tear them up or poke my eyes out' (#21). Matters are further complicated by the interaction between existential changes and more localized self-evaluations that arise against a backdrop of existential feeling. The depression itself is often cited as a reason for feeling guilty or ashamed, illustrating that reflective attitudes towards one's situation also have a role to play in experiences of guilt, shame, and the like: 'I'm ashamed of my illness, which in itself begins a self-perpetuating cycle of feeling depressed about the fact I'm depressed' (#21). Sometimes, the depression is conceived of as a punishment for existential guilt: 'When I am depressed I believe that I was just born this way and that I deserve it because my mother had an affair and I shouldn't have been born' (#186). This points to a more dynamic picture, where existential feelings dispose the person towards certain kinds of self-evaluation, which in turn have the potential to perpetuate or even exacerbate the feeling in question (a point I return to later in the chapter).

Themes such as guilt, worthlessness, shame, and self-hate can all be expressive of a single, unitary existential feeling. For convenience, I will continue to refer to this feeling as one of 'guilt'. A distinction is sometimes made between state guilt (an episodic feeling) and trait guilt (a disposition towards that feeling). State guilt is especially common in severely depressed subjects as compared to healthy control subjects, and occurs more frequently in depression than in chronic illness more generally. Trait guilt is also very common in those who are either suffering from depression or highly susceptible to it (see e.g. Ghatavi et al., 2002). What I seek to describe would probably be termed 'state guilt', but the distinction between psychological states and traits does not really capture it, as existential guilt is neither the experience of a transient psychological state nor a disposition towards that state. It is experienced as an enduring, all-encompassing way of being. There is some evidence to suggest that existentially guilty depression is not culture-specific (see e.g. Stompe et al., 2001). However, Jennifer Radden has argued that the prominence of guilt symptoms in accounts of depression is historically and culturally variable. After the appearance of Freud's essay 'Mourning and Melancholia', the themes of 'self-accusation' and 'self-loathing' became much more prominent in first-person accounts and in the more general literature on depression. Furthermore, in some cultures, 'guilt and self-accusation' do not feature as depression symptoms (Radden, 2009, p.161). Although I will concede that 'guilt' is most likely a contingent way of interpreting and expressing a type of depression experience, I will also make clear *why* that experience is so conducive to being construed as one of guilt.

Irrevocable Guilt

Recall that the recurrent themes of imprisonment, darkness, and being trapped do not convey a loss of physical space but of possibility space. In depression, there is no sense that things could be otherwise in certain kinds of significant way. So the depression itself is not experienced as a transitory state, a way of feeling, but as an inescapable way of being. This also amounts to a change in the experience of time, which I will describe more fully in Chapter 7. For now, suffice it to say that, without any practical orientation towards salient future possibilities, the dynamic between past, present, and future that we more usually take for granted is replaced by a predicament that seems eternal. Depression does not involve complete loss of temporal experience but an alteration in its structure. In some cases, future possibilities remain but only in the form of an imminent danger, in the face of which one is helpless. All experience is shaped by the feeling of passively waiting for some unknown and all-enveloping threat to materialize.

Why would this be experienced as 'guilt'? I have indicated that its conceptualization as guilt is not inevitable. Even so, there are several structural similarities between what I have just described and kinds of intentional experience that we would confidently label 'guilt'. Minkowski (1958, 1970) observes that our days are ordinarily distinguished from each other by how each day fits uniquely into a coherent, purposive life structure. Without any sense of purposes and projects, without things that are done and other things that remain to be done, every day starts afresh, no different from the one before. As there is nothing to distinguish one day from the next, there is no way of locating a sense of impending threat within a long-term temporal framework. It is therefore experienced as forever imminent but never realized.[7] The future is exclusively oppressive; it is no longer a dimension of possibilities for meaningful activity and offers no potential relief. Experience thus dwells in the past, in a domain of deeds that are fixed, as there is no possibility of ever compensating for them. Along with this, there is an inescapable and painful feeling of isolation from other people. Feeling 'guilty about something' likewise involves the following:

1. A focus on past deeds

2. Recognition of the effects of past deeds as unchangeable

3. Estrangement from others, in whose eyes one has done wrong

4. Anticipation of being harmed or punished

The difference is that existential guilt does not involve feeling guilty about anything in particular. Instead, experience as a whole takes on the form of guilt:

> One awful thing about my depression was the tremendous sense of guilt that I was unable to attach to any memory, or action or any part of myself. I was all feeling at that time and no thought—not real thinking, only a slow-motion kind of guilty rumination. Certainly I had no hope that the future would bring me relief, let alone happiness. (Patient quoted by Rowe, 1978, p.270)

Whereas intentional guilt is one of many emotional attitudes that one might adopt towards one's deeds, existential guilt involves no sense of there being such alternatives. Hope, pleasure, interpersonal connection, curiosity, and goal-directed action are gone from the world. The space of possibilities that

---

[7] This transformation can be interpreted in terms of what Heidegger calls 'thrown projection' [*geworfener Entwurf*] (1962, p.188). According to Heidegger, we are 'thrown' into the world, meaning that we find ourselves in a place that is not of our own making, where things present themselves as significant to us in a range of ways. Inextricable from this is the way in which we 'project' ourselves towards some of the significant possibilities that the world offers, understanding both ourselves and the things around us in terms of the possibilities we strive to actualize. This kind of depression, one might say, involves a change in the structure of 'thrown projection', where various kinds of possibility are removed from the world into which one is 'thrown', and with them the possibility of purposively pursuing anything at all. Passively waiting for some threat to be realized replaces the usual orientation towards future possibilities. See, for example, Tellenbach (1980) for an account of depression that draws on Heidegger.

remains is structurally similar to intentional guilt. A specifically focused feeling of guilt over deed p involves not feeling pleased about p, not being able to do q rather than p, and not feeling connected to others in virtue of p. Existential guilt involves the absence of precisely these *kinds* of intentional experience from one's world. One cannot 'feel pleased about something', 'feel able to do something meaningful', or 'feel connected to somebody'.

An important part of the puzzle remains though. Why, when one is confronted with an irrevocable past, is the response one of guilt rather than—say—pleasant nostalgia or complete indifference? Minkowski (1958) supplies the beginnings of an answer. He points out that the way we experience our past depends on the kinds of significance attached to remembered events. For instance, when we are pleased about what we have done, it appears to us as something to be built upon, pointing to possibilities for improvement and development. Good memories are often—if not always—shaped by a sense of where one is going, what one continues to aspire towards, or what one would like to happen again. Guilty deeds, on the other hand, are closed, complete, estranged from our aspirations. The only future possibilities they point to are acts of reparation, which do not further develop what was done but instead seek to compensate for something fixed and unchangeable:

> Once an error is made or a bad action committed, it remains engraved in the conscience, leaving palpable traces; from this point of view, it is static and a backward glance is enough to uncover it. On the other hand, the only remains of positive accomplishments or good acts is in the fact that we can do better in the future; such acts are really no more than bridges that we cross in our attempts to improve. (Minkowski, 1958, p.138)

The experienced completeness of a guilty deed is its estrangement from where one is going. To quote Fuchs (2003, p.231), guilt 'stops the movement of life and ties us to a moment in the past, which it presents at the same time as irretrievable to us'. As the depressed person is no longer going anywhere, no memories relate to an open future; everything is fixed, immovable. Hence memory as a whole takes on the same kind of structure as a guilty memory. However, all sorts of memories are utterly removed from our current pursuits and yet we remain indifferent to most of them, and so the account requires further refinement. First of all, we need to restrict ourselves to episodic memories, such as 'I first went to school at the age of four'. These are to be distinguished from non-episodic factual memories, such as 'the Empire State Building is in New York', and from memories of word meanings. (According to current terminology in psychology, non-episodic factual memory and memory of word meaning together comprise 'semantic memory'.) A further distinction is needed between impersonal episodic and personal episodic memories. An impersonal episodic memory involves recalling an event in a way that is not self-involving. Recalling a past event that one saw reported on the television news would be impersonal, while remembering one's first day at school would be personal. Remembering where one was when one heard a major news story and remembering how one was affected by it would also be personal memories.

We might well be indifferent to many semantic and impersonal episodic memories, but it is doubtful that we are ever wholly indifferent to personal episodic memories, other than perhaps in those cases where we adopt a detached, third-person attitude towards past deeds, recalling them in much the same way we would if they concerned someone else. Let us restrict ourselves to the category of personal episodic memories that are remembered in a first- rather than third-person way. To remember something in this way and at the same time experience it as closed, not related to any significant possibilities, is quite different from remembering a trivial, insignificant event that occurred during a television programme. The content of the programme was never integrated into one's life in the first place, and so it is not something that one could feel alienated from in the same way.

What would personal episodic memories be like if *all* sense of there being possibilities for significant future activity were absent from experience? All past deeds would take the form of closed, irrevocable occurrences. The possibility of one's past taking on any other form would be gone and all recollection would be similar in structure to guilty recollection.[8] Of course, guilt is not the only negative attitude we might adopt towards our past deeds. But even regret involves a sense that things could have been otherwise, and depends on there being values and aspirations that remain unrealized. We regret something in relation to something else that we value. So it is not just that one's past would appear as 'bad'; it would more specifically approximate the structure of guilt.

However, as we will see in Chapter 7, some depression experiences involve a future that is devoid of significant possibility and a past that is strangely *distant* rather than guilty. So a closed past and an empty future, although necessary for existential guilt, are not sufficient. It also involves a non-localized sense of threat, of a distinctively interpersonal kind. Many depressed people report feeling cut off from others, unable to 'connect', but this does not imply

---

[8] My position here is consistent with the view that 'autobiographically past-directed emotions' involve current emotional responses to remembered events rather than remembered emotions (Debus, 2007). One remembers one's past activities *through* the existential guilt, and therefore cannot summon past emotions that are incompatible with guilt.

that the world is altogether devoid of interpersonal possibilities. The feelings of worthlessness and wretchedness that often feature in first-person accounts of depression indicate an all-pervasive *way* of relating to others. In some cases, others are experienced only as threatening witnesses to one's own shortcomings: 'People change from being people who I love and am connected with to being hosts of a parasite—me. I can't see why anyone would like me, want me, love me' (#271). With this, the experience becomes one of existential guilt. Minkowski's discussion is focused around the experiences of one patient, who is said to suffer from 'schizophrenic melancholia'. The patient feels guilty *before others*, and thus retains some way of relating to them, but this is his only way. Consequently, they cease to be distinctive individuals and instead became indistinguishable persecutors, generic judges of his worthlessness:

> He no longer perceived the personal and individual worth of men; for him they were only faint, disfigured silhouettes cut out of the general ground of hostility. In fact, he was not persecuted by living men but by men who were transformed into persecutors and were only that. He no longer saw the total, complex life of the human being. Men had become schematic manikins. (Minkowski, 1970, p.189)

Guilt of this kind is a unitary modification of experience, a reconfiguration of the possibility space that implicates the interpersonal and the temporal, as well as one's sense of agency. However, it is just one form that the world of depression can take. And it is easy to misconstrue in terms of intense, wide-ranging, intentional guilt, given that it may be expressed in a range of more specific ways—as feeling guilty about what one has done, what one has not done, what one is, or what one has become. As Fuchs (2003, p.238) suggests, guilt feelings 'evoke a feeling of existential separation or expulsion, which means to be "guilty as such", and only secondarily do they materialize in presumed omissions or sins'. Such cases need to be distinguished from others where, in the absence of existential guilt, the depressed person feels guilty about specific things—about being unable to do things that she continues to recognize as important, letting people down, causing distress, or not being what she should be.

Alternative interpretations of guilt in depression, which assume that it involves a kind of intentional state, are therefore incompatible with what many sufferers describe. For example, Roberts (2001, pp.43–4) maintains that depression 'leaves one's evaluative outlook intact', on the basis that depressives 'normally suffer a great deal from their lack of ability to pursue their values. Strong painful feelings of guilt are extremely common in depressives'. On the contrary, we have seen that what he calls an 'evaluative outlook' can be altered quite dramatically. The guilt that many describe is not an intentional state directed at a series of omissions that are appraised in the light of intact values. It is a profound shift in the overall structure of experience, in the kinds of significant possibility that are available. When you feel guilty about something, you can still contemplate feeling otherwise, and you do not feel guilty about plenty of other things. In the case of existential guilt, no alternatives present themselves. When a person is judged to be guilty of something, there can be a cycle of guilt and retribution. She is blamed by others for doing wrong and thus alienated from them. Her associated feelings of guilt can ultimately help lead to recognition of wrong-doing, followed by reparation and redemption; 'healthy' guilt is part of a process (Bennett, 2002). Existential guilt is different. The loss of future possibilities includes that of redemption; the guilt is inescapable. It is not experienced as a contingent feeling that can be overridden by some course of action. In the absence of any conceivable alternative predicaments, it seems essential to one's being. For the sufferer, there is no possible world in which she is not guilty or will one day not be guilty. Her 'evaluative outlook' consists entirely of guilt.[9]

Existential guilt renders certain kinds of intentional state unintelligible, and this is what makes it more profound than experiences of intentional guilt. The existentially guilty person can assert 'I believe that I will not feel guilty one day', just as she can assert 'I will recover', 'there is hope', or 'things will get better', and she can also explain what is meant by these assertions. But being able both to put a tick next to a sentence and to define the relevant words does not add up to a capacity for genuine assent; she cannot summon up a sense of what the world has to offer through words alone. As we have seen, if a person cannot even remember or imagine what it is like to experience hope in relation to anything, then genuine assent to the proposition 'I have hope in relation to p' is impossible for any p. The same applies to statements such as 'I might not feel guilty one day' and 'I might recover'. However, there is a fine line between what is and is not intelligible. The depressed person can sincerely assert 'it is possible that one day hope will return to me', but she can only make sense of this as the abstract possibility that some individual without capacity h might come to have capacity h, an individual that happens to be her. She cannot envisage it as a possibility in the context of her own life, as something that 'might actually happen to *me*'. And sincere assent to claims such as 'I think I might get better one day' requires that they be understood in

---

[9] Fuchs (2003, p.239) describes the experience as follows: 'The melancholic is so identified with his guilt that he is guilty *per se*; this corresponds to an archaic, undifferentiated self-perception. He feels like being the center of a "guilt-world", in which everything becomes a sign of his omission. There is no forgiveness, no remorse or reparation in the future; being guilty comprises his total being'.

an engaged way, as possibilities for oneself rather than as possibilities relating to some entity that currently lacks some characteristic. Similarly, a person suffering from existential guilt of the kind I have described cannot think of herself as 'potentially not guilty, now or at some future time'. It should be stressed, though, that existential guilt and other kinds of 'experienced impossibility' are to be understood phenomenologically and not in causal terms. What a person takes to be impossible is in fact possible, and a predicament that seems irrevocable can be altered. The sense of irrevocability associated with an existential feeling does not reliably indicate how susceptible it actually is to various causal influences. Even a very short-lived existential feeling can present itself as eternal.

Varieties of Existential Guilt

So far, I have contrasted existential guilt with intentional guilt. However, as with despair and loss of practical significance, we can also discern different depths of existential guilt, and what I have described up to now is the most extreme form. Increasingly profound experiences of hopelessness and loss of significance can involve a widening of scope, where a sense that other people still have access to hopes, values and meaningful projects is also eroded. In contrast, the deepest kind of existential guilt is exclusively self-directed. This is not to say that it takes the form 'I am guilty and others are not; they have possibilities that I lack'. Rather, it involves the most pronounced sense of estrangement from all other people and thus of its being 'my' guilt. 'Our guilt' is not as deep, as it presupposes the possibility of communion with at least some people. Hence an estrangement that is partly constitutive of guilt is not so complete. This is quite compatible with the view that, for other aspects of the same existential feeling, such as hopelessness, greater profundity involves wider applicability. When others appear only as generic judges of one's guilt, they are not recognized as possessors of hope; the only significance they are receptive to is the significance of one's own inescapable failings. 'Our loss of practical significance' is similarly compatible with 'my but not our guilt', as a common loss of significance does not imply any sense of community between people while shared guilt does. We are guilty *together*, whereas a loss of practical significance just happens to afflict others too; it does not imply a relationship with them.

It is likely that certain forms of existential guilt in depression are experienced as shared with at least some others—they are 'ours'; 'we' are worthless. And, in some such cases, the guilt may still be experienced as irrevocable. However, there are also shallower kinds of existential guilt, where some sense of significant future possibilities remains, as does the appreciation that one could be otherwise. Even so, a sense of the past as complete, as largely dissociated from what possibilities one does have, still 'weighs one down'. Experience as a whole takes the form 'I am not what I should be' (rather than 'I am not all I could be', something that is required for aspiring hope). Possibilities such as that of 'feeling satisfied with an accomplishment' or 'content with one's current situation' are thus lacking from experience. This kind of guilt has the potential to drive action. Indeed, some of the most creative, committed people may well be afflicted by it. According to Heidegger:

> Freedom is only to be found where there is a burden to be shouldered. In creative achievement this burden always represents an imperative and a need that weighs heavily upon man's overall mood, so that he comes to be in a mood of melancholy. All creative action resides in a mood of melancholy [*Schwermut*] (1995, §44, pp.182–3)

But it is a short step from this to irrevocable guilt. An increasing sense of the past as fixed, of oneself as irredeemable, is at the same time a limitation on one's future possibilities: 'I cannot rectify that'; 'nothing I can do will change this'. As the burden of a guilty past builds up, the future constricts still further. So there is a fine line between a deepening feeling that 'I am guilty' and a feeling that 'I am irrevocably guilty'.[10] A descent into existential guilt, along these lines, is to be contrasted with a gradual loss of significant possibilities from experience. The guilty person is all too aware of the significance of things and has a heightened sense of obligation, but—perhaps in conjunction with bodily lethargy and loss of enticing possibilities—there is an increasing feeling that 'I can't do x' and 'I have failed to do x'. This eventually becomes so pronounced that failure and impossibility consume the future, while other kinds of possibility are lost. (I will further describe such experiences in Chapter 6.)

Forms of existential guilt can be interpreted and expressed in different ways. For instance, there is a noticeable connection between depressive guilt and themes that are central to a number of different theistic and non-theistic religions. Some have gone so far as to argue that guilt is central to all world religions (Westphal, 1984). It is certainly a recurring theme in Christianity.

---

[10] Heidegger (1962, Division Two, II) claims that guilt is an unavoidable correlate of our freedom. A being that directs itself towards the possible will inevitably fail to actualize certain possibilities; we are never all that we could be. What he calls the 'call of conscience' reveals our 'guilt' to us—our having failed to realize possibilities that are now lost. Heidegger's 'guilt' does not correspond to the existential guilt discussed here. Variants of what I call 'existential guilt' are *modifications* of the structure he describes.

In addition to Original Sin, there are many descriptions of inescapable worth-lessness and inadequacy before God, of being somehow less than one ought to be. Guilt is construed as part of one's essence, sometimes as something that cannot be surpassed. A guilt that we all share is not as deep as the deepest kind of solitary guilt, as shared guilt presupposes a communion with others that solitary guilt denies us. The guilt of communal religion is thus shallower than the deepest guilt that can arise in depression. However, religious think-ers have endured deeper forms of guilt too, a sense of utter estrangement from all humanity, accompanied by a relationship with God that takes the form of worthlessness and passivity before a source of all-encompassing dread and awe. One indicator of relative profundity is the extent to which one holds out hope for redemption.

Existential guilt in depression, whether or not it is associated with a reli-gious narrative, is not something that strikes the guilty person as in need of justification, as it is not an attitude adopted within the world but a way of being in the world. It might be construed simply as an existential feeling, something that does not rest on any kind of judgment (moral or otherwise) regarding one's deeds. Thus, although it is sometimes expressed and inter-preted in moral or religious terms, this is not required for the *feeling* of being guilty. That said, it is plausible to maintain that evaluative judgments and wider-ranging self-narratives are integral to experiences of *intentional* guilt. I have suggested that many intentional emotions are not simply 'states' or 'episodes' that appear and then disappear. They are processes that develop over time, where feelings and thoughts influence each other. And guilt is not a static emotional 'state' consisting of two separable 'components'. It has an integrated temporal structure, sometimes involving a lengthy process of estrangement and reintegration. This can involve interpretation and reinter-pretation of events and feelings by self and others, in ways that shape and regulate feeling. A similar point applies to existential guilt. Granted, more profound forms of guilt are experienced as static and irrevocable. They do not offer the possibility of change or significant re-interpretation. Nevertheless, the fact that they are experienced as impervious to one or another influence does not imply that they actually are. I have already noted that the kinds of feeling described here are not always construed in terms of 'guilt'. Rather, they are highly conducive to being interpreted and experienced in that way. So how, we might ask, does the way in which feeling p is interpreted influence how p is actually experienced—can we extricate an experience of existential feeling from its contingent interpretation? And do differing ways of interpret-ing p offer the potential to re-shape p in different ways? Conversely, how do existential feelings constrain the possibilities for their own interpretation?

Feeling and Narrative

Existential feelings are often interpreted and expressed through variably elaborate self-narratives, which tie together a range of themes. The term 'narrative' is used in many different ways. My concern here is with explicit autobiographical narratives of whatever length or sophistication, which relate life events in meaningful, chronologically structured ways. They can be written, spoken, told to others, or kept to oneself. And they can be enduring, transient, consistent, inconsistent, structured, or fragmented. Many self-narratives do not include explicit descriptions of first-person experience, but I will focus on those that do. Some of my remarks will apply only to these, but much of what I will say also applies to self-narratives more generally. Let us start by considering the more general relationship between existential feelings and their linguistic expression. Rowe (1978) claims that experiences of depression are inseparable from articulable propositions; depression centrally consists of a series of propositions that the depressed person assents to. This is in stark contrast to my own view. I have argued that existential feeling is presupposed by the possibility of belief (regardless of whether or not a belief is expressed linguistically), and that what look like attitudes towards specific propositions are often expressions of how a person finds herself in the world. However, Rowe does at least acknowledge the fundamental or 'profound' role that her 'propositions' play in our experience: 'There are propositions that we rarely bring into full consciousness or, when we do, we rarely question them, for we regard them as axiomatic in our structure of the world' (1978, p.236).

On one interpretation, certain 'axiomatic propositions', when articulated, just are expressions of existential feeling. Consider Wittgenstein's discussion in *On Certainty* of so-called 'hinge propositions', fundamental 'beliefs' of a kind immune from doubt. According to some commentators, Wittgenstein does not in fact take hinge propositions to be deeply held beliefs of a propositional kind. Instead, they are habitual tendencies that are presupposed by the possibility of adopting propositional attitudes (e.g. Moyal-Sharrock, 2005; Rhodes and Gipps, 2008). This is consistent with Husserl's view, as described in Chapter 2: you can only take something to be the case or otherwise having presupposed a different kind of certainty, a background of coherent 'confidence' that is not itself susceptible to negation because the possibility of negation depends upon it. To quote Wittgenstein (1975, p.18), 'if you tried to doubt everything you would not get as far as doubting anything. The game of doubting itself presupposes certainty'. Hinge propositions are, he says, the 'ground' for judgements of truth and falsehood (1975, p.27). Moyal-Sharrock (2005) construes them in terms of a practical 'trust' that the possibility of belief depends on. (This corresponds to the kind of trust described in Chapter 4, to which I will return in Chapter 8.) It is likely, however, that only some of Wittgenstein's hinge propositions fit this account. 'The earth exists' and 'there are physical objects' are good candidates, but propositions such as 'the earth is round' and 'I have a brain' fall into a different category. Whereas the former are expressions of something that is inextricable from the background style of experience, from the very possibility of perceiving and believing, the latter are deeply entrenched belief contents. Hence there is a distinction to be drawn here between our most confident beliefs and a confidence that makes belief possible.

The depressed person attempts to express something unfamiliar and troubling, rather than a comfortable sense of habitual certainty. He has to find words for this, and those words vary considerably. But what might at first look like several different evaluative attitudes that he adopts towards his experiences, his achievements, or his life as a whole often amount to different expressions of the same existential feeling. Take Tolstoy's autobiographical account of an existential crisis in *A Confession* (which will be addressed at length in Chapter 10). Tolstoy's despair is focused around the gradually emerging revelation that all life is irrevocably meaningless. It creeps up on him until the point where 'I felt that what I had been standing on had collapsed, and that I had nothing left under my feet. What I had lived on no longer existed; and there was nothing left' (1882/2005, p.14). What he describes is a felt change in how he *finds himself in the world*, which gradually takes on the guise of an articulate thought:

> I could not even wish to know the truth, for I guessed of what it consisted. The truth was that life is meaningless. I had, as it were, lived [...] till I had come to a precipice and saw clearly that there was nothing ahead of me but destruction. (Tolstoy, 2005, p.15)

Tolstoy's revelation that 'life is meaningless' is not something that can be separated from how he finds himself in the world. It conveys an existential feeling, a sense that the world is irrevocably bereft of the kinds of possibility needed to go on living.[11] In cases like this, existential feeling and articulate thought content are so closely related that the latter is little more than an expression of the former. The point applies not only to depression experiences but to existential feelings more generally, in psychiatric illness and elsewhere.

---

[11] See also Wynn (2012) for the view that certain 'beliefs', including—for many—a belief in God, are actually expressions of existential feeling.

For example, reflecting on experiences of derealization that have affected him for many years, Stephen Weiner (2003, p.371) writes:

> I certainly feel that my experience of derealization has had great consequences for my ability to make plans and carry them out, not because I slide into incongruous and discontinuous ego states, but because the worth of any endeavour is always being called into question by my strong feeling of solipsistic despair. This feeling has almost, I must admit, attained the status of a firm conviction, that because nothing truly exists, all effort is futile.

What he describes here is a kind of existential feeling, one involving a feeling of conviction that lends itself to expression in the form of a content-specific belief. It is not a belief about an existential feeling or an evaluation of it, but an attempt to relate the feeling. However, even when a self-narrative expresses an existential feeling in this way, there remains plenty of room for interpretation and elaboration. For instance, Rhodes and Smith (2010) describe how the 'pit' or 'hole' that is so common in depression narratives can be conveyed in more specific ways, drawing on memories, fears and symbols that reflect a person's biography. A first-person account that they discuss compares the pit of depression to the one used by Buffalo Bill in the film *The Silence of the Lambs*, with the added ingredient of rising water. So, although the world of depression inevitably lends itself to confinement metaphors, these can be more concrete, elaborate and idiosyncratic. Nevertheless, such interpretations amount to more or less embellished attempts to convey an underlying existential feeling. The route is *from* the feeling *to* its conceptualization and articulation.

However, the relationship between an existential feeling and how it is explicitly conceived of (in narrative form or otherwise) is not always a one-way street from the feeling to its conceptualization. When interpreting first-person narratives in terms of existential feeling, it can be difficult to tease apart existential feelings from other ingredients of experience, such as trains of thought, specifically focused perceptions, and self-evaluations. Consider William James's claim that religious and metaphysical doctrines are rooted in feeling: 'in the metaphysical and religious sphere, articulate reasons are cogent for us only when our inarticulate feelings of reality have already been impressed in favor of the same conclusion' (James, 1902, p.74).[12] On one account, existential feeling—of one type or another—comprises a sense of reality and belonging, which is then interpreted and conveyed in terms of explicit religious and philosophical doctrines. These doctrines 'rest on top

---

[12] See also Ratcliffe (2008, Chapters 7 and 8) for a detailed account of James on emotion and feeling.

of feelings', and exactly the same feeling can underlie a range of superficially divergent linguistic expressions. On another account, what James calls the 'over-beliefs' (culturally and historically contingent ways of interpreting a core feeling) somehow shape the feeling, maybe giving it a more specific content. The feeling crystallizes *into* something articulable, rather than enduring unchanged beneath the narrative that it motivated. I do not wish to claim that existential feelings are isolable *components* of experience, which exist in a purified form independently of whatever else accompanies them. More generally, it is doubtful that the interpretation and expression of feeling is always a matter of construing and conveying pre-formed experiences. It has been argued that expression, linguistic or otherwise, serves to individuate and even partly constitute certain feelings (e.g. Campbell, 1997; Colombetti, 2009). Hence, regardless of whether or not a self-narrative includes explicit attempts to express, communicate, and/or interpret feeling, it may well have some influence on the nature of the experience, a point that also applies more specifically to the relationship between existential feeling and its expression.

In some cases of existential feeling, it is plausible to maintain that the feeling cannot be cleanly separated from its interpretation. Suppose you encounter someone who complains of having 'the feeling of being surrounded by arseholes'.[13] This could well be symptomatic of an existential feeling involving a global sense of uneasiness, disconnectedness, and distrust. But, even if this is so, the feeling is phenomenologically inseparable from how it is understood and expressed by the person, something that may also influence how she responds to it, as well as how she relates to other people.[14] She might take it that she feels this way because she is indeed 'surrounded by arseholes'; the feeling reflects the reality of her situation. This, in turn, influences how she feels. Having accepted that her feeling is reliable, she may be content to engage

---

[13] Thanks to Jan Slaby for this example, which is the first thing he spotted when he typed 'the feeling of being' into Google, a method I once used to look for descriptions of existential feelings (Ratcliffe, 2005).

[14] It is not entirely clear what being phenomenologically 'separable' actually amounts to. On one account, no two experiences had by one person at the same time are separable, at least when they arise in a singular consciousness with a certain degree of unity. On the other hand, take the case of listening to something on the radio and, as you do so, experiencing a slight pain in your foot. The two contents are distinct, and it also seems that there are two distinct kinds of experience: *hearing* something and *feeling* pain. Granted, one may affect the other, but it is plausible to maintain that the pain's presence or absence does not substantially alter the experience of 'listening to *x* on the radio'. This is what I mean by 'separable' here. So the inseparability claim is that one could not subtract the interpretation of a feeling while (a) continuing to experience the same kind of feeling and (b) experiencing the feeling as having the same *content*.

with the world *through* the feeling, rather than reflecting on it and attempting to somehow distance herself from it and from the behavioural inclinations associated with it. From a dynamic perspective, at least, the feeling and its interpretation are entangled.

Existential feeling should therefore be regarded as an inextricable *aspect* of experience, rather than a dissociable *component*, to adopt a distinction made by Hobson (2010). In the case of a 'feeling of being surrounded by arseholes', there might well be an existential feeling aspect, but it does not suffice to individuate something so specific; the experience also has a contingent content. However, this does not imply that the distinction between existential feeling and other aspects of experience is irretrievably blurred. By analogy, the distinction between the three internal angles of a triangle is quite clear, even though they are indissociable. We can distinguish existential feeling from self-narrative and other aspects of experience in a clear way by means of abstraction; describing something in isolation does not imply the possibility of its isolated existence. This requires us to adopt the right level of description (set out in Chapter 2). While the existential structure of an experience might involve an 'all-pervasive sense of interpersonal estrangement', a 'feeling of being surrounded by arseholes' is too specific and blurs the boundary between experiential form and a more specific content.

The interplay between existential feeling and self-narrative becomes further apparent once we acknowledge the extent to which people rely on narrative in order to make sense of and regulate their experience and behaviour (to pick up on a theme of Chapter 1). The point is not specific to illness narratives. Nowhere is it more evident than in Albert Speer's prison diaries, which were written during twenty years of incarceration at Spandau, after his sentencing at the Nuremberg War Crimes Trials. Speer describes his writing as 'one concentrated effort to survive'. He writes that his diary is an 'attempt to give form to the time that seemed to be pouring away so meaninglessly, to give substance to years empty of content'. Diaries, he remarks, are 'usually the accompaniment of a lived life', whereas his 'stands in place of a life' (Speer, 1975/2010, xi–xii). Two themes can be discerned here. First of all, the *project* of writing the diary is itself something to fill the time with, and imposes a meaningful structure on it. Second, the *content* of the diary gives narrative form to a life that is otherwise bereft of meaningful change and longer-term teleological structure. The alternative, according to Speer, is to surrender oneself to existential collapse, to a way of inhabiting the world in the context of which structured, purposive activity of any kind is unintelligible.

Self-interpretation can thus shape existential feeling, perhaps via several different routes. For instance, a feeling could be interpreted in a way that induces

dread, which then affects the feeling, partly by influencing its ongoing interpretation. According to Jaspers (1963), this dynamic is at play in experiences
of delusional atmosphere. The person does not understand what is happening
to him and has a terrifying feeling of indeterminacy, which fuels a quest for
certainty in the form of the delusional narrative that eventually crystallizes.
This narrative is cultivated by an experience but also alters the experience,
rendering it more determinate. More generally, conceptual understandings
of situations and events have the potential to affect existential feeling. Take
the experience of distressing news 'sinking in'. Initial recognition of what
has happened might involve loss of various intentional state contents, such as
believing that p, hoping for q, expecting that r, and so on. Often, one gradually forms new hopes, new expectations, and new projects, thus adjusting to
a changed situation. However, disappointment or sorrow of this kind sometimes develops into something else. A series of disappointments can lead to
gradual erosion of confidence, which affects how the person meets further
disappointments. Eventually, she might reach a state where something is lost
from the world—a sense that the future offers certain kinds of possibility, a
sense that things are worth striving for.[15]

Although self-narratives (as well as more localized conceptualizations and
evaluations of one's feelings) can—to some extent—regulate existential feeling, the capacity for narrative also presupposes existential feeling. Of course,
the content of one's feelings will be reflected in the content of one's autobiographical narratives, but existential feeling also shapes narrative *form*. Many
depression narratives are written after a period of depression, but those written at the time are constrained by the loss of possibility. As Byron Good
(1994, p.155) notes, the majority of self-narratives, including illness narratives, oscillate between different points of view. They are open to diverse
self-interpretations and alive with possibilities: 'stories of illness and healing

---

[15] See Stephan (2012) for an account of how existential feelings are regulated. Stephan
regards existential feeling regulation as more problematic than I do. He would, I think,
reject the view that conceptual thought can influence existential feeling. That said, I am
not sure *how* understandings of events shape existential feelings. A problem we face in
attempting to offer a phenomenological account is that, in some cases, an intentional
state with content p affects existential feeling q in such a way as to remove the conditions of intelligibility for intentional states of that type. But how could an intentional
state somehow 'act upon' its own conditions of intelligibility? It is not clear to me that
much more can be said from a phenomenological perspective—it simply happens, just
as existential changes can happen when one is sick, tired or intoxicated. Perhaps, at this
point, we need to switch to a non-phenomenological approach. For instance, there is a
neurobiological story to be told.

experience which represent quite distinct and often competing forms of com-
posing the illness are present in narratives precisely because they maintain
the quality of subjunctivity and openness to change'. He adds that this form
is absent in 'tragic and hopeless cases', and this is what we find in depression.
There is a loss of narrative openness, an inability to entertain certain kinds
of possibility that reflects the loss of an open future. This loss also manifests
itself in terms of specific factual and evaluative beliefs that feature repeatedly
in depression narratives, such as the belief that recovery is impossible and the
view that the future offers nothing good. In more extreme cases, the person
cannot imagine how things could ever be different from the present or believe
that they ever were different. Hence the existential feeling shapes its interpretation insofar as it entails the loss of a certain kind of narrative capacity. As
one author remarks, 'people in the middle of depression are beings who have
to live, for a while, without a story, which is why it feels as though you've lost
your soul' (Lewis, 2006, p.96).

To conclude this chapter, I will offer a tentative account of another kind of
narrative disturbance, one that I think occurs in at least some cases of depression. Here, the person *needs* a narrative, principally one about where she is
going and how she is going to tackle various tasks, but she cannot formulate
one because there is no sense that the future could be any different. However,
what results is not an absence of narrative thought. Instead, there is a cacoph-
ony of disordered thoughts as she struggles to form a coherent story that cannot take shape. Thoughts go round and round without any efficacy, like a car
engine that is out of gear. Such an experience is suggested by the following
DQ responses:

> #14....my head is filled with so many thoughts I can't ever sleep. Just hundreds and
> hundreds of thoughts whirling around in my head, with no function or order. It's
> complete chaos.

> #23....when I have depression, my mind just feels overly active with all these dif-
> ferent thoughts spinning round in my head, but at the same time my mind feels
> completely blank of any feelings or emotions. I don't know if that makes sense, but
> it does to me.

> #37. Thoughts are jumbled, repetitive, extreme.

> #134. I find a weird combination of thinking too much and not being able to think
> about anything. I don't usually dwell on the past but when I am depressed things just
> pop into my head. However, ask me what I want for lunch or what time something
> needs to happen and there is nothing there.

> #224. Insane whirling repetitive thinking which is completely incapable of finding a
> solution and over-complicates and throws up road blocks at every turn. Can't focus
> or read, sometimes can't even watch TV as requires too much concentration.

The thoughts involved are generally negative ones about the past and the self, along with others that concern problems to which solutions never materialize. The person cannot entertain the possibility of anything good happening to her and so she cannot construct a future-oriented self-narrative in which problems are successfully dealt with, or a past-focused narrative that allows for the possibility of rectifying or mitigating mistakes. But she can envisage the bad—failure in its many guises, along with shame and guilt. So the more she thinks through her problems, the worse things get. The only new possibilities that she uncovers are bad ones, resulting in a spiral of hopelessness, worthlessness and sometimes self-loathing:

> #28. I can't think about anything positive, just negative thoughts. I only think about my own problems and they keep going round and round my head with no let up and no escape.

> #179. It's like a jumper unravelling; you pull at that stray thread and the thing unravels, you know you should stop pulling the thread or the whole thing will fall to pieces, but you hate that loose end that proves the thing is unravelling anyway so you keep on pulling.... You can't help yourself...

This kind of rumination is one way in which existential guilt might arise. Feelings constrain self-narrative, but the person still feels compelled to impose narrative order. The narratives she tries to concoct reveal only the bad, until she finds herself in a world that offers nothing but danger, failure, and guilt. I do not wish to suggest that narrative has no positive role to play in depression. People offer all sorts of different accounts of what caused their depression. A complicated history of life events is often involved, including parents leaving or divorcing, lack of parental care, abuse, bereavement, not being loved by anyone, going through a divorce oneself, or being neglected, bullied, or disliked. Others emphasize illness or accident and, regardless of the focus, the problems often date back to childhood. For some, depression is a brain disease, and many appeal to family history or genetic dispositions. Others attribute it to stress, and some state that their depression is postnatal or tracks the menstrual cycle. A few say that they simply do not understand what has happened to them.[16] It is likely that at least some such accounts have a role to play in steering the course of a depression. Suppose a person comes to accept that her depression is somehow her fault:

> #16. I know depression is an illness but at the same time I feel like I caused it. The doctor explained that it could be because of genetic reasons because my biological dad had bipolar and his mum did too. Also my psychologist believes that because I feel like I am to blame for the violence caused by my biological [dad] towards me

---

[16] All of these explanations appear in DQ responses.

and my mum, which started when she was pregnant with me, so I have always felt to blame because of that.

#137. There is tremendous guilt for me in depression—I'm weak, not like others who cope, therefore it's my fault.

Loss of an open future lends itself to a self-narrative that is past-oriented, pre-occupied with a life history riddled with failure and no longer amenable to re-negotiation in the light of future projects and goals. However, although narrative capacity is restricted to varying degrees in depression, and shaped by the kinds of existential feeling that are typical of depression, people still interpret their predicaments in ways that are, to an extent, contingent and malleable. The combination of 'self-loathing' and 'I caused it' together lead to a depression narrative according to which one deserves one's depression and is forever condemned to it, a conviction that is surely a further impediment to recovery for some people. This points to questions such as 'When and to what extent can certain kinds of narrative help sustain, alter, or rebuild a person's capacity for feeling?' and 'How are others able to assist in the construction and adjustment of such narratives, by drawing on imaginative resources that the depressed person lacks?' The empirical research that is needed to answer questions about the efficacy of intervention at the level of self-narrative can be informed by a better appreciation of the mutually constraining relationship between self-interpretation and kinds of existential feeling. Different existential feelings constrain self-narrative to varying degrees and in different ways, and are therefore likely to be susceptible to different forms of intervention. And a more nuanced account of the kinds of existential feelings involved in depression offers the potential to distinguish forms of experience that would otherwise be grouped together, including intentional and existential forms that are superficially similar but in fact profoundly different.

Chapter 6

Agency and Free Will

A consistent theme of my discussion so far is that depression experiences involve a sense of impossibility. Guilt is irrevocable, the possibility of hope is gone, and the world of depression is inescapable. All of this is inextricable from an alteration in the person's experience of agency. In this chapter, I offer an account of the phenomenology of agency in depression, focusing on why action seems impossible rather than just difficult. I suggest that there is a change in the 'experience of free will'. Although it is often assumed that we have such an experience, it is far from clear what it consists of. I begin by arguing that this lack of clarity is symptomatic of our looking for it in the wrong place. Drawing on themes in Sartre's *Being and Nothingness*, I propose that the sense of freedom associated with action is not—first and foremost—an episodic 'quale' or 'feeling' that is experienced as internal to the agent. Rather, it is embedded in the experienced world; our freedom appears in the guise of our surroundings. Then I show how this allows us to make sense of what people with depression so often describe: a diminished ability to act that is at the same time a transformation of the experienced world. As with other aspects of existential feeling in depression, there are several different variants.

Loss of Agency in Depression

People with depression often report an impaired ability to act. This not only affects actions that involve forethought or effort. Even habitual and undemanding activities, like making a cup of tea or having a shower, can seem overwhelmingly difficult and beyond one's abilities:

> When I'm depressed, every job seems bigger and harder. Every setback strikes me not as something easy to work around or get over but as a huge obstacle. Events appear more chaotic and beyond my control: if I fail to achieve some goal, it will seem that achieving it is forever beyond my abilities, which I perceive to be far more meagre than I did when I was not depressed. (Law, 2009, p.355)

Given that people describe feeling unable to initiate action in the way they once did, depression seems to affect what we might call the *phenomenology of free will*. Action seldom ceases altogether, but sufferers describe a feeling of being somehow diminished that permeates all their experiences and activities: 'My existence was pared away almost to nothing' (Shaw, 1997, p.27). Activities are often experienced as somehow different, oddly mechanical, and detached. For instance, in his *Autobiography*, John Stuart Mill describes how he did things 'mechanistically', 'by mere force of habit'. Various routines persisted only because he had been 'so drilled in a certain sort of mental exercise' that he could 'still carry it on when all spirit had gone out of it' (1873, pp.139–40). Even habitual action had lost its usual 'tone'; it was bereft of a sense of vitality and spontaneity.

The question of how depression affects the ability to act has not received much attention from philosophers. However, it is addressed by Roberts (2001), who proposes that depressed people fail to act because of an inability to satisfy their desires, due to loss of positive affect. The depressed person contemplates doing q, imagines that doing so will bring no relief from negative feeling, and therefore does not do q. This applies to all actions, and so the inclination to act is stifled. The point is not that we more usually act *in order to* experience a hedonic effect. Rather, when we act in order to achieve q, the sense of having done so successfully is partly constituted by experiencing feeling p in relation to q. In the absence of any anticipated feeling of type p, there is no sense of being able to achieve anything by bringing about q, no sense of anticipated satisfaction.

A serious problem for this view is that many people with depression not only decline to act; they say that action seems impossible. Realizing that one will not get any satisfaction from an action is not the same as regarding it as beyond one's abilities. Furthermore, it is plausible to maintain that motivation and anticipated satisfaction often come apart in the course of everyday life. For instance, when writing a long reference for somebody, one might do so out of duty, without anticipating or obtaining any sense of satisfaction. To accommodate such cases, it might be added that we also act in order to avoid anticipated negative feelings, such as guilt. But what about cases such as picking up a piece of litter that somebody else has dropped? One might do this because it strikes one as the right thing to do, but without anticipating any sense of satisfaction or—for that matter—any negative feeling in the event of one's not doing so.

Examples like these are far from decisive, given that they can always be reinterpreted in ways that are consistent with the 'anticipated satisfaction' hypothesis. In the case of picking up litter, it could simply be maintained that the anticipated feeling is a subtle one. However, we can also draw on neurobiology to support a distinction between motivation and anticipated reward. According to Berridge (2007), current evidence suggests that the neurotransmitter dopamine plays an important role in motivation or 'incentive salience', but is neither necessary nor sufficient for 'hedonic "liking"' or learning to anticipate outcomes. Motivation and reward are thus dissociable. We might gain satisfaction from something and also anticipate doing so, but remain unmotivated. Conversely, we might feel motivated to do something without anticipating or achieving any satisfaction. Berridge's conclusions are based largely on studies with rats, and I do not want to suggest that our phenomenology corresponds in any obvious way to the behavioural capacities of rats. Nevertheless, if the motivational system of a rat is complicated enough to distinguish between motivation, reward and anticipated outcome, it seems reasonable to assume that ours is too, and that the phenomenological distinction between being motivated to act and anticipating the positive effects of one's actions is a legitimate one to draw. 'Depression', I will show, encompasses a range of experiences, which implicate anticipated outcome and motivation in subtly different ways. Changes in the structure of anticipation can affect motivation. Sometimes, one is unable to contemplate the possibility of positive change and consequently loses any motivation to act. But, contrary to Roberts' account, this need not involve imagining a future state of affairs, given that one's current situation is experienced as lacking the relevant kinds of possibility. And there are other cases where a sense of significant possibility remains, a sense that it would be better if certain things were done. Even so, there is no 'enticement' to act, and action may even present itself as impossible.

To better appreciate how depression affects the phenomenology of free will, the approach I will adopt is to first characterize an intact experience of free will and then ask what is absent, diminished, or different in depression. It seems plausible to maintain that there is some such experience. Indeed, it lies at the heart of philosophical debates over free will and determinism. A belief in libertarian free will, it would seem, originates in an experience of free action. As Viktor Frankl (1973, p.14) remarks, most of us have an experience of free will, one that we assume to be veridical:

> Man's freedom of will belongs to the immediate data of his experience. These data yield to that empirical approach which, since Husserl's days, is called phenomenological. Actually only two classes of people maintain that their will is not free: schizophrenic patients suffering from the delusion that their will is manipulated and their thoughts controlled by others, and alongside of them, deterministic philosophers. To be sure, the latter admit that we are experiencing our will as though it were free, but this, they say, is a self-deception.

Experience of free will is also presupposed by debates concerning whether or not free will is an illusion. If we did not have an experience of free will, we could not have an illusory experience of it. For example, Libet (2004) not only assumes that we have an awareness of willing something to happen but further claims that the 'conscious will to act' can be timed. As others have observed, it is far from clear what the alleged experience amounts to (e.g. Holton, 2009). And not everyone accepts Libet's assumption that actions are experienced as initiated by 'volitions'. For instance, some claim that the phenomenology is more consistent with 'agent-causation' approaches, according to which agents rather than volitions are the causes of actions. But, if there is an experience of agent causation, what does that consist of? Again, the matter is unclear, prompting Nichols (2004, p.491) to dismiss the idea of such an experience as 'phenomenologically implausible'. So there is a tension between the widespread intuition that we experience our actions as free and the elusiveness of that experience. I will not compare the virtues of the various candidate experiences that have been proposed, which include mental causation, agent causation, and the sense of effort (see e.g. Bayne and Levy, 2006). Instead, I will suggest that the experience's elusiveness is symptomatic of our looking for it in the wrong place. Our sense of acting freely is not primarily something we experience as internal to ourselves, an episodic feeling associated with the initiation or performance of certain actions. Instead, *all* actions (along with any feelings or 'qualia' that might be associated with acting or being about to act) presuppose an experience of freedom. This experience consists simply of 'the world'—the sense that we are free is integral to how we experience our surroundings. I will go on to show how this view enables us to understand what people with depression so often describe: an impaired ability to act that is inextricable from 'living in a different world'.

The Phenomenology of Agency

What kinds of action do we experience as 'free' in the relevant sense? If we can establish that much, then we will at least know where to look in order to characterize the experience. The sort of action that Libet (2004) instructed his experimental subjects to perform—flicking a wrist without any forethought—is not a good candidate. Lowe (2008, p.85) points out that they were effectively asked '*not* to exercise their will' and instead to let the urge somehow 'creep up on them unawares'. Furthermore, it is arguable that free will is not merely a matter of initiating bodily movements. When we perform goal-directed actions, such as reaching for a pen, crossing the road, or drinking from a glass of water, every movement of a finger, hand, arm, or leg does not comprise a discrete free action. That would be the wrong level of description. If there is an experience of free will, it is associated with purposive activities, such as 'crossing the road in order to go to the shop' (Gallagher, 2006). Flicking a wrist is not a typical free action but a movement that would ordinarily contribute to such an action, one that has been extricated from its usual context.

Let us concede that certain behaviours contribute to actions, rather than being actions, and that others, like flicking a wrist, are dubious candidates for free actions. That still leaves us with many different candidates. Consider the following:

1. Thinking through a problem when there is not much at stake, deciding to do something, and then doing it.
2. Making a choice that will have a significant effect on one's life, with which various conflicting emotions are associated.
3. Performing a one-off goal-directed action without any forethought, such as picking up a glass and drinking its contents.
4. Unreflectively performing a habitual routine, such as cleaning one's teeth in the morning.
5. Making an impulsive ostensive gesture, in order to draw a companion's attention to something exciting.
6. Expressing anger at someone.
7. Saying 'phenomenology', rather than 'experience' in a sentence where either word would have sufficed.

It is debatable how many different kinds of action there are and what distinguishes all of them from (a) a cluster of closely related actions, (b) an action component, and (c) a behaviour that is neither an action nor an action component. The above list is not intended to be exhaustive or to reflect a uniquely appropriate taxonomy. My aim is merely to illustrate the wide variety of actions and accompanying experiences. Heading to the bathroom to brush one's teeth is different, in many respects, from asking someone to marry you. What kinds of action are associated with an experience of freedom? Perhaps it is exclusive to those that involve making a *choice*. It is difficult to pin down the scope of choice. Although it could be restricted to (1) and (2) above, it seems odd to say that I did *not* choose to clean my teeth, perform a gesture, or say a word. The intuition remains that I *could have done otherwise* in these cases. And there is a simple phenomenological argument against the view that our experience of freedom consists of a 'magic ingredient', added only to certain kinds of action. In short, we do not experience ourselves as mechanistically determined robots that are occasionally moved by a burst of freedom, thus making a subset of our activities stand out from all others. Our experience does not incorporate a clear distinction between certain actions, which are 'free', and all other behaviours. In what follows, I will defend the view that all of our actions are experienced as free. This is consistent with what depressed people describe. Their impaired ability to act concerns not only those actions that are preceded by deliberation or choice, but also activities that are ordinarily habitual, unthinking, and effortless: 'To get out of bed at midday was an ordeal' (anonymous, in Read and Reynolds eds, 1996, p.35).

I will draw on Sartre's discussion of freedom in *Being and Nothingness* in order to argue that the experience of freedom is neither an inchoate internal feeling nor an episode that accompanies some instances of action. Rather, it is an ordinarily constant background to all our activities. Our choices *presuppose* that we are free to act, rather than constituting an experience of freedom. Because our actions are experienced as free even when we do not explicitly *choose* them or *will* them to occur, I will refer more often to our sense of 'freedom' than to 'free will'. Freedom, I will argue, is a way of experiencing the world. I do not deny that our experiences of agency have additional features, some of which are episodic and/or internal to the self. My point is that these occur against the backdrop of a presupposed world, and the core experience of freedom is integral to that world. Other aspects of the phenomenology of agency may well be quite heterogeneous (which further explains why the sense of free will is so hard to pin down when the emphasis is placed upon something experienced as internal to the agent).

Will in the World

A first step towards characterizing the phenomenology of freedom is the acknowledgement that world-experience includes a sense of the possible. In Chapter 2, I extracted from Husserl's work the view that (a) perceptual experience includes various different kinds of possibility, some of which are significant to us in one way or another, and (b) perception of worldly possibility is inseparable from our bodily phenomenology—we experience our surroundings through our feeling bodies. Once this is accepted, we can see how the experience of freedom associated with action is integral to the experienced world. The kinds of possibility that the world offers include 'I can'. The *possibility* of my doing p or doing q is *there*, built into my surroundings. And this kind of possibility is phenomenologically distinguishable from others, such as 'p could happen', 'p could happen to me' or 'someone else could do p'. Our being presented with the 'I can', along with other kinds of possibility that it is distinct from, is what constitutes our experience of freedom. Perhaps the best statement of this view is Sartre's, and I will focus on four claims he makes about freedom:

1. The experience of freedom involves being presented with a world that offers various kinds of possibility, including 'I can'.

2. All action is free; action preceded by reflective choice is only one kind of free action.

3. The experience of freedom is inextricable from our bodily phenomenology.

4. The fundamental project that gives meaning to all of one's actions is itself a choice.

I will accept (1), (2), and (3), but will reject (4). Turning first of all to (1), Sartre emphasizes at various points in *Being and Nothingness* that the experienced world is imbued with the possible. Consider his description of looking up at a cloudy sky and perceiving the threat of rain:

> The possible appears to us as a property of things. After glancing at the sky I state, 'It is possible that it may rain.' I do not understand the 'possible' here as meaning 'without contradiction with the present state of the sky.' This possibility belongs to the sky as threat; it represents a surpassing on the part of these clouds, which I perceive, toward rain. (1989, p.97)

He further indicates that the experience of being free is a matter of being presented with possibilities. When we act, we do not perceive a purely factual state of affairs, think about the discrepancy between it and some preferred situation, and then experience an internal mental state of 'desire'. A current situation appears to us as *lacking* in some way and thus solicits a certain kind of action (Sartre, 1989, p.433). It is also clear from Sartre's account that, however much the world might call for a certain action, that action still appears as something we *could* do, not something we are compelled to do. Take his well-known example of walking along the edge of a precipice and feeling afraid. Sartre stresses that my fear is a way of experiencing my surroundings; they appear as offering the 'possibility of my life being changed from without'. Hence the precipice also invites me to act in a certain way; it 'presents itself to me *as to be avoided*' (Sartre, 1989, pp.29–30). However, moving away from the edge is not experienced as something I *must* do. And the revelation that nothing compels me to act in this way consists, Sartre says, in a feeling of 'anguish':

> Vertigo is anguish to the extent that I am afraid not of falling over the precipice, but of throwing myself over. A situation provokes fear if there is a possibility of my life being changed from without; my being provokes anguish to the extent that I distrust myself and my own reactions in that situation (1989, p.29).

He also maintains that I am free even when I am not *reflectively* aware of my freedom in this way. My unreflective experience of freedom consists in the simple fact of the world's offering significant possibilities that I might actualize, such as backing away from the cliff, and offering them as

possibilities rather than inevitabilities. Action is experienced *as* the actualization of worldly possibilities, and this applies to unthinking, habitual
action too: 'the consciousness of man in action is non-reflective consciousness' (Sartre, 1989, p.36). One might argue that the experience of possibility is merely epistemic; it is a matter of ignorance over what will happen
rather than an experience of freedom. Some of the possibilities we experience do reflect lack of knowledge, but it would be phenomenologically
implausible to maintain that 'I can do *p* or *q*' takes that form. The experience is quite different from 'I don't know whether *p* or *q* will happen next'.
And, even if one knows full well what one will do, the relevant course of
action still presents itself as one possibility amongst others, none of which
one *has to* actualize.

For Sartre, the kinds of significance that experienced entities have are
symptomatic of the projects we are knowingly or unknowingly committed
to. Insofar as I strive to be a good philosopher, a book may appear enticing, a
talk interesting, and a negative review of my work hurtful. Our projects thus
shape not only the possibilities for action that the world offers but various
other kinds of significance too. Even significant events that we have no control over depend—in a way—on our freedom. A being that cared for nothing,
that strove for nothing, could not be obstructed, threatened, or disappointed.
Things affect us in these ways only because we already have certain concerns,
and we choose those concerns by choosing the projects we pursue. Actions
respond to worldly possibilities that reflect our projects. These projects are
dependent on further projects, and so on. Hence what constrains our actions
is itself symptomatic of our freedom.[1]

As we saw in Chapter 3, Sartre maintains that the experience of worldly
possibility is essentially bodily in character. He also offers a transcendental
argument to the effect that having a body is a necessary condition for thought,
action, and choice:

> In fact if the ends which I pursue could be attained by a purely arbitrary wish, if it
> were sufficient to hope in order to obtain, and if definite rules did not determine the
> use of instruments, I could never distinguish within me desire from will, nor dream
> from act, nor the possible from the real. (1989, p.327)

If our capacities were unlimited, to wish would be to be to get, and the
distinction between desire, choice, and action would break down. Having

---

[1] Sartre also acknowledges that our possibilities are shaped and thus, in some way, 'constrained' by a social world of shared meanings. However, he says that these constraints
are not experienced as limits. We do not miss possibilities that were not sewn into the
experienced world to begin with (Sartre, 1989, p.531).

a body, and with it a contingent set of capacities, is required for the ability to distinguish between wanting, having, desiring, needing, willing, and acting. As Sartre puts it, 'the body is the contingent form which is taken up by the necessity of my contingency' (1989, p.328). In other words, freedom requires the limitations imposed by a body but does not require those limitations to take any particular form. However, the experience is not determined solely by our bodily capacities. Bodily fatigue, for example, is experienced as a way in which the 'surrounding world' appears, but how exactly it is experienced depends on what projects one is committed to (1989, p.454).

Sartre suggests that all of our activities and projects, all of the ways in which we find things significant, can be traced back to an original project that is chosen: 'all these trivial passive expectations of the real, all these commonplace, everyday values, derive their meaning from an original projection of myself which stands as my choice of myself in the world' (1989, p.39). I reject this last claim on phenomenological grounds.[2] I argued in Chapter 2 that all of our projects ultimately presuppose a structure that is not chosen. Whether it is x, y, or z that one encounters as frightening, enticing, or useful reflects the projects one has chosen to pursue. But, in order to have any sort of project, one must have the capacity to find things significant in these kinds of way. Only if one is already capable of experiencing threat can one find a particular entity threatening, and only if one already has a sense of being able to actualize meaningful possibilities is one able to have any kind of project. Access to these kinds of possibility is not chosen. The phenomenology of freedom does not originate in an ungrounded choice but in a pre-given space of possibility, a space that is susceptible to various kinds of change. Though I depart from Sartre's position here, this does not preclude endorsement of his other claims. I agree with Sartre that the phenomenology of freedom is a matter of experiencing one's actions as responses to significant worldly possibilities, that freedom is not restricted to reflective choices, that body and world are phenomenologically inseparable, and that many of the possibilities we perceive are symptomatic of projects that frame our activities. Furthermore, freedom does extend to some of those projects that form a habitual backdrop to our activities. People sometimes do make radical choices that change the structure of their lives.

---

[2] Indeed, just about everybody who has discussed Sartre's 'original choice' rejects the idea. For instance, Merleau-Ponty (1962, pp.441–453) claims that it is our 'habitual being in the world' that gives things the significance they have, and that the significant situation we find ourselves immersed in when we choose is not itself a choice.

This approach can be applied to depression, and I will suggest that experiences of inability in depression can be plausibly interpreted in terms of the following.

1. The sense of freedom associated with action is principally a matter of possibilities that are integral to the experienced world.
2. The possibilities we experience reflect our projects.
3. Worldly possibilities are inextricable from bodily dispositions.

The experience of freedom is sewn into a 'way of finding oneself in the world' that is presupposed by action, rather than being attributable primarily to a kind of episodic feeling that precedes or accompanies certain actions.[3] Depression involves a change in the *kinds* of possibility that are integral to experience, amounting to a diminishment of freedom.

A World without Will

In existential forms of depression, there is a change in the feeling of being able to act, which is also a change in how the world as a whole appears. The same existential feeling can be described in several different ways, in terms of how 'self', 'agency', 'freedom', 'body', and/or 'world' are experienced. All are inextricable aspects of a single, unitary way of 'finding oneself in the world'. So far as the 'self' is concerned, diminished agency is not experienced as the temporary loss of capacities that one contingently possesses. Openness to certain kinds of possibility is inseparable from a 'core' sense of self, of being a cohesive locus of experience and agency. Contraction of the possibility space therefore amounts to an experienced erosion of self (at least in those cases where there is an experience *of* loss, lack or absence). The kind of 'self-experience' I have in mind here is consistent with what others have referred to in terms of the 'minimal self' (see e.g. Gallagher, 2000; Zahavi, 2005, pp.105–6; Hohwy, 2007). It is not a 'content' of experience. Rather, it is inseparable from the having of a unified experiential world that offers possibilities for perception and action, a world that the intelligibility of having experiential contents depends upon. This sense of self is 'diminished' in depression, rather than 'disrupted' or 'fragmented'. The latter experience is more typically associated with schizophrenia diagnoses (a point I will return to in Chapter 10).[4]

---

[3] As Merleau-Ponty (1962, p.162) puts it, 'will presupposes a field of possibilities among which I choose'.

[4] See also Svenaeus (2013) for the view that depression impacts upon this core experience of self.

As emphasized in earlier chapters, most autobiographical accounts of depression describe a radical change in all experience and thought, one that also implicates the ability to act:

> When you are in it there is no more empathy, no intellect, no imagination, no compassion, no humanity, no hope. It isn't possible to roll over in bed because the capacity to plan and execute the required steps is too difficult to master, and the physical skills needed are too hard to complete. [...] Depression steals away whoever you are, prevents you from seeing who you might someday be, and replaces your life with a black hole. Like a sweater eaten by moths, nothing is left of the original, only fragments that hinted at greater capacities, greater abilities, greater potentials now gone. (Quoted by Karp, 1996, p.24)

References to 'stealing away whoever you are' and 'preventing you from seeing who you might someday be' could be interpreted in terms of losing one or more projects that are central to a life. Things appear significant in the ways they do partly in virtue of the possibilities we seek to actualize through our projects. Hence, with the loss of those projects, the entities and situations we encounter do not offer what they once did or solicit activity in the ways they did, resulting in a loss of the inclination to act. We can only look back and recall a time when the world was alive with possibilities that have since gone. The abandonment of a life-shaping project need not be self-initiated; all sorts of events could conspire to end it. For example, a life might be dedicated to the upkeep of a rare artefact that is then reduced to ashes by vandals.[5] So, one way of construing the inability to act in depression is in terms of the loss, self-initiated or otherwise, of projects upon which the significance of however many experienced entities, situations, and events depends. With this, there is a diminished sense of being presented with possibilities for action.

This account most likely does apply to some cases of diagnosed depression. Such an experience would also involve losing all of the hopes that depended on the projects in question. And there might also be intentional guilt feelings, focused on the effects that a loss of projects, self-initiated or otherwise, has had or is likely to have on others. But other depression experiences involve a different kind of loss. What is missing is not the practical significance of however many entities. That *kind* of significance is gone from the world. It is important to distinguish two forms this can take. In one type of case, a sense of there being worthwhile projects and significant scenarios remains, but the world ceases to entice, to draw one in. So there is a feeling of being unable to act, even though one retains various concerns and appreciates that certain actions are

---

[5] There is also the issue of normativity to consider—whether and when self-initiated abandonment of a project is appropriate and when it is inappropriate or even pathological.

appropriate in the light of those concerns. The world can lose varying degrees of enticement. It might be that nothing draws one in to the *extent* that it once did: 'when I'm depressed I find it very hard to perform routine tasks. Motivation is a big problem, though I find if forced then once I get going I'm generally fine' (#20). However, it could be that nothing entices at all anymore. And, in the most extreme case, the sense that anything ever *could* entice is absent from experience. Without any invitation from the world, any 'pull' on us from our surroundings, effortless action is no longer a possibility. Everything seems curiously distant, disconnected, amounting to an all-pervasive loss of motivation:

> When you're depressed, it feels as though there is a huge distance between you and things, which are inert, unresponsive to your wishes. Now that I was feeling better, a pen would leap into my hand, soap seemed to cover me of its own accord, the towel would be in exactly the right place for me to pick it up. Instead of being the slave of the objects around me, I was part again of an active world in which I could participate. (Lewis, 2006, p.225)

When the world fails to entice, things still appear significant in other ways. So the person may still 'want' to act, and there is a sense in which she remains motivated. But there is another sense in which motivation is lacking: a will to act, a drive towards action, is gone from experience and so she feels unable to respond to significant possibilities, even though she still cares. She therefore feels helpless, maybe worthless.

Loss of practical significance from the world is a different kind of privation. Here, a sense of anything being potentially relevant to any kind of project is eroded or lost. Everything the person encounters is stripped of the possibilities for action that it was previously imbued with. So she not only feels unable to act in such a way as to bring about significant outcomes; no sense remains of there being any significant outcomes. With this, enticement is gone too. The predicament is described with remarkable clarity in the following first-person account:

> ...it was as if the whatness of each thing—I'm no good at philosophical vocabulary—but the essence of each thing in the sense of the tableness of the table or the chairness of the chair or the floorness of the floor was gone. There was a mute and indifferent object in that place. Its availability to human living, to human dwelling in the world was drained out of it. Its identity as a familiar object that we live with each day was gone. [...] the world had lost its welcoming quality. It wasn't a habitable earth any longer. [...] It became impossible to reach anything. Like, how do I get up and walk to that chair if the essential thing that we mean by chair, something that lets us sit down and rest or upholds us as we read a book, something that shares our life in that way, has lost the quality of being able to do that? (Quoted by Hornstein, 2009, pp.212–3)

When all experienced entities lose their practical familiarity, their significance, the world no longer includes possibilities for action, not even possibilities that present themselves as 'impossible to actualize' due to an absence of enticement from the world. But 'practical significance' at least remains intelligible. The person quoted above goes on to say 'I never fell to that extreme, of not knowing that other ways of being existed. I always knew, through all those years, that I was trying to find my way back, that there was another way to be' (p.214). Even when faced with a global loss of experienced practical significance, one might be able to contemplate the *possibility* of finding things significant again and pursuing some as yet unformulated project. And, in some cases, an appreciation that things continue to be significant for other people is also retained (a predicament that corresponds to a 'loss of hope', of the kind where one still recognizes that others live with hope). However, more profound losses involve an inability to comprehend the possibility of anything being practically significant for anyone:

> But in among the bad and worse times, there were also moments when I felt, if not hope, then at least the glimmerings of possibility. [...] It was like starting from the beginning. It took me a long time, for example, to understand, or to re-understand, why people do things. Why, in fact, they do anything at all. What is it that occupies their time? What is the point of doing? During my long morning walks, I watched people hurrying along in suits and trainers. Where was it they were going, and why were they in such haste? I simply couldn't imagine feeling such urgency. I watched others throwing a ball for a dog, picking it up, and throwing it again. Why? Where was the sense in such pointless repetition? (Brampton, 2008, p.249)

This description of the 'return of possibility' serves to make salient what was previously diminished or lost: a sense of what it is for someone to act purposively, to find things significant and respond to them accordingly. Activities such as playing with a ball or hurrying to a destination had become strange, unfamiliar, bereft of meaning.

The depressed person therefore experiences her situation *as* something she cannot act upon. In some cases, this may be wholly attributable to a loss of enticing possibilities or practical significance. In others, however, active engagement with significant possibilities that entice one to act is replaced by passive anticipation of the arrival of some unavoidable threat. So a form of significance that opposes action becomes all-enveloping, a shape that the whole world takes on.[6] The sense of impossibility that many describe is at least partly attributable to this. Consider the following interview excerpt:

---

[6] Law (2009) offers the complementary view that, in depression, a change in how one perceives the world does not *cause* loss of motivation. Instead, perception incorporates motivation. He adds that the change need not be understood only in terms of loss. Something could also be *added* that blocks action. Experience of the world as threat plays just such a role.

> I lie in bed for ages dreading getting in the shower and then when I'm eventually in the shower I end up being in there for ages dreading getting out. [...] The feeling of dread isn't a fear or dread about something specific happening, it's more like feeling disabled in some way, like the effort and the idea of moving onto the next thing whatever that is, feels too overwhelming. [...] It's almost like I am there but I can't touch anything or I can't connect. Everything requires massive effort and I'm not really able to do anything. Like if I notice something needs cleaning or moving, it's like it's out of reach, or the act of doing that thing isn't in my world at that time...like I can see so much detail but I cannot be a part of it. I suppose feeling disconnected is the best way to describe it.[7]

There are two things going on here, working together. The world is bereft of any positive enticement; it no longer draws one in and seems distant, detached, not quite there. In conjunction with this, everything is enveloped by a distinctive kind of significance that only certain things previously had, amounting to a paralysing and inescapable dread.

Some maintain that anxiety and depression should not be regarded separately and that they have been artificially separated by current diagnostic practice. For instance, Shorter and Tyrer (2003, p.158) observe that 'the firewall between anxiety and depression ignores the fact that the commonest form of affective disorder is mixed anxiety-depression'. In reflecting on the phenomenology of agency, we can see that it is possible to have a depression experience without anxiety. One could lose enticing possibilities, or significant possibilities more generally, without their being replaced by anxious anticipation. However, where a depression experience does involve anxiety, it would be wrong to regard it as an additional *component*, which can be extricated from an accompanying experience of depression. There are various scenarios to consider. In some cases, it could be that erosion of enticing possibilities makes other kinds of possibility more salient, revealing a sense of threat that was already there but is now all that remains. In others, the experience of anxiety could be partly or wholly constitutive of the loss of other kinds of possibility; a world where dread is all-pervasive is a world where things cannot entice one to act in a confident, habitual, effortless way. So the sense of inability could— but need not—consist partly or wholly of dread. In another scenario, the person first loses significant or enticing possibilities and only later becomes anxious. For instance, she might lose enticing possibilities while retaining a sense of 'what needs to be done'. A growing feeling of all-enveloping failure then leads to anxiety; all experience takes the form 'given my concerns,

---

[7] From a conference presentation by Outi Benson (SANE), entitled 'Using the grounded theory method to explore emotional experience associated with self-cutting' (July 2010). See also Horne and Csipke (2009) for a shorter quotation from the same interview.

I ought to do p or need to do p, and I am not doing p, which will lead to bad things happening'. Although this could be described in terms of the 'addition' of anxiety to an already established experience of depression, it should instead be construed as a further shift in existential feeling, in 'how one finds oneself in the world'. Anxious depression involves a distinctive configuration of the possibility space, rather than an 'anxious configuration' that is added onto a pre-existent 'depression configuration'. The combination of the two amounts to a different kind of inability experience, a different sense of what the world has to offer. Hence, although depression does not invariably involve anxiety, this does not give us reason to suppose that anxious depression is any less phenomenologically unified.

The sense of threat varies in character. There is the feeling of being in imminent danger oneself: 'I feel too scared to move, like I have to sit in one place and not move and I'll be ok then' (#325). This involves an inescapable sense of helplessness and passivity. It is analogous to watching the ground approach as you fall. The future offers only a certain kind of significant possibility: something horrible is about to happen and you can do nothing to stop it. Another kind of experience is that of the world as fundamentally bad. This does not have the same immediacy. However, it can be equally pervasive, and it similarly undermines the experience of being able to act in order to bring about positive change: 'The world seems a bleak, cold and threatening place. What I would normally see as a challenge seems like an insurmountable problem. My whole perspective becomes negative, and I am unable to see the good and the potential in anything' (#347). Several different combinations of threat, loss of enticement, and loss of practical significance can thus add up to an experience of action as overwhelmingly difficult or impossible. The 'I can't' becomes the inescapable form of one's world.

First-person descriptions of diminished agency in depression also illustrate the inseparability of world-experience and bodily feeling, as well as making clear the relationship between bodily experience and hopelessness. The feeling that 'I can't' is a kind of bodily experience and, at the same time, a way in which the world appears:

#22. Everything seems 10 times harder. I had to do everything in such tiny steps. Just the simple task of getting out of bed or leaving a building would be a huge deal. I would have to tell myself 'first get into a sitting position. Then we'll worry about the rest of it afterwards'. I would see everything as such an ordeal, all these little things bundled into one huge thing. I just felt like there was this massive problem and I had no idea what to do about it.[...] Things seem almost impossible. Just getting out of bed is difficult. [...] It was an effort to do things like have a shower and get dressed. Everything was so difficult. It would take a lot of encouragement for me to begin to do anything.

> #26. It's a struggle to get out of bed and make a drink. I can only usually get a glass of squash, it's too much effort to stand there and wait for the kettle to boil to make tea. [...] your whole body struggles to move and [...] moving it is like pushing your way through treacle.

Different kinds of bodily experience can be distinguished. An experience of everything as 'more difficult and less enticing', involving a feeling of fatigue and heaviness, differs from an experience of anxious, helpless passivity. And both differ from the kind of bodily experience associated with a loss of practical significance from the world, where even a 'feeling of being unable to act in the way that one ought to' is absent: 'When life becomes pointless and your body seems to be on a permanent go slow, normal routine goes out the window as the effort just seems too much and pointless' (#34). In cases like this, the feeling of impossibility is not so pronounced, as a diminution of practical significance lessens the experienced tension between wanting to act and being unable to act. There is simply 'nothing to be done' and thus no sense of feeling unable to do things that need to be done.

Hence the following distinctions need to be drawn in order to understand the various experiences of diminished agency that feature in depression:

1. A loss of some fundamental project. The world no longer offers certain possibilities for action and nothing has yet replaced them. However, one does not lack an appreciation of what it *would be* for the world to offer such possibilities, and one also recognizes that others retain them.

2. A loss of enticing possibilities. The world might still include meaningful projects but its allure is gone and it no longer solicits action. There are different degrees of loss.

3. A loss of practical significance from experience. This comes in varying degrees too. The most extreme form is the complete absence of any sense that anything could be significant for anyone, amounting to a world that is bereft of the usual sense of freedom. This also involves (2).

4. An all-enveloping feeling of passivity before some threat, which varies in degree and character. This can contribute to (1), (2), and (3).

Returning to the theme of Chapter 5, (1) to (4) are all compatible with intentional guilt, the only exception being a variant of (3) where nothing at all is experienced as mattering, and so there is nothing to feel guilty about. (1) is incompatible with existential guilt, given that there is no existential change. But (2) and (3) can both involve forms of existential guilt. In (2), the person retains a sense that things matter, not just to her but to others too. She experiences herself as unable to actualize significant possibilities, as incapable, as letting others down. This might well be interpreted in terms of guilt, especially when combined with (4): 'I am irrevocably not what I should be'. But the most profound form of existential guilt described in Chapter 5 involves an extreme form of (3), in conjunction with a variant of (4). Practical significance has gone from the world and so the person does not find herself incapable of doing something that should be done. Instead, there is nothing left to be done, no possibility of remedying past failings. Other people appear only in the guise of potential threat, giving the fixed past a more specifically 'guilty' form. My account of freedom also complements the distinctions drawn in Chapter 4. Experience (1) maps onto loss of a system of 'hopes', while (4) involves loss of trust in the world and other people. Demoralization and loss of active hope are variants of (2), and the most profound losses of hope involve (3). What I called 'loss of aspiring hope' does not translate so easily, given that the person still feels perfectly able to act. But a certain kind of significant possibility is unavailable to her, and so it is to be construed as a less profound and more specific from of (3).

A diminished sense of freedom in depression thus takes several different forms, all of which are inextricable from experiences of hopelessness. Some also amount to experiences of worthlessness and guilt. Common to all of the existential forms is a loss of certain *kinds* of possibility from the world. This seldom stifles activity completely. Certain habitual behaviours may continue, albeit against the backdrop of a radically altered sense of the world and one's relationship with it. One may also act in response to a feeling of threat, cowering and retreating from situations that offer nothing else. Even so, what remains is a distortion and impoverishment of the more usual experience of freedom, of the self as a locus of agency.

Hence we can employ a broadly Sartrean interpretative framework in order to illuminate alterations in the experience of freedom and agency that occur in depression. Insofar as that framework coheres with first-person testimony and makes sense of otherwise obscure phenomena, it is corroborated in the process. But we should also be open to the possibility of revising and refining our phenomenological account as we engage with experiences of depression. Sartre insists that even the most exceptional circumstances leave our freedom intact. For example, he writes that 'the red hot pincers of the torturer do not exempt us from being free' (Sartre, 1989, p.505). However, reflection on experiences of depression indicates that matters are more complicated. The structure of our experience of freedom is changeable, and can be eroded in a number of different ways. By studying first-person accounts of depression, we can begin to describe some of these and, in so doing, further clarify what an intact sense of freedom consists of.

This is at odds with Sartre's own view. In his *Sketch for a Theory of the Emotions*, he offers an account of 'melancholy', according to which the 'potentialities of our world' initially remain intact but our means of actualizing them are obstructed. For example, one might lose one's car due to financial problems and therefore require an alternative means of transport in order to achieve various goals. Sartre proposes that melancholy is a way of avoiding such life adjustments by 'transforming the present structure of the world, replacing it with a totally undifferentiated structure'. It results in a world that altogether lacks significance and no longer solicits action: 'I behave in such a manner that the universe requires nothing more from me' (1939/1994, pp.43–4). This, he maintains, does not compromise our freedom; it is in fact an exercise of freedom.[8] Even if something along these lines were accepted, it could only account for the first of the variants described above, where one loses certain core projects and, with them, a range of ways in which things appeared significant. It does not account for (2), where one is *unable* to find anything enticing. And, in the case of (3), it is not just that however many things lose their significance; certain *kinds* of significant possibility lose their *intelligibility*. Whereas (1) is compatible with intact freedom, cases (2) and (3) amount to an alteration in the phenomenological structure of freedom, regardless of whether or not they also involve (4).

I will conclude the chapter with a brief digression. How, one might wonder, does any of this relate to the question of whether we actually are free? I have suggested that the principal ingredient of freedom is a sense of being able to actualize, through our activities, possibilities that are experienced as belonging to the world. But the fact that we experience ourselves and the world in this way does not imply that possibilities really reside in the world or that, when we act, we do actualize possibilities. One could maintain that, so far as the metaphysics is concerned, the phenomenology is irrelevant. Alternatively, one could attempt to formulate an argument for the reality of human freedom on the basis of phenomenology. In brief, it is arguable that, without a sense of there being worldly possibilities that we might actualize, we could not inhabit the kind of world that empirical enquiry itself presupposes and attempts to describe. An ordinarily taken-for-granted 'sense of reality' would be lacking. One would be unable to take anything at all to be 'the case' or 'not the case', to even make sense of the distinction between what 'is' and what 'is

---

[8] Another approach that construes depression as freely chosen is that of Solomon (1993, p.237), who proposes that 'our depression is our way of wrenching ourselves from the established values of our world, the tasks in which we have been uncritically immersed, the opinions we have uncritically nursed, the relationships we have accepted without challenge and often without meaning. A depression is a self-imposed purge'. This might apply to a 'loss of hopes' or 'loss of some fundamental project', but not to changes in the kinds of possibility one is open to.

not'. Any result of empirical enquiry denying that we actualize worldly possibilities would therefore undermine its own intelligibility, and so one could not coherently deny that we have freedom in the sense described here. This seems to be Sartre's position: 'scientific knowledge, in fact, can neither overcome nor suppress the potentializing structure of perception. On the contrary science must presuppose it' (1989, p.197). *If* this is correct, then most of us are free most of the time, and any attempt to maintain otherwise is ultimately self-defeating.[9]

---

[9]   See Ratcliffe (2013c) for a more general argument to the effect that the world, construed as a possibility space, is presupposed by the intelligibility of empirical enquiry.

Chapter 7

Time

The kinds of existential change that I have described all implicate the experience of time in some way. Losses of hope involve the absence of certain kinds of possibility from the anticipated future and, in more extreme cases, from any imaginable future or remembered past. The conviction that one cannot recover is similarly bound up with what the future offers, as are experiences of diminished agency. And the most profound form of existential guilt involves a past that is frozen in place by the impossibility of redemptive change. Experiences of hopelessness, guilt, diminished agency, and bodily conspicuousness, along with various characteristic belief contents, might appear to be distinct 'symptoms' that interact causally. However, I have argued that they are inextricable aspects of unitary phenomenological structures—configurations of possibility. To illustrate this, I have approached existential changes in depression from a number of different directions, describing their various aspects and how they relate to each other. All of these changes can also be conceived of in terms of time and, in this chapter, I address some of the different kinds of temporal experience that arise in depression. I start by considering the view that time slows down when one is depressed, and argue that depression often involves alterations in the overall structure of temporal experience, rather than just the experienced rate of temporal 'flow'. After that, I distinguish some of these alterations, with an emphasis on how the future is experienced. Then I turn to the past. In the process, I further address the question of what distinguishes a guilty past from other ways of experiencing the past that are equally compatible with a 'closed future'. The chapter concludes by briefly reflecting on whether the kinds of temporal experience considered here are specific to forms of 'depression', focusing on temporal disturbances in schizophrenia, somatic illness, and grief.

Varieties of Temporal Experience in Depression

A common theme in published and unpublished first-person accounts of depression is that of time slowing down or even stopping. For example:

> I'd watch, incredulous, as putting cereal in a bowl took forever. Sitting downstairs became a marathon of endurance because there was no escape from the dullness of each second, which had stretched so that it seemed like hours. I had no way of

screening out boredom, so it made me scream internally. The ordinary afternoon light refused to change, it was going to stay like that all day and I'd never be able to move again and God why couldn't it do something instead of just continuing. (Lewis, 2006, p.14)

#24. Time goes so slowly when I'm feeling really bad.

#26. Time seems to drag. A day feels like a year.

#38. Things seem much slower, time drags.

#49. [Time] goes very, very slowly. Like I remember lying awake at about 4am in my [...] room and it was going so slowly, all I had to do was get through to the morning so I could get some help and it seemed almost impossible just to get through those few hours because it was taking so long.

It might seem that time consciousness in depression can be characterized fairly easily: it involves an increase in the perceived duration of events, something that is also describable in terms of the rate at which time 'flows'. It could be added that this is consistent with diminished agency. When one is engrossed in activity for an hour, the hour seems to pass more quickly than when one is sitting and waiting. So a world of pervasive disengagement and passivity would be one where time drags. Some suggest that this is exactly what happens. For example, Vogeley and Kupke (2007, p.162) claim that there is a 'systematic change in velocity', which leaves the 'basic temporal structure' intact. They propose that changes in the experience of time that occur in depression are therefore less extreme than those that occur in schizophrenia. In schizophrenia, the overall *structure* of temporal experience is affected, rather than just the *rate* at which time passes. Depressed subjects consistently over-estimate time intervals, thus supporting the view that depression involves an experience of time slowing down (Vogeley and Kupke, 2007; Ghaemi, 2007). However, this does not preclude the possibility of there being additional changes in some or all cases of depression. Indeed, it could be that altered experience of duration is symptomatic of changes in the *structure* of time, in how past, present, future, and the transition between them are experienced. And this is what we find when we look carefully at first-person accounts:

#17. I just felt very detached from time, it simply didn't matter.

#30. Yes, days go past slower and more boring feeling like everything's going to drag on. On the other hand can feel like life going too fast and the years are flying by and start getting depressed thinking not long to live now etc.

#34. When depressed, time seems to slow down, and to a certain point can become irrelevant. It is easy to lose track of days without realising it.

#45. When I am depressed I feel like time goes slowly, yet at the same time I feel like I—or anyone else—has hardly any time to live at all. It feels as if time is running out.

#54. When I am depressed I don't seem to notice time, it just doesn't matter to me, it all seems to blend into a mass of nothing. [...] Time loses significance.

#98. I have no concept of time when I am depressed.

#112. Time becomes insignificant. It passes and that's all that matters.

Remarks such as these suggest that there is more to the experience than a change in experienced duration. For some, although time slows down, there is also the feeling that it is running out, that death is approaching at high speed. Others report a feeling of detachment from time—they are outside time; it has become irrelevant, insignificant, or meaningless. I will suggest that differences such as these reflect different kinds of experience, and that time consciousness in depression is heterogeneous. Of 133 DQ respondents who answered the question about time, 21 stated that they had noticed no change at all in temporal experience, and some of them were quite insistent about that. Others described phenomenological disturbances that were difficult to distinguish from more commonplace experiences: 'Time I am spending doing something I consider unpleasant (such as work or chores) seems to go by very slowly, while time I spend in sedentary mode (on the couch, watching TV) seems to go by very quickly' (#171); 'Time is elastic when I have depression' (#179). So it is likely that some cases of diagnosed depression do not involve changes in the experience of duration or in the overall structure of temporal experience. And it is arguable that some of those cases where a 'slowing of time' is mentioned do not involve an existential change but something we all experience when bored and/or waiting for something. Depressed people tend to be rather disengaged from their surroundings and are therefore more prone to experience time in this way. However, I will argue that many cases of depression involve more profound disturbances in the structure of temporal experience.

There has not been much phenomenological discussion of time in depression or, indeed, of any other aspect of depression (compared to schizophrenia, which has received far more attention from phenomenologists), but temporal experience in depression is discussed by Eugene Minkowski (1970), Erwin Straus (1947), Hubertus Tellenbach (1980), Martin Wyllie (2005), and Thomas Fuchs (2001, 2003, 2005, 2013b), amongst others. Taking some recent work by Fuchs as my starting point, I will argue that temporal experience in depression is heterogeneous, even if we restrict ourselves to a subtype such as 'major depression'. Given that how we experience time is inseparable from, and also central to, the more general structure of experience, this further supports the view that there are importantly different kinds of depression experience.

Implicit and Explicit Time

In a series of papers, Fuchs (2001, 2003, 2005, 2013b) addresses temporal changes that occur in depression and, more specifically, 'melancholic depression' (as described by Tellenbach, 1980). In the process, he makes some useful distinctions, which I will critically discuss and further develop here. Most important, for current purposes, is the distinction between implicit and explicit time. When I am absorbed in writing, I do not think about time but inhabit it; time is implicit. In contrast, when I am waiting for a bus and keep looking at my watch, I become explicitly aware of temporal phenomena such as 'lateness'. Fuchs (2003, 2013b) maintains that this distinction corresponds to that between the lived body [*Leib*] and the corporeal body [*Körper*]. The corporeal body is an object of experience or thought, whereas the lived body (as discussed in Chapter 3) is that *through which* we experience, think and act. According to Fuchs, we are oblivious to our corporeal bodies when comfortably immersed in activity. It is when things go wrong that the body becomes conspicuous—when our actions meet with unexpected failure, when we are uncomfortable or in pain, when we struggle or fail to complete some task, when we feel socially awkward or ashamed. Similarly, implicit time is associated with absorption in activity, and explicit time with feeling disengaged from our projects.

Fuchs acknowledges that a clear-cut distinction between implicit time, which is experienced when our projects go smoothly, and explicit time, which is experienced when they break down, is overly simple. Even when I am immersed in activity, I usually retain at least some attentiveness to time. I may be absorbed in giving a lecture but occasionally glance at the clock. And everyday conversation is often like this too. Even when it proceeds fairly smoothly, we are aware of temporal phenomena such as overly long pauses and untimely interruptions. It is also arguable that one can be *absorbed in explicit time*, as when an athlete waits for the whistle that will start an important race. This is consistent with a concern raised in Chapter 3: the contrast between uncomfortable, disengaged bodily conspicuousness and comfortable, engaged inconspicuousness is not sufficiently discriminating. Nevertheless, I think there is still a rough distinction to be drawn between explicit time, where temporal properties are objects of experience, and implicit time, which shapes experience but is not an object of experience. And this distinction is a helpful one when it comes to interpreting temporal experience in depression.

Fuchs suggests that depression involves disturbances of both implicit and explicit time. He distinguishes two aspects of implicit time: its 'affective-conative momentum' and what Husserl calls its 'protentional-retentional' structure (Fuchs, 2013b). By 'conative' drive, Fuchs means a temporal orientation that we ordinarily take for granted, which also comprises a disposition towards activity. It is not a matter of having explicit desires or motives, but of feeling drawn towards a meaningful future in a manner that such attitudes presuppose. However, the appeal to Husserl requires further explanation. 'Protention' and 'retention' are inseparable from what Husserl calls the 'horizonal' structure of experience. As we saw in Chapter 2, a horizon is not a static structure. There is a dynamic process of anticipation and fulfilment: as certain possibilities are actualized, others appear, and so on (Husserl, 1973, 2001). This process is inseparable from the experienced 'flow' of time. By 'protention', Husserl means an experience of anticipation that gives us a variably determinate sense of what will happen next. It is not 'added on' to an independently constituted experience of the present. Our sense of entities *as present* depends, in part, on experience having this anticipatory structure. Husserl adds that our experience of the immediate past is likewise inseparable from the present. Once a possibility is actualized, it is not simply 'present', after which it is 'gone' or experienced as a 'fading present'. Experience includes 'retentions', present experiences of events *as* having just passed (e.g. Husserl, 1991, p.89).

Protention and retention are not to be regarded as separate 'components' of temporal experience. Retention shapes protention; what we anticipate and how we anticipate it (as certain, uncertain, doubtful, determinate to varying degrees, and significant in various ways) is shaped by what has just passed. The experienced flow of time involves a structured interplay between protention and retention. An oft used example is that of listening to a melody. Even if you haven't heard it before, there is a sense of roughly what will come next, as illustrated by the surprise you feel when a note is out of tune. This expectation also shapes how a present note is experienced. Notes that have just passed are experienced in the present but *as* having passed, and *as* that out of which the present has arisen.[1] My focus here will be on protention more so than retention, on the anticipated actualization of various kinds of possibility.

Fuchs proposes that schizophrenia involves disruption of Husserlian 'passive synthesis' (the ordinarily effortless achievement of finding ourselves in a cohesive world that contains enduring entities of various kinds, some of which we experience as present). The structured interplay of possibilities breaks down and experience becomes disordered, fragmented. Melancholia, in contrast, is a matter of 'intersubjective desynchronization' and 'disturbance of conation'. With this, ordinarily implicit time becomes explicit. So there is no disturbance of passive synthesis in melancholic depression: the 'constitutive synthesis of

---

[1] See Gallagher and Zahavi (2008, Chapter 4) for a good summary of Husserl on time consciousness.

inner time consciousness remains intact'; 'what is lacking instead is the conative dynamics' (Fuchs, 2013b, p.98). With loss of conation, the depressed person experiences the future as lacking openness; it is no longer a domain of
potential activity. Minkowski offers an account along similar lines. Drawing
on the work of Bergson, he calls this drive towards the future the 'élan vital'. It
is not a matter of first finding oneself in the world and then experiencing some
sort of mental quale that somehow induces activity. As Minkowski (1970, p.38)
describes it, 'I feel myself irresistibly pushed forward and see the future open in
front of me'; 'I tend spontaneously with all my power, with all my being, toward
a future, thus achieving all the fullness of life of which I am usually capable'.
Straus (1947) refers to the same thing as a state of 'becoming'. It is something
that all of our experiences and activities ordinarily presuppose, something that
is easy to overlook when a sense of being at home in the world is undisturbed.

Fuchs is critical of earlier phenomenological approaches, such as that of Straus,
for being too individualistic. He observes that our experiences and activities are
ordinarily synchronized with those of others, something we are reminded of on
those occasions when we experience our own actions or the actions of those we are
interacting with as too early or too late. Depression, he suggests, involves disruption of a 'basic feeling of being in accord with the time of the others, and to live
with them in the same, intersubjective time'. Although loss of synchrony is commonplace, depression is distinctive as it involves a 'complete desynchronization'
(2001, pp.181–2). Fuchs (2003) adds that desychronization and loss of conation add
up to a fixed past from which there is no hope of redemption, and thus to a pervasive sense of irrevocable guilt (of a kind I described in Chapter 5). This account
captures at least some experiences of major depression, including some of those
that might be labelled 'melancholic'. However, I will show that the category 'major
depression' also accommodates a range of other changes in the structure of temporal experience. In the process, I will challenge Fuchs' claim that melancholia—
and depression more generally—affects conative drive but does not disrupt passive
synthesis. I will argue that more severe forms of depression can involve loss of
practical significance rather than just conation, and will also suggest that different
degrees and kinds of conation can remain even when practical significance is lost.

Loss of Significance

If we follow Husserl, what Fuchs calls 'conative drive' is integral to the pro-
tentional structure of experience and plays a role in passive synthesis. Husserl
describes the perceptual 'allure' of 'enticing' possibilities, and he does so
under the heading 'analyses concerning passive synthesis' (Husserl, 2001).
And, in Chapter 6, I showed that conation does not have a wholly internal phenomenology. It consists largely of a subset of experienced possibilities, those

that entice us. Some of these draw us in perceptually, amounting to a kind of curiosity that permeates world-experience, whereas others solicit and sustain goal-directed activities. Although Husserl emphasizes perceptual enticement, I suggested in Chapter 2 that the inclusion of goal-directed enticement in the horizonal structure of experience is consistent with his account, perhaps even implied by what he does say. Enticing possibilities of both kinds are integral to our experiences of entities and situations, as well as to our more general sense of belonging to a world. In the absence of enticing possibilities, things 'look' strangely different, distant, and there is a feeling of being 'not quite there', cut off from everything and everyone. I also distinguished enticement from something closely associated with it: the ability to find things practically significant. Only some of the things that I find practically significant at a given time actually draw me in. For instance, I can recognize the significance of a hammer without feeling drawn to pick it up and start hammering nails into a wall. Depression, I suggested, can involve a loss of significance, rather than just enticement.

Does a loss of practical significance similarly affect what Husserl calls 'passive synthesis'? The answer is surely yes. Passive synthesis does not become unstructured, as Fuchs suggests that it does in schizophrenia. Even so, something is missing from its structure. By analogy, removing the roof from a building is not as dramatic as blowing it to pieces. Even so, there is a major structural change. Likewise in depression, experience retains a coherent structure but an aspect of that structure is missing. Loss of practical significance also amounts to a profound change in temporal experience. Without any sense that things could ever be significantly different, a kind of anticipation that more usually permeates the present is lost. So the experience of significant possibilities being actualized, which characterizes the transition from future to present to past, is lost too. The immediate and long-term future offers only 'more of the same'; there can be nothing new.[2]

Now, it could be maintained that losing conative drive is an inevitable symptom of losing practical significance. If nothing appears significant, then nothing appears enticing, as there is nothing for the drive to act upon. Indeed, I suggested in Chapter 6 that a loss of significance *can* amount to a loss of

---

[2] Various others have suggested that something like this occurs in depression. For instance, Wyllie (2005, p.180) remarks that 'every situation normally contains the possibility of change; if the future is closed, the possibility of change is denied'. And Straus (1947, p.257) states that depression can involve a 'pathology of becoming' and that 'with a standstill of becoming future is rendered inaccessible'.

enticement and conation too. However, this does not *have to be* the case. There are three potential scenarios to consider:

1. Drive is lost, along with practical significance.

2. Things still appear enticing and so drive remains, although it is undirected, cut off from any ordered system of significant possibilities.

3. Enticing possibilities are lost but other aspects of drive linger on. What is left of conation becomes a conspicuous bodily agitation, rather than the allure of the world.

The second of these may well capture an experience of mania, where one is caught up in the present, leaping from one thing to the next without any orientation towards the longer-term future. There is either a loss of fundamental projects or a more profound loss of certain kinds of significance, but there remains a positive enticement to act. So there is a feeling of being 'busy', 'productive', or doing something 'important', but one that has been decoupled—to varying degrees—from an enduring network of cares, concerns, commitments, and projects. Binswanger (1964, p.130) describes more extreme forms of the 'manic mode of being-in-the-world' as active but unfocused in exactly this way:

> His so-called hyperactivity which, in the onset of illness, is often still a stimulus for outstanding achievement, projects, scientific or artistic works of every kind, gradually turns into an aimless, meaningless, empty busy-ness. What we call the seriousness of living turns into a game. [...] Everything is 'handy' for the patient, is at once 'handled' and 'played away'. So he is continually on the move.

The manic person thus lives in an enticing present. It draws her in, but in a way that is unconstrained by longer-term projects and associated systems of significant possibilities that would otherwise inhibit her from acting in response to the immediate allure of things. As in experiences of depression, her sense of the future is impoverished by an erosion or loss of practical significance. Binswanger (1964, p.132) goes on:

> A self that does not live into the future, that moves around in a merely playful way in the here and now, and, at best, still lives only from the past, is but momentarily 'attuned', not steadily advancing, developing or maturing, is not to borrow a word, an existential self.

We can think of this as an extreme form that 'loss of aspiring hope' could take, where the person lacks a sense of there being longer-term, self-transformative possibilities, to such an extent that the concerns she does have are unstructured. They are hostage to fleeting enticements that come and go from one moment to the next. She is 'active' in the sense that her environment constantly calls for action, but there is another sense in which she is 'passive'. What solicits her to act is not shaped by projects of her own; she is pulled in by her surroundings like a puppet on strings. This is not to suggest that these enticements need be inconsistent with each other or random; much the same things could draw the person in at different times. The point is that any consistency is not attributable to enticements being embedded in longer-term and wider-ranging systems of significant possibility.

Predicament (3) is consistent with descriptions of some so-called 'mixed states', which go by names such as 'anxious' or 'agitated' depression. In Chapter 6, I described a kind of existential change where things still appear significant but the world lacks enticement. The person still 'wants' to act, but in ways that she experiences as impossible; the world does not draw her in—it appears somehow alien to the possibility of action. This can involve retention of something that contributes to 'drive' or 'conation' but is insufficient to summon action on its own. Consider an analogous experience, one that will be familiar to many authors. You are sitting in front of your computer with the aim of writing something. You need to get it done soon, and you also want to get it done. So you prepare to start writing, but it doesn't happen. Instead, you check your email, attend to other less pressing tasks, or resort to distracting yourself with the Internet. On one account, you lack motivation; loss of enticing possibilities in relation to task x is loss of the motivation to perform task x. Nevertheless, you really do want to complete the paper, you envisage a future state of affairs where it is complete as better than one where it is not, and you experience an increasingly pronounced sense of bodily agitation as you waste hour after hour. Sometimes, it just does not happen—the situation does not draw you in. Without any enticement, what remains of motivation is insufficient to spur you into action. Now, think of a world that offers only this kind of experience—an appreciation that things need to be done, a sense of being unable to act, and an unpleasant, bodily feeling of tension and urgency. It would amount to a kind of 'agitated' depression.

In the case of (3), the world is bereft of significance as well as enticement, but this sense of being called upon to act lingers on, an 'action-readiness' without any intelligible outlet. I described something like this in Chapter 5, but with more specific reference to 'agitated' thought processes. There is a felt need to act upon one's situation in some way. In a world from which the possibility of meaningful change is absent, this involves 'urgent', unstructured, racing thoughts, as well as a more general feeling of agitation. One cannot rest, even though there is nothing to be done. It is worth noting that mixed states, involving mania or hypomania and depression, are arguably more common than 'pure manic and depressive states' (Ghaemi, 2007, p.122). Several types have been distinguished, and perhaps the most comprehensive inventory is still that of Kraepelin (1921, Chapter VI), who distinguishes 'mania', 'depressive or anxious mania', 'excited depression', 'mania with poverty of thought', 'orthodox depression', 'manic stupor', 'depression with flight of ideas', and 'inhibited mania'. Hence it is plausible to maintain that (1) to (3) are all forms of experience that occur, rather than mere phenomenological possibilities, and also that there are further distinctions to be drawn. I have already emphasized the phenomenological heterogeneity of depression, something that renders a clear-cut distinction between unipolar depression and mixed states unsustainable. Mixed states encompass various different configurations of the possibility space, which cannot be distinguished in a principled way from the sum of all those other configurations that are labelled simply as 'depression'. Some depressive configurations are no less different from other depressive configurations than they are from some mixed configurations. Consider a depression experience where practical significance and conation are both lost. This is structurally closer to a mixed state where significance is lost but some aspect of conation lingers than it is to a depression experience where conation is altogether lost but practical significance remains. Hence the broad phenomenological distinctions that I have drawn can equally be employed to interpret mixed states.

Experiences (1) to (3) all involve changes in the sense of time and, more specifically, the future. In (1), there is just sameness; there is no anticipation of significant change. In (2), there is an unstructured, short-term allure. And, in (3), there is a feeling of urgency without any outlet.[3] The effects of existential changes such as these on implicit time are not restricted to the short-term experience of temporal flow, the transition from one moment

---

[3] It might also be possible to understand 'borderline personality disorder' and associated experiences of 'borderline depression' in these terms. (See DSM-5, p.664, for a description.) Borderline experience is said to involve shallow and turbulent emotions, especially in the interpersonal domain. Both shallowness and turbulence could be construed in terms of lacking a coherent, consistent sense of significant possibilities, of a kind that would otherwise regulate feeling and behaviour by allowing the formation of long-term projects and commitments. As with mania, the person lives in the present and her emotions therefore seem 'shallow'; they are not securely embedded in a structured, meaningful system of cares and concerns. The distinction between this and mania may hinge, at least in part, on the greater prominence in borderline experience of bodily agitation and a sense of interpersonal threat. See Stanghellini and Rosfort (2013) for a phenomenological description of borderline depression that is consistent with some of these suggestions, insofar as it emphasizes a 'desperate' and aimless feeling of 'vitality' in conjunction with a pervasive sense of futility. Fuchs (2007) suggests that borderline personality disorder involves a '*fragmentation of the narrative self*' (p.381). This is also compatible with what I am suggesting, as it entails a loss of long-term teleological structure: the person inhabits the present in a way that is not constrained by a coherent future-orientation. However, it could also be that there is a loss of significant possibilities from experience, of a kind that self-narrative presupposes.

to the next. It is important to acknowledge another aspect of implicit time, which we might call 'teleological time'. As implied by my suggestions regarding mania, this is partly responsible for a longer-term grasp of temporal direction. Fuchs restricts the scope of implicit time to passive synthesis and conation. But distinct from both is a sense of the ongoing projects and commitments that render things significant to us. Of course, one might object that this appreciation of longer-term duration is not implicit at all; it is an explicit understanding of where we are heading. That would be implausible though. As I type these words, my activities are intelligible in relation to the project of writing a book, which is embedded in the project of being a philosopher, something that gives meaning to many of my daily activities. Although I am not explicitly aware of these projects as I act, they still render my activities intelligible and give me a sense of working towards something, of direction. As Heidegger (1962), Sartre (1989), and others have emphasized, the world that we take for granted in everyday life reflects our projects. To return to a theme of Chapter 6, the significance we experience as integral to things, a significance that structures our activities, is symptomatic of the projects we are committed to. Sartre offers the example of a crag that presents itself to a climber as impossible for him to climb:

> . . .although brute things [. . .] can from the start limit our freedom of action, it is our freedom itself which must first constitute the framework, the technique, and the ends in relation to which they will manifest themselves as limits. Even if the crag is revealed as 'too difficult to climb', and if we must give up the ascent, let us note that the crag is revealed as such only because it was originally grasped as 'climbable'; it is therefore our freedom which constitutes the limits which it will subsequently encounter. (Sartre, 1989, p.482)

The significance of the crag reflects the project that the climber is pursuing, and she does not have to make that project explicit for her world to be structured by it. A person might even be unable to conceptualize and articulate an implicit, long-term project that regulates his activities. Sartre (1989, p.570) therefore proposes a form of 'existential psychoanalysis', the aim of which is to uncover the fundamental but unacknowledged project that shapes a person's life. A loss of practical significance from the world would not only be an impoverishment of protention. It would also be a collapse of all the projects that give things their meaning and regulate activity, a loss of teleological time. This is just what some first-person accounts of depression appear to describe:

> #271. When I'm depressed, for the most part there is no time. The concept of time no longer exists. It's like living outside of time. There is no concern or even awareness of schedules, day or night, normality, commitments, birthdays, events—nothing. It's like being in a box with no holes or light—time just disappears.

It is therefore clear why some depressed people say that time has 'stopped'. The experience of temporal passage is partly teleological. It involves a sense of meaningful transition from one state of affairs to another, a kind of transition that presupposes coherent, enduring frameworks of cares and concerns. Their absence does not amount to a total loss of longer-term temporal direction; the person is still able to identify x as happening before y, y before z, and so on. Even so, there is a substantial change in the experience of temporal direction. Imagine a life that involved nothing but watching a spot trace a circle on a screen in front of you, over and over again, with no sense of there being any alternative to this pattern. There might still be an experience of anticipation and completion: 'it has not yet reached the top of the screen'; 'it is moving towards the bottom'. So some aspects of protention would remain. However, it is not clear that a longer-term sense of linear direction would be sustainable. Time would instead take a cyclic form. Unless some kind of teleological structure were imposed, making a particular cycle or number of cycles stand out in some way (for example, 'if it reaches ten cycles, I win some money'; 'if it reaches 100 cycles, something bad will happen'), there would be nothing to distinguish one cycle from the next, nothing to constitute an appreciation of 'having moved on'.

Something not unlike this can happen in depression. Of course, a variety of events occur during the course of a day, even when one is depressed. So depression differs in that respect. Even so, there is nothing to distinguish one day from the next—nothing stands out; nothing makes a difference. So time loses something of its longer-term direction and takes on a more cyclic form. Minkowski (1958, pp.132–3) describes the experience of one patient (also discussed in Chapter 5), for whom 'each day kept an unusual independence, failing to be immersed in the perception of any life continuity; each day began anew, like a solitary island in a gray sea of passing time'. Nothing matters and so there is no way of individuating days or putting them in a linear order.[4] This is not to imply that longer-term implicit time is more usually exclusively 'linear' as opposed to cyclic. It has both aspects. Many of our activities have their place in a repeating cycle, such as a week, a month or a year. And the various significances that things have for us reflect these cycles, as well as more linear teleological structures.[5] The point

[4] See Broome (2005) for a discussion of this kind of experience. He relates it to a scenario entertained by Nietzsche, the 'eternal recurrence of the same'.

[5] The extent to which a person's projects are linear or cyclic in structure is likely to vary. For instance, a life of farming may differ in this respect from obsessive pursuit of being the very best in an academic field. There is most likely social and cultural variation too, including differences associated with established gender roles.

is that, in some depression experiences, the cyclic aspect becomes more salient than the linear. Furthermore, it becomes salient in a different way. What we have are not meaningful cycles but cycles that are experienced due to a loss of meaning; it is 'the same again' because there has been an erosion of significance and, consequently, of any significant difference between the days.

Loss of Drive and Loss of Projects

Depression can involve a partial or perhaps even total loss of practical significance from the world, instead of or in addition to a loss of what Fuchs calls 'conative drive'. This does not apply to all cases though, and diminished conation is more central to others. In Chapter 6, I construed this in terms of the loss of enticing possibilities. I have since complicated things by suggesting that conation is not *wholly* constituted by enticement. Nevertheless, some depression experiences do involve a complete or near-complete loss of conation. There is a more extreme and prolonged version of the everyday scenario where we sigh wearily and say that we 'can't be bothered' to do something we previously regarded as worth doing. We might still 'care' but we do not—or perhaps cannot—summon the inclination to act. Rather than lacking the will to act at a particular time and in relation to a particular project, the depressed person lacks it altogether—it is gone from the world. Descriptions such as the following suggest something like this:

> I felt that I had nothing to look forward to, no interest in anything—in short I felt totally apathetic. I couldn't even be bothered to talk to my girlfriend or father, the two people who were closest to me. I had no interests at all. I wouldn't listen to the radio or stereo, or watch TV, never mind go out. I never even felt the desire to drink beer! (From a first-person account in Read and Reynolds eds. 1996, pp.35–6.)

I suggested earlier that Husserl would have regarded loss of conation as something that affects passive synthesis. However, it might be objected that enticing possibilities are not integral to our sense of what things are to or our sense that things are. I agree that we could still experience and identify objects in the absence of any enticement from the world. However, there would still be a profound change in the overall structure of world-experience. A world that was completely drained of its allure would appear somehow detached, not quite there, incomplete. Consider this description by William James:

> In certain forms of melancholic perversion of the sensibilities and reactive powers, nothing touches us intimately, rouses us, or wakens natural feeling. The consequence is the complaint so often heard from melancholic patients, that nothing is believed in by them as it used to be, and that all sense of reality is fled from life. They

are sheathed in india-rubber; nothing penetrates to the quick or draws blood, as it were. […] 'I see, I hear!' such patients say, 'but the objects do not reach me, it is as if there were a wall between me and the outer world!' (1890, p.298)

At least part of what is going on here is the complete or near-complete removal of enticing possibilities from the world; things no longer move one in the ways they did. This is inextricable from a diminishment of the usual sense of reality, from a sense of being *there*, situated in the same world as the entities one encounters. Insofar as this sense of reality is an achievement of passive synthesis, a loss of conation affects passive synthesis: objects are still recognized as 'what they are', but the sense 'that they are' is eroded. With this, an aspect of temporal flow is also lacking—the anticipation and actualization of enticing possibilities. And Fuchs is right to emphasize that such an experience also involves 'desynchronization'. The person still 'cares', in the sense that she has projects and commitments, but she watches the social world go by from elsewhere. The phenomenology of protention is less impoverished than it would be if she also lacked a sense of anything as significant. Even so, there is an all-encompassing feeling of detachment from activities, situations, and other people. When the person does act, she is not enticed to do so in the usual way. She is not quite there, not fully immersed in a situation, and things happen in a curiously mechanistic fashion:

> #117. Time is immaterial to me during a depressional episode. I lose track of time. I wonder what I've done all day when the children suddenly burst through the door from school. Time has gone by, but I have done nothing, even to think one thought seems to have taken all day. Everything around me seems to carry on with routines and time scheduled activities, it feels like I'm watching it all happen but am not a part of it: as though I'm inside a bubble. My living becomes mechanical, based on necessities to be done. Children need to be fed. Plates need to be washed, School clothes need to be clean, Everything else in life is put on hold.

I have distinguished two broad types of existential change, loss of significance and disturbances of conation, which come in varying degrees and take different forms. There is also a further experience to consider, one that I previously described in terms of a 'loss of hopes' and 'loss of projects'. Here, the person retains a grasp of what it would be to find things practically significant, but all or most of his projects have—for whatever reason—collapsed, and so hardly anything does appear significant. In addition, he retains a sense of teleological time; he appreciates that significant events unfold in the lives of others, and he is still able to find things significant in the context of his own life. This kind of experience could be associated with intact conative drive (in the form of a disposition to seek out and create new projects and possibilities), although it need not be. Where drive remains intact and the content of experience is affected rather than the form, we have something that might be described in a very similar way to losses of drive and significance—'nothing matters anymore'. But, as stressed by Minkowski (1970, p.224), superficially similar symptom descriptions can obscure profound phenomenological differences. And this is a case in point. So we return to the complaint that the diagnostic criteria for major depression in the DSM and elsewhere are insensitive to the considerable difference between losing however many possibilities of a given kind and losing the kind itself. As all three broad types of experience almost certainly occur and are hard to distinguish on the basis of cursory descriptions of experience and behaviour, it is plausible to assume that they are often placed under the same category of 'major depression' or just 'depression'.

That diagnostic criteria fail to distinguish changes in experiential content from changes in the overall form of experience also accounts for why some of those with depression diagnoses report no noticeable alteration in their awareness of time. A loss of projects and hopes would not impact on the *form* of temporal experience. The person might be less engaged with the world than before, more inclined towards watching and waiting. Hence the perceived duration of events is—on the whole—greater. With this, there may also be a degree of desynchronization. Time 'passes him by'; he is adrift without his projects. While his 'personal future' offers the daunting task of finding new projects and new systems of meaning, 'they' remain cosily immersed in established activities. However, a content-specific desynchonization of this kind differs from a content-independent experience of estrangement from others, where kinds of significance and enticement are gone from the world. We can therefore distinguish existential forms of depression, where the overall structure of temporal experience (and experience more generally) has changed, from other diagnosed 'depressions' where the sense of time remains intact. As well as contributing to classification and diagnosis, this overarching distinction has the potential to inform neurobiological studies and pharmaceutical intervention. Seemingly similar but ultimately very different forms of experience are likely to have different neural correlates and be receptive to different kinds of treatment.

Time and Dread

The dread or anxiety discussed in Chapters 4, 5, and 6 is also inseparable from temporal experience. It contributes to a sense of impossibility, even where some significant or enticing possibilities remain. Consider an analogy with a kind of everyday experience. Suppose you go to visit the zoo with your children, especially hoping to see a tiger, but when you get to the zoo you see a sign that says 'zoo closed today'. What you feel is not simple disappointment, as when a team you support loses a football match. When that happens, the possibility has gone; there is nothing to be done about it. However, both the tiger and the possibility of seeing it remain, and they also remain enticing. So a degree of frustration lingers on despite the disappointment. As you look at the 'zoo closed today' sign, you recognize your own inability to actualize something that is both physically possible and desirable. Seeing the tiger presents itself as 'possible, but not amongst my own possibilities'; it is experienced as 'blocked', rather than just disappointed.

Something like this can happen in depression. However, it is not that specific activities are blocked; the blockage is global, inescapable. Everything and everyone appears oppressive, menacing, threatening, in a way that prevents one from acting. The sign says 'world closed'. In cases where practical significance and conation remain, there is a sense of being unable to actualize possibilities that continue to present themselves. The experience is more extreme when conation is lost, when there is no positive tendency towards action that might counter it. When practical significance is eroded too and one lacks a long-term, teleological future, the all-enveloping experience of threat can amount to what is often described as a feeling of impending death. Many first-person accounts of depression relate such an experience. For example, Solomon (2001, p.28) remarks that 'what is happening to you in depression is horrible, but it seems to be very much wrapped up in what is about to happen to you. Amongst other things, you feel you are about to die'. As Minkowski observes, without the usual impetus towards the future (the élan vital), 'the whole of becoming seems to rush toward us, a hostile force which must bring suffering' (1970, p.188). For one patient, he says, it was 'as if there were absolutely nothing between the present moment and death except the fruitless unfolding of time; this fills her with terror' (1970, p.304). The moment of one's death seems imminent because there is no significant temporal order in which to place it. More generally, Minkowski suggests, there is a tension in how we experience the future. The future is a realm of self-transformative possibilities that we might actualize; it is 'expansive'. On the other hand, every moment brings us closer to death:

> . . .in life we march toward the future and we march toward death; and these two marches, while seeming to be congruent, are in reality completely different from each other. The one is composed of that which is great, infinite, and positive in the future, the other of that which is excluded, limited, and negative in it. (1970, p.137)

When the expansive future is lost, when conation and significance are gone, all that remains of the future is the increasing proximity of one's unavoidable extinction.[6] This allows us to make sense of seemingly paradoxical statements to the effect that time moves more slowly and yet more quickly. There is a change in the structure of protention, which no longer includes the anticipated actualization of significant and/or enticing possibilities. Without significant change, every moment seems to go on forever; there is no possibility of reprieve. The 'slowing down' thus relates to short-term, previously implicit time. When it comes to long-term time, however, there is a feeling of impending threat. Nothing of consequence stands between one's current state and the realization of that threat, as the future promises only more of the same. Hence it seems imminent, an experience that is often conceived of more specifically in terms of approaching death.

Nothing captures the experience better than the closing scenes of *Macbeth*. I am not suggesting that the character Macbeth should himself be interpreted as suffering from depression, but that the world of depression and the situation he finds himself in towards the end of the play are structurally very similar. Macbeth already has a past that takes the form of irrevocable guilt; he can never undo or compensate for his deeds. Then, news of his wife's death prompts a revelation of the timeless, irrevocable futility of all human life:

> Tomorrow, and tomorrow, and tomorrow
> Creeps in this petty pace from day to day
> To the last syllable of recorded time,
> And all our yesterdays have lighted fools
> The way to dusty death. Out, out, brief candle.
> Life's but a walking shadow, a poor player
> That struts and frets his hour upon the stage,
> And then is heard no more. It is a tale
> Told by an idiot, full of sound and fury,
> Signifying nothing.

> *Macbeth, Act 5, Scene 5.*

Shortly after this, Macbeth's future takes the form of Birnam Wood creeping up towards Dunsinane. All that remains for him is the realization of an imminent threat that surrounds him. Its precise nature is unclear, hidden by the

---

[6] There is an interesting contrast between this account and what Heidegger says in *Being and Time* about recognition of mortality and the authentic pursuit of projects. Heidegger maintains that existential anxiety is not incompatible with purposive striving. Indeed, it offers the potential for an 'authentic' form of engagement with one's life, a way of inhabiting time that reconciles the possibility of purposive activity with an appreciation of one's finitude. So far as I can see, there is no reason to rule out Minkowski's alternative conception of temporal experience: perhaps the future has a twofold structure, and the two aspects can never be fully reconciled.

trees, but it promises to end a life that has been stripped of all its possibilities. This is the world of severe, anxious depression—a place bereft of meaningful pursuits, where the future takes on the guise of inchoate, all-encompassing, and imminent menace.

Although my emphasis has been on changes in an ordinarily implicit sense of time, it is important to acknowledge the role of explicit time too. Fuchs (2013b) observes how aspects of temporal experience that are more usually implicit become explicit in depression. So changes in implicit time are also changes in explicit time. An obvious comparison is with boredom: when nothing significant happens to absorb one's attention, one becomes increasingly aware of the passage of time.[7] But, unlike boredom, a loss of all practical significance does not leave one waiting, as there is nothing to wait for. So the experience is akin to boredom without reprieve. The world says 'there can be nothing but this', and so the experience includes an explicit awareness of time, a painful sense of being condemned for all eternity. A future that takes the form of dread is similarly explicit; it appears as a conspicuous threat, rather than a medium that one inhabits while striving to actualize possibilities. And, where there is loss of more localized projects, one can be all too aware of having lost them and of the impact on one's life. As for conative drive, it is not just absent—its absence can itself be salient. A sense of action as impossible is also something that one is very much aware of; situations offer something that at the same time presents itself as unrealisable.[8]

Creating the Past

Ways of experiencing the future are also ways of experiencing the past. 'Protention' is inextricable from 'retention', and so a privation of the former impacts on the latter. Retention involves experiencing an event *as* having just passed, where a significant possibility may or may not have been actualized. In a world without that kind of possibility, the sense of significant transition is absent. The distinction between what is coming and what has just passed is therefore

---

[7] See Heidegger (1995) for a detailed phenomenological analysis of boredom. Heidegger's analysis of temporal experience in boredom resembles, in some respects, what I have said about depression, given that boredom is essentially temporal and more profound forms involve the absence of certain kinds of possibility from experience. See Ratcliffe (2010b) for further discussion.

[8] I suggest that explicit time be subdivided into (i) experience of temporal properties and (ii) narrative time, where the latter involves organizing one's experience of time into a coherent, linear pattern of inter-related life events. Fuchs (2013b) similarly refers to 'personal-historical or biographical time' as something that orders and unifies explicit time.

less pronounced; the future offers only more of the same. The phenomenological difference between protention and retention lessens and time does not 'flow' in quite the way that it once did, an experience that is sometimes described in terms of the spatializing of time: 'Time is like an alternate reality to me, when I am going through a depressive mood. It's like time and space seep together. It's hard to distinguish between the two during those times' (#51). Other kinds of significant difference can be heightened, as in experiences of all-enveloping dread. There is a pronounced sense that 'something bad is coming', and retention takes the form 'it hasn't happened yet'. But there remains a privation of temporal transition, given that other forms of significance and/or enticement are lacking. Depression also involves changes in how the longer-term past is experienced:

> Our views of the past vary with the changes in our state of becoming. Looking backward on a good day we see the past as a territory which we left behind us or as a solid ground which supports us; on a bad day, however, we experience the past as a burden which crushes us. (Straus, 1947, p.257)

By 'view', Straus does not mean an explicitly formulated position concerning some subject matter. Rather, he is referring to how we experience the past *through* our orientation towards the future. The same point is made by Minkowski (1970, p.157): 'as long as a breath of life is in us, we see past works synthesized into a compact mass which seems to have only one end: that of making us go further'. Events in our past are only experienced as relevant, as mattering, insofar as we are heading somewhere. Furthermore, *which* past events are significant and *how* they are significant to us depends on where we are heading (and vice versa—the dependence is mutual). It is for this reason that Sartre (1989, pp.497–9) claims there is a way in which we 'choose' our past:

> …the past as 'that which is to be changed' is indispensable to the choice of the future and […] consequently no free surpassing can be effected except in terms of a past, but we can see too how the very nature of the past comes to the past from the original choice of a future. […] all my past is there pressing, urgent, imperious, but its meanings and the orders which it gives me I choose by the very project of my end. […] It is the future which decides whether the past is living or dead.

As we saw in Chapter 5, when the past is no longer experienced in the light of a significant future, it is encountered as dead, closed. This can amount to existential guilt, of a kind described by Minkowski and Fuchs.[9] However, I also noted

---

[9] The experience is also described by Straus (1947, p.258): 'The blocking of the future throws the depressive patient back to the past. Thence he hears a terrible judgment pronounced, a judgment which knows no appeal. For his guilt the depressive faces ultimate reprobation, eternal punishment. In depressive delusion, history is experienced in its absolute irrevocability, the past as unpardonable guilt, the future as inevitable catastrophe, the present as irreparable ruin'.

that 'the past as guilt' is not always a central theme in first-person descriptions of depression, even very severe depression. According to some accounts, the past is distant, somehow far away, rather than something that bears down on the person as guilt. Straus (1947, p.255) quotes the following reports: 'Everything seems ages ago'; 'I can't remember the last morning; yesterday is as remote as events years ago'; 'Everything I have done seems like a long time ago; when the evening comes and I think back over the day, it seems years away'. Such experiences are equally understandable in terms of a future bereft of possibility. Past events that are more relevant to our current situation and where we are heading are 'closer' to us, more 'alive', than those that are removed from our current concerns. Without any potential for significant change, any sense of teleological direction, all of one's past is a settled past, a distant past.

Why do some people experience this and others guilt? A key difference is the presence of dread in guilty depression. A fixed past appears in the form of guilt or wrong-doing when it is experienced through an all-pervasive sense of threat, especially when that threat takes a personal form. However, this still does not add up to guilt. The past could instead be experienced as simply 'horrible', a catalogue of suffering and misfortune:

> #199. Time is backwards and all I can think about is the past, all the horrible things that happened—but when I'm happy I don't think about those things at all. I think that my life was pretty good so far and that I survived a lot of things and I'm really strong. But when I'm depressed all I can think about is the horrible things that happened and I exaggerate them so much plus I feel that I have to be perfect and pure. I have to be better than others. I really focus on this when I'm depressed. I have to be more conscientious and kind and go to great lengths to be helpful because I know that 90 percent of people don't. Most people can't be bothered to help others and they are a big disappointment but I can. I can do more than others.

If dread is insufficient to distinguish a horrible past from a more specifically guilty past, what does the difference consist of? There is a clue in the passage I have just quoted (even though the predicament it describes is not as extreme as some, given that there remains the possibility of striving to be better). The author feels a need to be 'perfect and pure' in *contrast* to others, who cannot 'be bothered' and are a 'big disappointment'. Hence the experience does not involve a sense of one's own guilt but of *others* being bad. In recalling the past, the emphasis is on unpleasant events, in which other people no doubt had some role to play. A guilty past involves something slightly different. The depressed person feels irrevocably lacking, and she experiences the threatening presence of others as directed at her deficiencies; it is 'my fault' rather than 'theirs'. Such an experience can involve either of the following: (1) significant possibilities remain in the absence of enticing possibilities, and so things are experienced as 'to be done' but at the same time impossible to do; (2) agitated conation lingers on in the absence of significance or enticement, amounting to a feeling of inchoate urgency that vaguely approximates the evaluation 'I am irrevocably incapable of doing what is demanded of me'. However, as I suggested in Chapter 5, the existential structure of these experiences does not render their construal as guilt inevitable, a point that will be further addressed in Chapter 8.

It is not that experiences of depression affect one's experience of the past *and* also one's experiences of the future. The two are inseparable and, for many, there is an erosion of the distinction between past, present, and future. Loss of significance, I have noted, can affect experiences of past and future in similar ways. One cannot contemplate the possibility of things ever being different, at least not in a positive way, and this incomprehensibility extends into the past as well. One cannot recall what it was like to find things significant; they were not and could not have been any different from how they are now:

> When you are depressed, the past and future are absorbed entirely by the present moment, as in the world of a three-year-old. You cannot remember a time when you felt better, at least not clearly; and you certainly cannot imagine a time when you will feel better. Being upset, even profoundly upset, is a temporal experience, while depression is atemporal. Breakdowns leave you with no point of view. (Solomon, 2001, p.55)

This blurring of the difference between past and future contributes to the experience of time as somehow static. If you listen to a dripping drainpipe for half an hour while waiting for a bus, the next few drops are experienced as *more of the same*, rather than as a departure from the last thirty minutes. Although the tap drips, nothing *happens*; there is change but no significant change. In the absence of a sense that anything is or could be practically significant, all temporal experience is like this. The future is just more of the past, and does not offer the possibility of any significant deviation. Some describe feeling as though they are dead or that they have ceased to exist: 'I do not exist any more. When someone speaks to me, I feel as if he were speaking to a dead person. [. . .] I have the feeling of being an absent person. In sum, I am a walking shadow' (quoted by Minkowski, 1970, p.328). Such remarks relate to erosion of the transition from future to present to past. Experience of being in the present consists, in part, of our actualizing meaningful possibilities and being affected by things in ways that matter. Without any sense of there being significant possibilities, the present would appear structurally similar to the past in some respects: complete, unchangeable, and closed to activity. This experience of being confronted with the *present as past* is something that one might well be inclined to describe in terms of being dead or a ghost—it feels as though one is not there, that one is surveying something complete, that one has become a disconnected witness to a life that is over.

A different way of experiencing the past can arise in conjunction with a loss of projects and/or a loss of conative drive. In the absence of any preoccupation with future possibilities, one may increasingly come to re-inhabit past possibilities instead. So the past is not distant or closed; it is unusually salient, significant. In W. G. Sebald's semi-autobiographical novel, *The Rings of Saturn*, the author completes a book project and decides to take a long and directionless walk through the Suffolk countryside. So, from the outset, there is a peculiar lack of future-oriented drive or projects. As the novel progresses, he becomes absorbed in the significance of past events—the past draws him in. In the process, it progressively reveals itself as an inevitable cycle of misery, horror, and tragedy, provoking a feeling of repetition and sameness:

> Scarcely am I in company but it seems as if I had already heard the same opinions expressed by the same people somewhere or other, in the same way, with the same words, turns of phrase and gestures. The physical sensation closest to this feeling of repetition, which sometimes lasts for several minutes and can be quite disconcerting, is that of the peculiar numbness brought on by a heavy loss of blood, often resulting in a temporary inability to think, to speak or to move one's limbs, as though, without being aware of it, one had suffered a stroke. Perhaps there is in this as yet unexplained phenomenon of apparent duplication some kind of anticipation of the end, a venture into the void, a sort of disagreement, which, like a gramophone repeatedly playing the same sequence of notes, has less to do with damage to the machine itself than with an irreparable defect in its programme. Be that as it may, on that August afternoon at Michael's house I felt several times, either through exhaustion or for some other reason, that I was losing the ground from under my feet. (2002, pp.187–8)

One could perhaps experience the world in a past-oriented way for an indefinite period, where the past is alive with a significance the future lacks. But the culmination of what Sebald describes is a sense of inevitability that engulfs past and future. The kinds of significance that past events embody become increasingly restricted, until there is only the inescapable repetition of horror, suffering, and futility—one can anticipate nothing else. This amounts to a sense of timelessness and inevitability. Some people with depression describe a similar kind of experience, although I do not wish to suggest that it can originate only in this past-focused way:

> #161. I see my whole life in one frame. I can see centuries before and of the people who have already been here and gone. Of how people in the future will look back on the time that I have lived in when I am long gone. It just makes all aspirations and goals completely pointless. All the troubles and things people worry about are pointless.

To summarize, I have suggested that 'depression' can involve a range of subtly different changes in the structure of temporal experience. To better understand them, we can apply a broad distinction between loss of practical significance, loss of drive, and loss of life-projects, as developed in Chapters 4 and 6. All of the following phenomenological changes are consistent with a diagnosis of 'major depression' and/or 'depression' more generally (where the latter includes 'mixed states'):

1. Loss of some or all of one's projects, with or without (2) and/or (4).

2. Partial or complete loss of conative drive/enticing possibilities, with or without [(1) or (3)] and/or (4).

3. Loss of the sense of things as practically significant for oneself and perhaps for others too, with or without (2) and/or (4).

4. A sense of passivity before an impending threat, which can participate in any of (1) to (3) above.

This is much like the list in Chapter 6, but it also makes clear that (3) does not imply (2). It thus acknowledges a variety of experiences where enticing possibilities or some other aspect of conation linger on, despite a loss of the significant possibilities that coherent projects and other commitments depend upon.

Ways of Being in Time

In suggesting that 'depression' encompasses several different forms of temporal experience, I do not want to insist that any of them are *specific* to depression. As noted, some cases of diagnosed depression most likely involve experiences of time that are no different, or not much different, from what we might call 'everyday' experiences. All of us experience time differently when bored, frantic, tired, or awaiting some occurrence with great fear of excitement. We might look back on some event and remark on how distant it seems or, alternatively, how it feels like yesterday. Nevertheless, cases of depression that involve changes in the *structure* of temporal experience (most likely the majority of depression experiences) are different. 'Everyday' variations in temporal experience do not include such pronounced existential changes. But what about kinds of experience associated with other illnesses?

One question to consider is whether different kinds of temporal experience are involved in depression and schizophrenia. We should be wary of associating specific forms of experience with specific diagnostic categories. These categories were formulated partly on the basis of phenomenological considerations, but without the aid of detailed, systematic phenomenological study of the relevant phenomena. However, there does seem to be a qualitative difference between the kinds of temporal experience involved in depression and some of those associated with schizophrenia. In short, the former have an impoverished structure, whereas the latter involve structural disruption. Fuchs (2013b) emphasizes fragmentation in schizophrenia, a *breakdown* of passive synthesis. Vogeley and Kupke (2007, p.162) also maintain that there is an 'unsystematic disruption' in schizophrenia, whereas mania and depression involve more consistent changes. And Minkowski (1970, p.284) suggests that 'time entirely breaks down' in schizophrenia, while other illnesses involve a 'modification' of temporal experience. Drawing this distinction is quite compatible with allowing that the two kinds of change can occur together, that fragmentation can be accompanied by the consistent loss of certain kinds of possibility. I will further discuss the comparative phenomenology in Chapter 10.

What about temporal experience in somatic illness? Serious, chronic, somatic illness is often comorbid with depression and, as discussed in Chapter 2, it is difficult to disentangle the two phenomenologically. Setting aside comorbidity, an important difference between somatic illness and those forms of depression involving a loss of practical significance is that, although the ill person might stop looking ahead, she retains a capacity to do so. Furthermore, activities such as getting one's affairs in order may remain significant, and the pursuit of a 'good death' can itself become a project. Even so, serious illness can have a profound effect on one's sense of the future as a realm of significant projects, and might lead to a loss or abandonment of life projects that closely resembles non-existential 'depression' experiences. However, it is not clear that it *has to* resemble them. For example, Carel (2008, pp.124–5) describes a way of learning to 'dwell in the present' in response to illness, which differs markedly from depression. It can, she says, be 'liberating to live in the now. It is liberating to be freed from having to plan, to make a future, to strategize'.

It is also difficult to draw boundaries between those depression experiences that involve loss of conative drive and certain somatic illness experiences. For instance, the associated desynchronization that Fuchs emphasizes is something that can arise in illness more generally. Good (1994, p.126) describes experiences of pain in chronic illness as follows: 'Time caves in. Past and present lose their order. Pain slows personal time, while outer time speeds by and is lost'. Hence 'I feel like the world is passing me by'. This feeling of watching the world go by and inhabiting a time cut-off from that of other people can amount to a desynchronization just as pronounced as what many depressed people describe.[10] More generally, I do not think the distinction between temporal experience in depression and in other forms of illness is a clear one. As I argued in Chapter 2, some forms of depression experience are phenomenologically indistinguishable from some forms of so-called 'somatic' illness experience.[11]

However, it should not be assumed that, in all cases where differences in temporal experience appear unclear, there is no difference to be discerned. Seemingly similar experiences can have different existential structures. To illustrate this, I will conclude my discussion of time by examining a first-person account of profound grief. In the book *Lived Time, without its Flow*, Denise Riley (2012) describes how, for some years after the unexpected death of her adult son, her overall sense of belonging to the world was profoundly altered. She focuses specifically on temporal experience and states that time stopped 'flowing'. How are we to understand this? Riley refers to 'that acute sensation of being cut off from any temporal flow that can grip you after the sudden death of your child' (p.7). So the emphasis is on being removed from a temporal world, from a community of people for whom time still flows, rather than on a simple absence of flow. There is, she says, a 'sensation of having been lifted clean out of habitual time' (p.10); 'of living outside time' (p.45). We might think of this in terms of a loss of projects. But Riley is quite explicit that the experience involves loss of something more than that, something that the intelligibility of projects depends upon, and the intelligibility of narratives too. The possibility of putting things into words in a meaningful, chronologically structured way presupposes a sense of temporal order that was absent from her world:

> ...to live on after a death, yet to live without inhabiting any tense yourself, presents you with serious problems of what's describable. This may explain the paucity of accounts. To struggle to narrate becomes not only an unenticing prospect, but structurally impossible. (p.57)[12]

---

[10] See also Toombs (1990) for some interesting remarks on how chronic, severe pain affects the experience of time.

[11] We might also wonder about the relationship between depression experiences and ageing. It is in fact rather naïve to contrast depression with a singular, 'everyday' way of experiencing time. A child's sense of the future surely differs from that of an eighty-year-old. To quote William James (1902, p.151), 'How can the moribund old man reason back to himself the romance, the mystery, the imminence of great things with which our old earth tingled for him in the days when he was young and well?' Perhaps the structure of depression differs too. Indeed, *some* experiences of ageing may be very similar to a slow descent into depression—future possibilities contract, one's body becomes more conspicuous, the significance of things diminishes and the past is ever-more complete.

[12] Hence Riley's account was, of course, written after the period it describes.

One might respond by expressing some scepticism about the claim that time stopped flowing. After all, in Chapter 1, I raised a number of concerns about the reliability of memoirs as phenomenological resources. However, once it is acknowledged that experience incorporates a changeable sense of the possible, what Riley describes strikes me as quite amenable to interpretation. Profound grief can but does not always involve—amongst other things—a loss of the sense that anything could ever be significantly different from the present in a positive way. This affects long-term experience of time because there is no longer a teleological sense of direction, of moving or even being able to move 'forward'. It also affects short-term experience, as the transition from moment to moment does not include a sense of meaningful change. Things still change but nothing of any consequence happens. Hence there is no experience of short- or long-term temporal direction, involving the ongoing actualization of possibilities against a backdrop of cares, concerns, commitments, goals, and projects. It is 'meaningful change' rather than 'mere change', Riley indicates, that is responsible for the aspect of experience we call the 'flow', 'passage', or 'movement' of time.

Given what I have said so far, it might sound as though this experience has the same existential structure as a form of depression where practical significance is lost, but it does not. Both involve loss of openness to a meaningful future, but a consistent theme in Riley's account is the retention of an intense second-person connection; she continues to relate to her son, to be with him, in a way that is incompatible with purposive immersion in a world that he is absent from: 'imagined empathy seals your sense of stopped time' (p.41). Desynchronization from the social world, loss of a significant future, and the absence of 'temporal flow' are all inextricable from *being with* someone who is no longer part of that world. Grief experiences differ in all manner of ways, but the theme of some sort of enduring interpersonal relationship with the deceased is a consistent one. Culturally entrenched narratives about gradually 'letting go' following a bereavement conflict with the observation that grief usually involves maintaining a long-term, personal relationship with the deceased, albeit one that varies in character and evolves in a number of ways (Klass, Silverman, and Nickman, 1996). Existential depression, in contrast, involves feeling estranged from everyone, unable to 'connect'. Hence it differs from a sense of social disengagement that stems from retention of a personal relationship. Even so, what Riley describes amounts to a kind of existential shift: it consists in a bodily *feeling* that is at the same time a sense of being dislodged from the world: 'This state is physically raw, and has nothing whatsoever to do with thinking sad thoughts or with "mourning". It thuds into you. Inexorable carnal knowledge' (p.21). This 'feeling' structures all experience and thought; it is an altered sense of the possible, a loss of the open future.

Interpersonal experience is therefore central to the phenomenological difference between grief and depression. Given that experiences of grief can develop
into depression experiences of kinds that I have described, the boundary is
no doubt blurred. However, even those cases that might be termed 'complicated' grief involve retention of an interpersonal relationship. As we will see in
Chapter 8, in existential forms of depression, the possibility of a certain kind of
second-person relation is gone from the world. One can no longer direct oneself
towards others in that kind of way, the living or the dead.[13]

---

[13] See also Pies (2013) for the view that the intersubjective phenomenology of grief differs
importantly from that of depression. We can draw such distinctions without taking
sides in debates over whether, when, and why grief is to be deemed 'pathological'.

Chapter 8

Other People

The interpersonal has been a consistent theme throughout my discussion so far. The 'prison' of depression is 'mine and mine alone', and experiences of hopelessness are often similarly self-specific: others have hope and the depressed person is cut off from them, marooned somewhere else. The same applies to temporal experience: others inhabit a time where significant change is possible; she does not. Experiences of diminished agency often take the form 'I can't do something that they can' or 'I can't do what I'm supposed to do, or be what I'm supposed to be, to the detriment of others'. Guilt also has an interpersonal structure: one feels guilty before others. And losses of practical significance involve the interpersonal in a range of ways. We encounter other people against the backdrop of our various cares, concerns and commitments, which shape how we relate to and interact with them. Most projects have an interpersonal structure: we collaborate with others, often to achieve shared goals; we act for others; and we act because others ask or require us to do so. There is a sense in which even the most solitary projects implicate others. They are experienced 'mine', in a way that depends on a contrast with other projects that are 'ours' or 'for the sake of others'. Where existential changes are involved, the overall *structure* of interpersonal experience and relatedness is affected, rather than how one experiences or relates to specific individuals. The depressed person does not encounter anyone in quite the way he once did.

In the first part of this chapter, I offer an account of what it is to experience and relate to someone *as a person*. Following that, I describe how interpersonal experience is affected in depression. My overarching claim is that distinctively *interpersonal* possibilities are inseparable from the experience of an open future, from the appreciation that certain kinds of significant change are possible. A sense of 'my possibilities' is partly constituted by (a) my feeling able to enter into certain kinds of interpersonal relation, and (b) my actually doing so. Hence we cannot fully appreciate the closed, static world of depression unless we recognize the inseparability of interpersonal experience from world experience more generally. As with bodily feeling, guilt, despair, diminished agency, and temporal experience, I show that interpersonal experience in depression has several variants. All of these can be understood in terms of losing 'self-transformative' possibilities. I also propose that an erosion of interpersonal 'trust' is central to many of them, thus building on the discussion of trust in Chapter 4.

Depression and Estrangement

J. H. van den Berg (1972, p.105) remarks—very plausibly, in my view—that 'loneliness is the nucleus of psychiatry'. It is certainly a salient theme in most autobiographical accounts of depression. For example:

> ...I felt an immense and aching solitude. (Styron, 2001, p.45)

> I thought I had no hope of ever making it back to that place I called life. I thought, too, that I was the only one who felt that way. Depression feels like the most isolated place on earth. No wonder they call it a disease of loneliness. (Brampton, 2008, p.1)

A closely related theme is that nobody else understands one's predicament:

> #15. ...my friends are supportive but struggle to know what to say.

> #34. I find other people irritating when depressed, especially those that have never suffered with depression, and find the 'advice' often given by these is unempathetic and ridiculous.

> #153. Nobody understands or loves me.

This sense of not being understood is not a phenomenologically isolated 'judgment' that can be distinguished from a prior experience of depression; the two are inseparable. In earlier chapters, I argued that most depression experiences involve existential changes, and are therefore difficult to understand and describe. This partly explains why many people state that depression is somehow 'ineffable'. However, the kind of 'understanding' that is taken to be lacking on the part of others is not primarily a matter of being able to conceptualize and articulate depression experiences. There is a *feeling* that they do not understand, which could equally be described as a feeling that they are unable to 'relate to' or 'connect with' the depressed person. What is missing is the potential for certain kinds of interpersonal relation. Regardless of whether or to what extent others actually do understand his experience, he does not *feel understood*. A pervasive sense of estrangement features consistently in first-person accounts of depression, but it takes different forms. The theme of incarceration involves isolation from other people and from the world more generally. With this, others may appear not quite real or, in extreme cases, strangely impersonal, mechanical. Other themes, as we have seen, include guilt, shame, worthlessness, and dread. In all cases, though, there is a sense of disconnection from the interpersonal world. This is illustrated by the following passage from Plath's *The Bell Jar*:

The two of them didn't even stop jitterbugging during the intervals. I felt myself shrinking to a small black dot against all those red and white rugs and that pine-panelling. I felt like a hole in the ground. [...] It's like watching Paris from an express caboose heading in the opposite direction—every second the city gets smaller and smaller, only you feel it's really you getting smaller and smaller and lonelier and lonelier, rushing away from all those lights and that excitement at about a million miles an hour. (Plath, 1966, p.15)

Here, the experience of social isolation is inseparable from that of feeling cut-off from the world more generally and somehow diminished as a result. The self does not detach from the interpersonal world unscathed, to become a passive but fully intact spectator. The sense of self is eroded as the potential for certain kinds of interpersonal engagement is lost, something I will interpret in terms of a lack of access to distinctively interpersonal kinds of possibility.

In order to understand how interpersonal experience is affected in depression, we must also understand what is affected: what is it to experience and relate to someone as a person? Of course, our answer to that question can be informed by reflecting on the phenomenology of depression. But, if we are to begin interpreting the kinds of experience that depressed people describe, we need to have at least some initial grasp of what distinctively *interpersonal* experience consists of. And a problem we face is that orthodox philosophical accounts of the interpersonal are of little help. I will suggest that the 'belief-desire psychology' they fixate on is peripheral or even irrelevant to the kinds of privation that depressed people describe. The relevant sense of 'understanding' and 'being understood' consists of something else. If we are to describe it, we have to get past entrenched ways of thinking about 'understanding other minds'. To do that, I will take my lead from Sartre's account in *Being and Nothingness*, according to which our awareness of being in the presence of another person involves a bodily response that is inextricable from a distinctive way of experiencing possibilities. I will concede that Sartre's more specific emphasis on *loss* of one's possibilities is too restrictive, while defending the more general claim. So again, we will see that bodily experience is inseparable from experience of the possible. At the same time, it will become clear how the interpersonal is integrated into the same unitary phenomenological structure that I have described in terms of the body, hope, guilt, agency, and time.

Experiencing Persons

Most recent accounts of interpersonal understanding in philosophy of mind, cognitive science, and developmental psychology take the principal achievement to be an ability to attribute beliefs, desires, and other kinds of mental state to people. The focus of debate is on whether this involves employment of a theory, an ability to 'simulate' the minds of others, or some combination of the two. So-called 'theory theorists' propose that an ability to understand the mental states of others (and perhaps one's own mental states too) depends largely or wholly on deployment of a systematically organized, domain-specific body of conceptual knowledge about types of mental state and how they interrelate, a largely tacit 'theory of other minds'. 'Simulation theorists', in contrast, emphasize an ability to use one's own mind as a model. One grasps other people's mental states by replicating those states, instead of drawing on a theory. More recent approaches maintain that theory and simulation are not mutually exclusive, and that a 'hybrid' account of some description is needed in order to capture our ability to attribute mental states (see e.g. Davies and Stone, 1995a, b).

The theory-simulation debate is centred upon the question of how a seemingly detached spectator attributes mental states to a third party, rather than that of how mental states are attributed in the context of interpersonal relations. Most of the contributors just assume that there is no relevant difference between the two situations: we use the same theory-simulation mechanism to attribute mental states, regardless of whether we are observing someone or interacting with him. Consequently, this approach does not address what people with depression describe, which is concerned more specifically with an ability to *relate* to others as *persons*. Theory and simulation theories do not have much to say about distinctively *personal* ways of relating. Indeed, some accounts are curiously impersonal: the other person is construed as a very complicated object of a distinctive type, which we deal with by drawing on domain-specific knowledge and skills.[1] Hence, even if it is conceded that these approaches succeed in identifying and explaining a circumscribed cognitive ability that we do indeed possess, they are of little use here. Furthermore, insofar as (a) depression involves experiencing oneself as irrevocably cut off from other people, unable to relate to them in a personal way or feel understood by them, (b) theory and simulation theories seek to capture what is central to interpersonal understanding, and (c) these theories offer little or no insight into the nature of (a), we can conclude that (d) their emphasis on belief-desire psychology and the mechanisms that enable it is seriously lacking.

It might be objected that recognizing and relating to someone as a person just *is* a matter of attributing mental states to her, perhaps more mental states or more sophisticated mental states than one would assign if one watched her from afar. However, in contrast to theory and simulation theories, some

---

[1] See Ratcliffe (2007) for a survey of 'theory' and 'simulation' accounts of belief-desire psychology, as well as a critique of both.

have argued that the concept of a 'person' plays a more fundamental role in our thinking about each other than 'minds' and 'mental states'. For instance, Strawson (1959) proposes that 'person' is a primitive concept; it is not derived from other concepts and therefore resists further analysis.[2] He points out that our thought does not respect a clear distinction between two kinds of entity—minds and bodies. It is not that one entity has arms and legs, while another has thoughts and feelings; the same 'I' has both mental and physical characteristics. Strawson adds that the properties attributed to persons do not divide neatly into 'mental' and 'non-mental' categories. He distinguishes M- and P-predicates, where the former are possessed by material things and persons, while the latter are specific to persons. For example, a rock and a person both have weight, but only a person has feelings of jealousy. Although jealousy might be an uncontroversial example of a 'mental state', other P-predicates, such as 'is smiling' and 'is going for a walk', straddle the two categories.

Even if Strawson is right, what he says does not imply that there is a distinctive *phenomenology* associated with encountering persons, but I think there is.[3] It is illustrated by those occasional moments of ambiguity when there is a flickering between personal and impersonal experiences of an entity. Consider looking at a waxwork, first taking it to be a person and then realizing it is not. There is a kind of 'gestalt switch', and occasionally a feeling of ambiguity that is not fully resolved. Perhaps, as Freud (1919/2003) suggested, such 'uncanny' feelings sometimes arise due to conflicting experiences of an entity as animate and, at the same time, inanimate. They can also be associated more specifically with the personal/impersonal distinction though. For instance, being stared at by a chimpanzee can produce an odd feeling of personal/impersonal indeterminacy, without any disturbance in one's appreciation of it as an animate organism.[4] As the waxwork example shows, we can of course be mistaken when we experience an entity as a person. But I am concerned with what the relevant experience consists of, regardless of whether or not it is veridical. One might object that there is no generic sense

---

[2] See Ratcliffe (2009b) for a more detailed discussion of Strawson's work and its significance for current debates about belief-desire psychology. See Lowe (1996) for a defence of the view that 'person' is metaphysically primitive. Others have defended a broadly Strawsonian view of persons in the context of developmental psychology (e.g. Hobson, 1993, 2002; Reddy, 2008).

[3] See also Laing (1960) for the view that we experience others as persons, a view that I mentioned in Chapter 1.

[4] I do not wish to rule out the possibility of non-human persons. For the purposes of this discussion, I remain agnostic over whether animals such as chimpanzees are properly regarded as persons.

of personhood involved in our experiences of others. I could experience a given person in any number of ways—I might be indifferent to her, uncomfortable with her, in love with her or afraid of her. And these experiences have little in common. However, I suggest that the diverse ways in which we experience, think about and respond to others also presuppose a more general appreciation of personhood. This is illustrated by the contrast with forms of anomalous experience where it is absent. For example, in *Autobiography of a Schizophrenic Girl*, Renee describes how others ceased to look like persons:

> I look at her, study her, praying to feel the life in her through the enveloping unreality. But she seems more a statue than ever, a mannikin moved by mechanism, talking like an automaton. It is horrible, inhuman, grotesque. (Sechehaye, 1970, p.38)

The complaint is not that a perceived property or set of properties has changed. Rather, a *feeling* of the personal, which does not depend on the perception of any particular physical property, is absent. This leaves Renee with a peculiar experience of others as physically unchanged and yet disturbingly different. What we find in depression is seldom so extreme. Plath (1966, p.136), amongst others, does describe an experience of other people as curiously inanimate: 'I felt as if I was sitting in the window of an enormous department store. The figures around me weren't people, but shop dummies, painted to resemble people and propped up in attitudes counterfeiting life'. However, what many depressed people report is feeling unable to relate to others in a distinctively personal way, rather than being unable to experience them as persons. It might appear that I have so far conflated the two, but the questions of what it is to experience someone as a person and what it is to relate to someone in a personal way are intimately connected. Consider the analogy of experiencing and relating to something as a coffee cup. Even if one's hands are tied behind one's back, one can still experience it as a coffee cup. Nevertheless, although one remains able to engage with it in certain ways (nudge it, move it across the table or tip it over), one is unable to engage with it *as* a coffee cup. To pursue the analogy further, suppose one lost all sense of what it is to engage with an entity in a cup-specific way—to pick it up and drink from it. This would plausibly erode one's experience of entities as cups, given that the ability to experience something as a cup is inextricable from an appreciation of the potential to relate to it as a cup. Of course, persons are importantly unlike cups. But the point of the analogy is to suggest that interpersonal experience similarly involves distinctive kinds of relational possibility. Hence an account of what it is to experience others as persons will also cast light on what it is to relate to someone in a personal way. In depression, access to specifically interpersonal kinds of possibility is eroded or lost. One might still experience others as persons, but at the same time feel unable to interact with them as persons.

In such cases, the possibilities are there but blocked, in a way that is comparable to experiencing a cup of coffee (while feeling tired and thirsty), when one's hands are tied behind one's back. However, other kinds of change in the possibility space also involve diminished and distorted experiences of the personal. The result need not be something so extreme as others looking like waxworks or mannequins, but at least something of the personal is lacking.

One might still insist that experiencing or relating to someone *as a person* depends, wholly or partly, on an experience of attributing mental states to him. Contrary to that view, Gallagher (2001, 2005) and others have argued that many interpersonal interactions are facilitated by a perceptual or perception-like appreciation of agency, embedded in contexts of shared practice, rather than by the explicit or even implicit attribution of propositional attitudes.[5] It would be implausible to insist that such interactions involve no sense at all of being with a person and that personhood is only established once propositional attitudes are assigned. Our advocate of belief-desire psychology could concede this, and maintain instead that appreciating personhood is a matter of recognizing that one *could* legitimately attribute propositional attitudes to an entity. In fact, even if we disregard Gallagher's view, the stronger position is untenable; we do not encounter seemingly inanimate entities, which are then suddenly imbued with personhood the moment we ascribe beliefs or desires to them. However, it is also doubtful that recognizing entities as legitimate targets for belief-desire attribution is fundamental to our grasp of them as *persons*, as it is not specific enough. We understand non-human organisms, institutions and even certain artefacts in such terms, without experiencing them in a personal way, and it is not clear where to draw the line between metaphorical and non-metaphorical uses.

One could instead appeal to a wider range of mental states. For example, Goldman (2006, p.20) points out that a comprehensive theory of interpersonal understanding or 'mindreading' will need to include a lot more than just beliefs, desires, and propositional attitudes more generally; there are 'other kinds of mental states: sensations, like feelings and pain, and emotions, like disgust and anger'. Why, though, should appreciating that an entity possesses these states involve a distinctive way of *experiencing* it? One answer is that we perceive their behavioural effects or perhaps even something of the mental states themselves, and that the relevant perceptual contents are what render experience of the personal distinctive.[6] However, the experience is not always

---

[5] See also Ratcliffe (2007) and Hutto (2008) for defences of this view.

[6] As noted in Chapter 5, it is arguable that perceivable expressions of emotion are partly constitutive of some emotions. If that is right, then some mental states are to some extent perceivable.

associated with perceived expressions, gestures, actions, words or, indeed, any consistent set of perceived properties. It can involve a diverse range of perceptual stimuli. I might hear the door creak, feel a touch on my back, or hear breathing, and be immediately struck by the feeling that *someone* is there.

Another option is simulation: maybe appreciating someone as a person is associated with a distinctive experience because it sometimes or always involves simulating his experiences and, by implication, having an experience. This would account for the experience's distinctiveness, as we do not ordinarily recognize other kinds of entity by simulating them. So, when you hear the creak at the door, you adopt—perhaps automatically—the perspective of a person at the door. It is unclear, though, how an experience of that kind could constitute our sense of being in the presence of *someone else*. As pointed out by Scheler (1954, p.10), recognizing something as a legitimate target for what is these days referred to as 'simulation' is an achievement that simulation presupposes. One would not attribute mental states of whatever kind to an entity (via simulation or theory) unless one already took it to be an entity of the type that possessed those states—a person. A further objection Scheler raises is that, although we recognize others as like ourselves in some respects, interpersonal experience equally involves an appreciation of their distinctness. We react to their experiences *as theirs* rather than our own: 'To commiserate is [...] to be sorry at another person's sorrow, *as being his*. The fact that it is his is part of the phenomenological situation' (Scheler, 1954, p.37). We respond to others' predicaments, rather than just replicating them, and our response is not always preceded by replication.[7]

A distinction is sometimes drawn between two types of simulation: there is explicit simulation, which occurs when we imaginatively and knowingly project ourselves into the physical situation or psychological state of another person, and there is implicit simulation, where replication of the other person's cognitive states is achieved via non-conscious processes. So, in response to what I have said so far, the simulationist could maintain that there need be no awareness of the simulation routine underlying the experience. 'High level' or explicit simulation is to be distinguished from 'low level' or implicit simulation (e.g. Goldman, 2006), and experiencing others as persons involves the latter. However, before attempting to account for a kind of experience in terms of low-level simulation, we first need to be clear about what the relevant experience consists of. In what follows, I will suggest that it involves a felt sense of *connectedness* to others, rather than replication of some aspect of

---

[7] See, for example, Zahavi (2007) for a good account of Scheler's work and its importance as a corrective to assumptions made by both theory and simulation theorists.

their psychology. And this is what is altered and diminished in depression. Perhaps the relevant phenomenological achievement does depend in some way on 'low-level' matching amongst other things, but an appeal to 'matching', 'simulating', or 'replicating' does not explain or even acknowledge the kind of relational structure that makes it distinctive. Hence simulation, in both its guises, is not so much mistaken as beside the point. My approach will also imply that interpersonal experience cannot be explained in terms of an implicit or explicit *theory*, as our sense of the personal is rooted in a distinctive kind of *feeling*. One concession I do make to simulation is that depression can be described as involving an inability to 'simulate' certain things. If a person lacks any sense of the possibility of significant change, she cannot, by implication, simulate anything significantly different. But this is to be understood in terms of a wider-ranging inability to imagine, which is embedded in a possibility space that equally affects perception, memory, expectation, and thought more generally. So an emphasis on 'simulating the minds of others' is too specific.

Persons and Possibilities

In his discussion and defence of simulation theory, Goldman discusses several ancestors of modern simulation theories, including the work of Adam Smith. His portrayal of Smith as a proto-simulationist is hard to resist.[8] However, consider the following passage, quoted in part by Goldman (2006, p.17), which also gestures towards something different:

> When we have read a book or poem so often that we can no longer find any amusement in reading it by ourselves, we can still take pleasure in reading it to a companion. To him it has all the graces of novelty; we enter into the surprise and admiration which it naturally excites in him, but which it is no longer capable of exciting in us; we consider all the ideas which it presents, rather in the light of which they appear to him, than in that in which they appear to ourselves, and we are amused by sympathy with his amusement which thus enlivens our own. On the contrary, we should be vexed if he did not seem to be entertained with it, and we could no longer take any pleasure in reading it to him. (Smith, 1759/2000, p.11)

The passage is revealing because it does not merely describe the simulation of one person by another, but also interaction between two people. And there are various things going on. One person certainly appreciates something of the other's experience, but that appreciation is at the same time self-affecting. Engaging with the other person's experience of the book changes and enriches one's own experience of it. Furthermore, it is not clear that there

---

[8] See, for example, Smith (1759/2000, p.4).

are two distinct experiences of the book co-existing in the same person: an experience of a dull book and a simulated experience of an exciting book. Rather, a book that previously seemed dull has had new life breathed into it through a shared experience. It is 'us' who perceive the book together, shaping each other's experiences in the process. Simulation alone fails to capture the relational and self-affecting character of the experience, which Smith (2000, p.10) describes in terms of the 'pleasures of mutual sympathy'. If we can understand what such experiences consist of, we will be better placed to interpret interpersonal experience in depression, given that depression often involves an experienced inability to enter into exactly this kind of interpersonal relation: 'There is the realization that you have never connected with anybody, truly, in your life' (#224).

One might suggest that the above example involves three separate steps: there is a simulation, which causes certain feelings or thoughts, and these then affect one's own experience of the book. However, interpersonal experience does not always respect linguistic distinctions between (i) a person's own experiences of the world; (ii) her appreciation of how someone else experiences the world; and (iii) kinds of feeling that might be causally associated with (i) or (ii). In many instances, the three are indeed separate occurrences but, when it comes to engaging with someone *as a person*, they are aspects of a single, unitary experience, not discrete perceptual and/or cognitive achievements that interact causally with each other. Interpersonal experience consists in a kind of bodily feeling that is at the same time (a) an acknowledgement of the other person as a locus of experience and activity distinct from oneself and (b) a change in how one experiences the world. To illustrate this, I will return to Sartre's *Being and Nothingness*.

For Sartre, our most fundamental sense of 'the other' (which I will instead refer to as 'a person') is not a matter of attributing internal mental states, analogizing, inferring, hypothesizing, deploying a theory, simulating, or anything of the sort. Instead, it consists of a non-conceptual feeling, a change in how one's body is experienced. Take his description of shame:

> I have just made an awkward or vulgar gesture. This gesture clings to me; I neither judge it nor blame it. I simply live it. I realize it in the mode of for-itself. But now suddenly I raise my head. Somebody was there and has seen me. Suddenly I realize the vulgarity of my gesture, and I am ashamed. (1989, p.221)

On one account, what happens here is that I first perceive the presence of another person, then reflect on what she has seen me doing, and finally feel shame. But this is not Sartre's view. He suggests that shame is a reflex-like reaction to a stimulus, which does not require prior recognition that someone is present or an evaluative judgement concerning the shameful nature of one's deeds. It is, he says, 'an immediate shudder which runs through me from head to foot without any discursive preparation' (1989, p.222). This feeling is not just *associated* with awareness of someone's presence; it *constitutes* that awareness. Put simply, one cannot feel ashamed without having a sense of being ashamed before somebody. What shame reveals, according to Sartre, is the relation of 'being-seen-by-another', 'the look' (1989, pp.257–8). There are two inseparable aspects to this: recognizing someone as a locus of experience and recognizing oneself as an object of her experience. 'The look' is not to be construed literally, as seeing a pair of eyes. It is not a matter of perceiving that one has actually been seen but of having the sense of being perceived. The latter is more abstract, and could be associated with any number of different perceived properties:

> Of course, what *most often* manifests a look is the convergence of two ocular globes in my direction. But the look will be given just as well on occasion when there is a rustling of branches, or the sound of a footstep followed by silence, or the slight opening of a shutter, or a light movement of a curtain. (Sartre, 1989, p.257)[9]

How could something be a change in bodily experience and, at the same time, a feeling of relating—in some way—to another person? Sartre's answer is that a change in bodily feeling can also be a change in one's experience of worldly possibilities, and a certain kind of modification of those possibilities just *is* our most fundamental sense of the interpersonal. As discussed in Chapters 3 and 6, Sartre maintains that we do not usually experience our bodies as conspicuous objects of experience. When I am involved in a project, my body is that through which I perceive and act upon things: 'My consciousness sticks to my acts, it *is* my acts' (1989, p.259). Entities are not experienced solely in terms of their actual features but also in terms of the significant possibilities that they offer me, and these possibilities are determined—at least in part—by a sense of my bodily capacities and dispositions. But how does the interpersonal fit into this picture? Consider Sartre's well-known example of peeping through a keyhole at somebody. The voyeur is absorbed in the perceived situation, in the project of spying. Then, as she hears a creak on the stairs, there is a sudden shift in how her body feels. It ceases to be an inconspicuous medium through which she perceives the

---

9 Even when the look *is* manifested by a pair of eyes, one does not perceive the eyes as objects but as openings onto the other person's situation, a situation in which oneself is included (Sartre, 1989, p.258). And the look presumably does not depend specifically on *visual* perception either, as it is essential to a sense of the interpersonal that people without sight also possess.

room and enters the foreground of awareness. As this happens, perception of her surroundings is altered too. The possibilities that the situation incorporates reflect her bodily dispositions and, as her body becomes object-like and awkward, those dispositions change. With this, the possibilities offered by her surroundings change too. Things *look* different, since significant possibilities that they previously offered, such as 'useable in the context of my current project', are lost.

According to Sartre, a feeling of being object-like amounts to a feeling of being the object of someone else's experience, of inhabiting a world that is now configured in terms of *her* projects and purposes: 'I grasp the Other's look at the very centre of *my* act as the solidification and alienation of my own possibilities'. This experiential shift is not primarily a matter of knowing or believing something. It is a change in a felt sense of one's relationship with the world. I do not simply 'know' that I am being looked at; I am 'suddenly affected in my being'; I 'live' it (1989, pp.260–263). What we have here is not a three-step process of recognizing the presence of someone, feeling ashamed and then experiencing the world differently; the three are one and the same.

Are there any grounds for accepting Sartre's view that (a) a change in our bodily phenomenology can at the same time be a change in possibilities that are integral to the perceived world and (b) some such change constitutes our sense of others as persons? We can do so without also accepting his more specific emphasis on a certain type of interpersonal encounter. It is routinely pointed out that Sartre's approach over-emphasizes confrontational relations. Merleau-Ponty (1962, p.361) complains that it best captures those awkward occasions when 'each of us feels his actions not to be taken up and understood, but observed as if they were an insect's'.[10] However, the more general view that this emphasis presupposes is, I think, right. And it is not specific to Sartre either. Indeed, Merleau-Ponty observes that 'no sooner has my gaze fallen upon a living body in process of acting than the objects surrounding it immediately take on a fresh layer of significance' (1962, p.353). There is a shift

---

[10] Sartre does acknowledge that even experiences like this do not involve a sense of being wholly object-like. The look does not extinguish an awareness, shared by both parties, of the objectified person's potential to set up a new system of possibilities: 'the Other-as-object is an explosive instrument which I handle with care because I foresee around him the permanent possibility that *they* are going to make it explode and that with this explosion I shall suddenly experience the flight of the world away from me and the alienation of my being' (Sartre, 1989, p.297).

in one's sense of the possibilities that things offer; now they are perceived as offering possibilities for someone else too.[11]

Interpersonal Relations and World Experience

Sartre emphasizes something that is not sufficiently acknowledged by simulation or theory theories: recognizing someone as a person is self-affecting, involving a change in one's experience of the possible. It takes various forms, some of which are quite different from what Sartre describes. Take Sartre's example of walking in the park and seeing a figure on a bench. You feel, he says, the pull of the world away from you and towards him. The park ceases to be a realm of significant possibilities *for you* and becomes *his* park, where you take your place among his objects (Sartre, 1989, p.254). Compare this to van den Berg's (1952, p.166) example of showing a guest around a town:

> ...one can learn to know another best by traveling with him through a country or by looking at a town with him. One who often shows the same town to different people will be struck by the ever new way in which this town appears in the conversation that is held about the sights during such a walk. These different ways are identical with the people with whom one walks, they are forms of subjectivity. The subject shows itself in the things...

Here, the significance of one's environment is not stolen by one's companion. The possibilities it offers are enriched by an experience of relating to him—new life is breathed into one's surroundings.[12] We do not live in a world of fixed possibilities; our relations with specific others reshape how things appear, sometimes fleetingly and sometimes in enduring ways. The interpersonal world is a dance of changing possibilities, some of which are experienced as 'mine', others as 'belonging to someone else', and others as 'ours', the three being inextricable. One retains an appreciation of the other person

---

[11] The view also has some empirical support. There is evidence to suggest that the experienced significance of entities depends, to a degree, on perception of what others are doing, and is influenced by factors such as their expression and direction of gaze. This effect is perceptual in nature, something we are unable to inhibit, and present from an early age (Gallagher, 2009, p.302).

[12] Leder (1990, p.94) offers a similar account of walking through a forest with a friend: 'we are cosubjectivities, supplementing rather than truncating each other's possibilities. I come to see the forest not only through my own eyes but as the Other sees it'. He calls this process 'mutual incorporation'. Such descriptions are complemented by work in developmental psychology. See, for example, Tronick et al. (1998) for the view that bodily, affective interaction between people can serve to somehow'expand' one's state of consciousness, a process that they claim is central to cognitive development.

as distinct from oneself and, with this, of certain possibilities being hers and others one's own. But the experience of *being with* that person also involves *our* having possibilities and our transforming a shared space of possibilities together. Elsewhere, van den Berg offers this observation:

> We all know people in whose company we would prefer not to go shopping, not to visit a museum, not to look at a landscape, because we would like to keep these things unharmed. Just as we all know people in whose company it is pleasant to take a walk because the objects encountered come to no harm. These people we call friends, good companions, loved ones. (1972, p.65)

Experience of our surroundings can vary considerably, depending on who we are with. It can be shaped by non-localized and pervasive feelings of discomfort, threat, vulnerability, openness, connectedness, ease, calm, safety, tension, or effortlessness. The other person need not say or do anything specific; the simple feeling of being with her can at the same time amount to enrichment or impoverishment of one's world. This feeling is not just a matter of connecting with other persons; it is an experience of connecting with them *as* persons.[13]

Given an emphasis on how we *affect* each other, it is clear that *interaction* between persons better exemplifies the structure of interpersonal experience than seemingly detached, unaffected contemplation of one party by another. Feelings of connectedness not only determine how we experience a person; they also shape how we interact with him. And these feelings can be enhanced or diminished, depending on how the interaction progresses. Several philosophers have emphasized that interpersonal understanding is not merely associated with interaction but somehow dependent on it (e.g. Gallagher, 2001; Hobson, 2002; Ratcliffe, 2007; de Jaegher and Di Paolo, 2007; Hutto, 2008). Although I am sympathetic to this emphasis, it should also be noted that the experience of interacting with another person need not be explicitly focused on him, or on the task of interpreting him. As indicated by van den Berg, it is often more a matter of how the *shared world* is experienced. There is a

---

[13] As Colombetti and Torrance (2009, p.509) observe, there is a 'basic level of feeling connected' to another person that characterises interpersonal relations, a feeling that varies in degree and quality. Others have pointed out that *feelings* of connectedness shape a child's relations with others from a very early age. To quote Trevarthen (1993, p.151), 'expressions of the self "invade" the mind of the other, making the moving body of the self resonant with impulses that can move the other's body too'. This, he says, remains the case in adult conversation, which 'is full of an immediate interpersonal vitality that goes beyond, or beneath, the words' (1993, p.159). For similar views, see Stern (1985), Hobson (1993, 2002), Gallagher (2005, 2009) and Reddy (2008).

non-localized feeling of being with someone, which continually shapes and re-shapes experience of one's surroundings when in his presence.[14]

A sense of others as persons is not constituted by interaction; we usually appreciate someone as a person before we initiate any kind of interaction with her. Even so, reflecting on the phenomenology of interaction can help illuminate experience of the personal. There are many kinds of interpersonal interaction. They do not just involve *different* ways of experiencing people; some involve *greater* receptivity to personhood than others. For instance, handing money to a cashier and saying 'thank you' does not involve the same level of personal engagement as looking into someone's eyes and sincerely saying 'I love you'. We can approach the structure of interpersonal experience by first identifying which interactions involve the most pronounced sense of the personal and then identifying what it is that distinguishes them. Appreciating someone as a person, I suggest, need not involve *actually* participating in the relevant relation. However, it does involve recognizing the *possibility* of doing so (along with that of entering into other relations that are comparatively lacking in one or another respect). To return to the earlier analogy, recognizing something as a cup need not involve actually drinking from it, but one would have no sense of what cups were if one did not recognize the possibility of drinking from them.

It has been suggested that *second-person* relations embody recognition of others as persons, to an extent that third-person 'I-she/he/it' relations do not (e.g. Gallagher, 2001). However, it is not enough to distinguish second-person interaction from third-person observation and to prioritize the former. First of all, some second-person interactions are rather impersonal compared to some third-person observations. Compare saying 'no thanks' to someone who attempts to sell you something on a busy street to watching one's child perform in a school nativity play. The former could amount to a habitual response involving almost no sense of interpersonal connection. One encounters a token of the generic social type 'salesperson', rather than a unique individual. In contrast, watching one's child perform involves both a strong feeling of connection

---

[14] See also Gallagher (2009) for a discussion of this distinction. He maintains that what de Jaegher and Di Paolo (2007) call 'participatory sense-making' is principally a matter of how we perceive our surroundings, whereas his own 'interaction theory' is concerned with how we understand and experience the other person, a distinction that de Jaegher and Di Paolo do not draw. That said, he also acknowledges that the two come together as a unitary process, where 'the presence of others calls forth a basic and implicit interaction that shapes the way that we regard the world around us' (2009, p.303). Indeed, I think the two are best construed phenomenologically as distinctive but inseparable aspects of a unitary experience.

and also a much greater sense of him as a specific individual, a 'who'. Unlike recognizing something as a coffee cup or a frog, an appreciation of being in the presence of a person is not just a matter of appreciating that a nearby entity belongs to one or another kind. In the cup or frog case, it does not usually make a difference that this is a particular cup or a particular frog; any individual would instantiate the kind equally well. Engaging with someone as a person is not like that. There is receptiveness to the fact that someone is a 'who', not just a 'what', which makes the experience quite different from that of encountering pragmatically indistinguishable particulars of whatever kind. So it does seem right to emphasize a certain *kind* of second-person relation, where one addresses a 'you' rather than scrutinizes a thing. However, we need to be more specific. Experience of the personal is not at its most pronounced in those second-person interactions where one is guarded, defensive, reserved, or uncomfortable, where one feels disconnected from the other person, or where she seems somehow lacking. We can also disregard those cases where an exchange is brief or regulated almost entirely by established social norms and roles.

In my view, a plausible description of the relation is offered by the Danish philosopher Knud Løgstrup (1956/1997).[15] He maintains, as I want to, that engaging with others as persons is principally a matter of being receptive to the fact that we have the potential to alter each other's world:

> By our very attitude to one another we help to shape one another's world. By our atti-tude to the other person we help to determine the scope and hue of his or her world; we make it large or small, bright or drab, rich or dull, threatening or secure. We help to shape his or her world not by theories and views but by our very attitude toward him or her. Here lies the unarticulated and one might say anonymous demand that we take care of the life which trust has placed in our hands. (1997, p.18)

He stresses that we have an unavoidable effect on others, as they do on us. Their gestures or expressions, however subtle, permeate us and influence our experience in ways that we cannot easily resist. It follows, Løgstrup says, that relating to someone as a person involves inescapable responsibility for her:

> A person never has something to do with another person without also having some degree of control over him or her. It may be a very small matter, involving only a passing mood, a dampening or quickening of spirit, a deepening or removal of some dislike. But it may also be a matter of tremendous scope, such as can determine if the life of the other flourishes or not. (1997, pp.15–16)

How does one 'shape' another's world? In referring to a world that can be large or small, threatening or secure, Løgstrup seems, like Sartre, to be refer-ring to the possibilities it offers. A felt sense of being with someone, which

---

[15] Thanks to Owen Earnshaw for pointing out to me the relevance of Løgstrup's work.

evolves as interaction progresses, is at the same time a change in the possibilities one's world offers. Specific possibilities might become more or less inviting—something that looked enticing before may appear less so now. But the phenomenological change is sometimes much more wide-ranging. Following an unpleasant encounter with someone, an air of threat or discomfort can pervade everything; the world as a whole takes on a different tone. Løgstrup's emphasis differs markedly from Sartre's. He identifies a kind of habitual, felt 'trust' as central to the interpersonal. Relating to someone as a person involves being open to the transformative possibilities she offers, rather than guarding against the possibility of one's world being harmed by her. The kind of trust in question is not a specifically directed attitude but a more general way of *finding oneself in the interpersonal world*:

> Trust is not of our own making; it is given. Our life is so constituted that it cannot be lived except as one person lays him or herself open to another person and puts her or himself into that person's hands either by showing or claiming trust. (1997, p.18)

For Løgstrup, a fully rich interpersonal relationship involves both mutual openness and a sense of mutual responsibility. It also involves at least a degree of vulnerability, as one could not be affected by someone in this sort of way without also rendering oneself more generally susceptible to her influence, to other kinds of relation. In addition, Løgstrup stresses that interpersonal relations do not reside in a social vacuum, freed from all norms and conventions. It is only against a backdrop of established norms that interactions can occur in a structured and secure fashion. Norms can facilitate evasion of interpersonal relations: one relates not to 'this person' but to 'this café waiter', in exactly the way that established norms prescribe. They also allow what Løgstrup describes as various 'perversions' of interpersonal relatedness, such as pleasing someone while avoiding an issue, indulging in mutual praise without any associated demands, and trying to change people without engaging with who they are. However, norms equally serve to regulate relationships, preventing a kind of affective over-exposure to each other: 'without the protection of the conventional norms, association with other people would be unbearable' (Løgstrup 1997, p.19).

I think something along these lines is broadly right. The vulnerability that Sartre focuses on is an aspect of the interpersonal but, as Løgstrup makes clear, there is a balance between this and an openness to self-transformative possibilities. And it is this balance that characterizes our richest engagement with others *as* persons. Our sense of being in the presence of a person consists in a felt receptiveness to the potential for engaging in a certain kind of relation, along with other kinds of relations that fall short of it in various ways.

I will now show how this view serves to make sense of changes in the structure of interpersonal experience that occur in depression, which centrally involve an inability to enter into exactly the kind of interpersonal relationship that Løgstrup describes.

Interpersonal Experience in Depression

Depression experiences generally involve a change in the overall structure of interpersonal experience. A common theme in almost every first-person account is the felt loss of interpersonal connection:

> Each person's tale of depression inevitably speaks to questions of isolation, withdrawal, and lack of connection. The pain of depression arises in part because of separation from others; from an inability to connect, even as one desperately yearns for just such connection. (Karp, 1996, pp.26–7)

The problem is not one of *actually* failing to connect with however many people, perhaps even everyone. Rather, a kind of interpersonal connection that many of us take for granted seems *impossible*, absent from the world. This is closely related to the more general theme of being trapped, imprisoned, cut off from the rest of the world by some impenetrable substance:

> I couldn't feel anything for [my husband]. I couldn't feel anything for the children. It was like being inside a very, very thick balloon and no matter how hard I pushed out, the momentum of the skin of the balloon would just push me back in. So I couldn't touch anybody, I couldn't touch anything.[16]

Impaired interpersonal relations are not an 'effect' of depression experiences but absolutely central to them. So it is a mistake to suggest, as the DSM does, that depression is merely 'accompanied' by 'impairment in social, occupational, or other important areas of functioning' (DSM 5, p.163). With the possibility of interpersonal connection gone from experience, the world no longer includes certain kinds of self-transformative possibility. It is diminished, closed, and static—one's current situation is no longer experienced as contingent, susceptible to certain kinds of change. This is why, in just about every autobiographical account, the theme of isolation in some inescapable and unchanging realm is tied up with that of being estranged from others. There are two general forms that the experience can take:

1. One retains the sense of what it would be to connect with others but feels unable to do so. This is attributable to a loss of enticement (one no longer

---

[16] Interview excerpt from healthtalkonline.org, available at: <http://healthtalkonline. org/peoples-experiences/mental-health/depression/experiencing-depression>. Last accessed 7 May 2014.

feels drawn into interpersonal situations, able to interact with others in the required way), to a sense of other people as somehow threatening (which blocks interaction even when one still feels drawn to seek out others), or to a combination of the two.

2. A more profound form of loss, where the sense of what it is to connect with others in a personal way is eroded or gone. They seem curiously distant and impersonal, an experience that is also compatible with their being threatening.

In both scenarios, a loss of interpersonal possibilities is inseparable from a more general shift in the kinds of possibility offered by the world. When one's current situation appears threatening and/or no longer enticing, an enduring sense of being able to connect with others, and thus of there being self-transformative possibilities, contributes to one's appreciation of that situation as contingent. So the difference between losing a system of enticing possibilities and altogether losing that *kind* of possibility is partly attributable to a change in the structure of interpersonal experience. The same applies to losses of significance. When one's situation lacks certain kinds of significance, the prospect of relating to others implies that of potential change, and so the absence of significance is experienced as contingent. However, if others cease to 'draw one in' or appear only in the guise of threat, that kind of change is experienced as impossible. The most profound form of loss is when an absence of significant possibilities from experience includes distinctively *interpersonal* possibilities. Here, one loses a sense of what it would even be to enter into a self-transformative relation with someone else. In all these cases, the relationship between loss of possibilities and erosion of interpersonal connection is one of mutual implication. Lack of access to certain kinds of possibility could not occur without an associated change in the structure of interpersonal experience, and vice versa. They are different aspects of a unitary way of 'finding oneself in the world'. I will first address some of those experiences that involve threat and loss of enticement, after which I will turn to more profound forms of privation.

What depressed people often describe is not just the absence of interpersonal connection. There is also a painful *feeling* of absence, a felt need for something that at the same time presents itself as unobtainable:

A paradox of depression is that sufferers yearn for connection, seem bereft because of their isolation, and yet are rendered incapable of being with others in a comfortable way. [...] Much of depression's pain arises out of the recognition that what might make me feel better—human connection—seems impossible in the midst of a paralyzing episode of depression. It is rather like dying from thirst while looking at a glass of water just beyond one's reach. (Karp, 1996, pp.14–16)

We can understand this in the following way: The person still anticipates experiencing the possibility of interpersonal connection when in the presence of certain others, and she 'needs' this kind of connection, as her world is impoverished without it. However, whenever she encounters another person, the kind of relatedness she anticipates and/or needs is not experienced as possible. Indeed, it may be experienced *as* impossible—the world appears as a place from which it is altogether gone. The feeling of global estrangement is thus constituted by retention of an anticipatory structure, but without any prospect of fulfilment. So we have a reversal of Sartre's claim that the other is the 'death of my possibilities'. Other people do not just offer the potential to take away my possibilities. The world is experienced as a dynamic space of significant and enticing possibilities in virtue of our potential and actual relations with them. One's sense of the possible is in fact eroded by a *lack* of access to what Sartre describes in terms of possibility-death.[17]

The sense of being cut-off from others and unmoved by them concerns certain *kinds* of interpersonal relation, those involving emotional communion, effortless conversation, and the like. Other kinds of interpersonal possibility, such as that of being threatened, may remain. As discussed in Chapters 4 to 7, many depressed people describe an all-encompassing sense of threat or impending doom, something that is often more specifically interpersonal in character. All that others are perceived to offer is a distinctively *personal* form of threat, which might be experienced more specifically as derision, dismissal, ridicule, condemnation, aggression, or shame. Hence, although some losses of interpersonal possibility in depression are to be contrasted with Sartrean possibility-death, the two occur together in other cases. Loss of interpersonal connection drains the world of its openness, while a sense that others offer only harm adds to an experience of meaningful action, positive change, and hope as absent from the world.

Many first-person accounts repeatedly mention feelings of being vulnerable, exposed, threatened, or unsafe. For example: 'A law clerk friend invited me to a party one Saturday night, and I went. The noise and bright social talk were almost physically painful. Standing in that crowded room holding a beer, I felt like some poor creature that had been boiled and peeled' (Thompson, 1995, pp.231–2). Such experiences are similar, in some respects, to something

---

[17] Despite Sartre's emphasis on others as threatening rather than enabling, he does seem to recognise that they are a source of possibility too, as exemplified by his remark that 'to die is to lose all possibility of revealing oneself as subject to an Other' (1989, p.297). In fact, as noted in Chapter 2, depressed people sometimes describe the experience as akin to a living death.

that R.D. Laing (1960) describes in connection with paranoid schizophrenia. Laing remarks on how 'in psychotic conditions the gaze or scrutiny of the other can be experienced as an actual penetration into the core of the "inner" self' (p.113). He quotes one patient as saying, 'I can't go on. You are arguing in order to have the pleasure of triumphing over me. At best you win an argument. At worst you lose an argument. *I am arguing to preserve my existence*' (p.45). Here, the more usual experience of mutual influence is replaced by one-way influence from other to self, and the openness-vulnerability balance is tipped towards an extreme: there is only vulnerability, with nothing to counter it. The other person does indeed become the death of one's possibilities, an existential threat before which one is passive and defenceless. In such a case, there is also a diminished sense of others as persons. They are reduced to their roles in conveying threat, and *who* someone is becomes of little consequence. Laing further observes that, more usually, the experience of being perceived by someone else is not a matter of threat; it is something that human existence requires:

> The need to be perceived is not, of course, purely a visual affair. It extends to the general need to have one's presence endorsed or confirmed by the other, the need for one's total existence to be recognized; the need, in fact, to be loved. (p.128)

Consequently, if one cuts oneself off from others in order to escape from the feeling of being threatened, one loses a life-affirming connectedness in the process.[18] Although depression experiences sometimes have a similar structure, what people describe is usually less extreme. The depressed person retains a sense of what it would be to connect with others, a possibility that cannot be actualized because they offer only threat, whereas the experience described by Laing also involves loss of the sense that people could offer anything other than threat. Furthermore, depression experiences are often not quite so passive. Some first-person accounts also describe feelings of hostility, which may be directed at specific others or others in general.[19] The theme is not so prominent in many published memoirs (perhaps because it

---

[18] One might worry that the experience Laing describes is partly or wholly an artefact of his own interpretations. But such concerns are, in my view, unwarranted. People with schizophrenia diagnoses sometimes describe exactly this kind of change in the structure of interpersonal experience. See Ratcliffe and Broome (2012) for a discussion. Laing is not the only one to have applied a Sartrean approach to the phenomenology of schizophrenia. See, for example, Lysaker, Johannesen, and Lysaker (2005, pp. 343–344).

[19] See Csordas (2013) for an interesting discussion of the close connection between depression and anger in the depression experiences of some adolescents.

is unpalatable to readers and/or authors), but feelings of anger, resentment, and suspicion are more conspicuous in other accounts, including many DQ responses:

> #158. To paraphrase Sarah Kane 'depression is anger, it's where you are and who you're blaming and I'm blaming myself'. It's very much anger and distress turned inwards, a constant battle with your own mind. It's rarely rational and always destructive.[20]

There is something right about Freud's account in the famous essay 'Mourning and Melancholia' (an account that he does not intend to apply to all experiences of 'melancholia', just those that involve guilt and self-loathing). In brief, Freud suggests that there is a 'splitting' of the ego, whereby one becomes both the subject and the object of criticism. He makes the more general observation that self-reproach often amounts to a veiled criticism of others: the woman who pities her husband for putting up with her is actually criticizing him (2005, p.208). Drawing on this, he proposes that melancholia involves losing a 'love object', finding oneself unable to direct one's ambivalent and negative emotions towards that object, and re-directing them at oneself. The self becomes a simulacrum of the other, and revenge takes the form of self-torment. What this gets right is the close connection between hostility towards others and hostility towards oneself. Some first-person accounts emphasize the former, some the latter, and others both. And, regardless of whether negative attitudes are explicitly directed at self or other, they often implicate both: I am worthless/you see me as worthless; I am guilty/you judge me; I am hurt/you have hurt me; I am alone/you have abandoned me. Nevertheless, there are two broad (although admittedly overlapping) kinds of experience, one where the hostility is turned inwards and another where it is turned outwards. Both, I suggest, arise in the context of having lost what Løgstrup calls interpersonal 'trust'. One feels passive, incapable, vulnerable, and threatened. Encounters with other people no longer offer the possibility of change for the better. There is only the prospect of their further eroding one's already impoverished sense of belonging. The experience is not specific to however many individuals; one experiences others only in the guise of potential danger. Even so, one might continue to *anticipate* the possibility of other kinds of interpersonal relation.

When this kind of interpersonal experience occurs in conjunction with feeling unable to act, when enticing possibilities are lost but things are still recognized as personally and interpersonally significant, others may be

---

[20] The reference is to Sarah Kane's play *4.48 Psychosis* (Kane, 2000).

experienced as disapproving voyeurs of one's failings. In another type of case, the possibility of encountering anything as enticing is gone from experience *because* the world offers only threat, a threat that takes on a more specifically interpersonal form. Here, others are more likely to be experienced as the problem, the source of one's alienation. Faced with a sense of all-enveloping threat and vulnerability, the person seeks comfort from others but finds, in every instance, that they fail to offer what she seeks, what she needs, what they ought to offer. Thus, whether negative emotional attitudes are self-directed or other-directed is partly symptomatic of a depression experience's existential structure. To return to a theme of Chapter 5, it is likely that differences in emphasis are also attributable in part to how an existential change (which is not fully determinate in this respect) is interpreted. The person feels alienated from others, unable to relate to them, and she also feels lacking in some way. But whether this is then construed, and indeed experienced, in terms of her own shortcomings or theirs is to some degree contingent. So what Freud says is right, to the extent that some depression experiences involve self-directed negative emotions that could just as well be directed at others, but the underlying structure of the experience does not take the form of an implicit revenge strategy. Instead, one or another determinate interpretation progressively coagulates out of an existential feeling, and may then serve to further shape that feeling. Moreover, it is not always the case that negative emotions are either directed at the self *or* at others. Self-directed and other-directed attitudes of much the same kind frequently co-exist, with first-person narratives vacillating between the two.

In Chapter 4, I suggested that many depression experiences involve a weakening of existential trust. What I described was not exclusively interpersonal but wider-ranging. However, interpersonal trust has an important role to play in the sustenance and repair of trust more generally. Other people offer self-transformative possibilities, including that of changing one's sense of what various situations offer so as to rekindle feelings of safety, of being at home in the world. In many cases of depression, the possibility of entering into such relations is absent from experience. Either the possibility of calling for help is gone or it remains but presents itself as unanswerable. The sense that others offer only threat is therefore inextricable from a more pervasive feeling of being unsafe, of there being nothing one can or ever could depend upon. Regardless of whether the depressed person emphasizes her own failings or those of others, the common underlying structure often involves loss of the kind of trust described by Løgstrup. A tipping of the trust-vulnerability balance towards vulnerability gives interpersonal experience a different structure, one that is inseparable from the more general way in which one 'finds oneself in the world':

> #21. I can feel very paranoid and unsafe, like I'm on the verge of being attacked, mocked, the subject of any kind of negative attention.

> #45. When I'm depressed I feel like my relationships are less stable and I trust others a lot less. I try to avoid people, as they seem angry and irritated at me, and like they don't want me around. I feel like a burden to others and don't want to cause anyone unnecessary distress.

> #66. The world appears to be a frightening place full of people who are bad and threatening.

> #150. I withdraw from people when I'm ill and feel an outcast but even when I'm better I feel an outcast because it's always there and [I] find it hard to trust people enough to let my guard down.

> #179. I find it extremely difficult to trust anyone; it feels like they have all 'guessed' there is something wrong with me and now they are all conspiring to get me 'sorted out' i.e. remove me from normal society so that I don't affect everyone around me with my awful, scary madness.

The themes of estrangement, vulnerability and fear often feature alongside a continuing need for other people:

> #21. I feel very separate from people, fearing that if I talk about how I'm feeling they'll reject or disapprove of me. And yet, on the flipside of that, I can become very clingy and over-reliant on people, particularly my boyfriend, and fear that without him I'll somehow disappear. Seeing people becomes a huge chore, so I avoid friends, but then get upset when I'm not invited to things, feeling rejected and left out.

A feeling of being incapable, when combined with alienation from others and a sense of them as disapproving or threatening, is sometimes experienced as guilt. However, the theme of being 'worthless' or 'burdensome' is usually more prominent. The word 'burden' appears in many first-person accounts, often repeatedly: 'I feel like I'm being a burden and that they only put up with me because they feel they have to' (#107). This 'feeling of being a burden' can also be expressed in terms of other people's attitudes. That 'I am a burden to them' also says something about their treatment of me:

> #53. I feel like family members are angry with me when I'm depressed. When I think about it when I'm not depressed, I realize they are probably not—they are just concerned and frustrated. But when I'm depressed I feel like people blame me. I also feel like people don't take me seriously when I'm depressed, and like people dislike me and are secretly talking about me.

> #106. My family and friends don't show me support. They think I'm just lazy and I should pull myself together.

In some such cases, it may be that the depressed person's assessment of others' attitudes towards her is largely accurate. But regardless of what others actually say and do, they will be interpreted as unsupportive, and this is because they are *experienced* as unsupportive. They no longer offer the kinds of possibility that the person seeks. Those possibilities are gone from the interpersonal world. Consequently, people *look* unsupportive. Some first-person accounts describe feeling more specifically 'paranoid', an experience that is to be understood in the same way. Others appear to behave in ways that cannot be sincere, as they are no longer experienced as offering the kinds of possibility that would be associated with honest expressions of support and concern. In the absence of those possibilities, their well-meaning utterances can only appear disingenuous. The depressed person may then start to wonder what their real agenda is, and the options she considers are constrained by the possibility space she already inhabits:

> #124. I become paranoid. People don't like me, I'm a burden, they become patronizing because they know I can't cope. When they care, it's because they have to—and their happiness always seems to be in spite of me, never because of me, and I know I get in their way. Those I don't see often feel like they're from a different life and they're moving quicker than me. They're effort. They're intense.

> #129. People in general seem more hostile and uncaring when I am depressed and more likely to make fun of me or criticize me.

> #166. I think people are just being nice to me out of guilt or obligation. I take offence at random comments and see these as purposeful digs at me because I am inadequate and they're getting annoyed with me. Any or most attempts to be nice to me are assumed to be false and lies. Pity or some perceived obligation to tolerate me.

> #168. I feel like they're talking about me and planning and having fun behind my back and not including me because I'm horrible.

Although a range of specifically focused perceptions and evaluative judgments are at play in such cases, they arise in the context of global changes in the structure of interpersonal experience, changes that vary in structure. Even without the trust required to initiate and regulate interpersonal encounters, one might still need others, and continually seek out something that repeatedly presents itself as impossible. Alternatively, the sense that certain kinds of possibility cannot be actualized may be so pronounced that the prospect of achieving interpersonal connection seems utterly futile. One therefore retreats from the social world, even though some sense of what it would be to connect with others remains, along with a profound feeling of isolation. In both scenarios, the inability to connect can take the form of 'blockage', where one retains a sense of certain kinds of relational possibility but finds oneself unable to actualize them because others offer only threat. However, there can also be loss of enticement without threat. The person seeks out others but they fail to draw her in, to solicit the kind of interaction she seeks. So she feels cut off from them, but not because of other kinds of possibility that they do offer. And, where the loss of interpersonal enticement is especially profound, she will no longer seek out interpersonal connection. The possibility of looking for something is gone from the world, as well as that of actually finding it. Hence there is considerable variety. In fact, one way of thinking about interpersonal experience in depression is to consider all of those ways in which one might feel estranged from a particular individual or alone in his presence: shame; guilt; vulnerability; detachment; discomfort; lack of any shared, meaningful context; unworthiness. Then imagine a world where other people in general offer only one or another combination of these experiences.

The kinds of interpersonal experience that I have so far described also involve some degree of what Fuchs (2001) calls 'desynchronization' (discussed in Chapter 7). There is a pronounced awareness of lacking something that others have, of being detached from a social world where they go about their business, interacting effortlessly with each other:

> #22. It seems like everyone is having an amazing time and you're the one missing out. It's so easy to beat yourself up and think there's something wrong with you. It feels like no one else has ever experienced anything like this before, like you're all on your own.

> #41. [The lives of other people] are just going on while mine has stagnated.

> #112. I feel like the world is happening around me and I am standing still, almost like in a haze.

> #231. It feels as though I am on a small ice floe drifting away from the main floe.

However, the category 'major depression' also includes other, more profound privations of interpersonal experience. These involve a diminished sense that there *are* other people and, by implication, a less pronounced feeling of being 'cut off from other people'. Rather than anticipating or at least recognizing possibility *p* but feeling unable to actualize it, appreciation of what it is to experience *p* is gone. One loses a sense of what it would even be to participate in certain kinds of interpersonal relation, something that impacts upon one's experience of others *as* persons. I described a variant of this in Chapter 5, where others are bereft of their particularity and appear as nothing more than generic judges of one's guilt. Some expressions of 'feeling worthless' similarly point to a diminished sense of others as persons. Sometimes, others are mentioned only in their role as voyeurs of one's own worthlessness, and are described in an oddly generic way. It does not matter 'who' another person is, if all she can offer is the same kind of condemnation offered by everyone else. So there is a notable paucity of references to particular individuals and their attitudes; 'friends and family' become part of an undifferentiated 'they':

> #280. They seem distant, inaccessible, critical, hostile. I find it much harder to understand their points of view and they seem to struggle to understand mine. I look at friends and family in a different way. Because I don't understand how they could possibly like somebody I hate so much (me), I feel like I am a burden to them. I also feel that seeing them is in a way a burden on me. It feels too overwhelming to be around others with my distress and like a chore to attempt to be sociable or hide how I'm feeling and if I don't hide how I'm feeling I feel intense guilt for putting it on them. I feel lonely if I withdraw but it feels hard to be around people.[21]

Though diminished experience of others as persons may involve guilt or worthlessness before a generic other, there are other cases where threat and vulnerability are absent but others still seem oddly distant and impersonal; they 'look' different from how they once did. Minkowski (1970, pp.329–330) quotes this account by a patient suffering from some form of depression:

> When I go out, the men that I see give me the impression of being phantoms. When I hear their voices, I am surprised that they are able to speak. I am astonished, and I admire others' ability to do things. [...] I have the feeling of being alone. Conversation with someone seems to me something from far away, airy, intangible. My words no longer correspond to my thought. I am condemned not to be understood.

Here, there is also association between a loss of felt connection with others and an impaired sense of their being persons, but the estrangement does not take the more specific form of guilt or worthlessness.

Throughout this chapter, I have emphasized changes in the 'structure of interpersonal experience', which affect how everyone is experienced. However, this is not to imply that all others are experienced in exactly the same way. More usually, how we experience and relate to particular individuals varies considerably. For example, how one relates to one's child is quite different from how one might relate to a work colleague. In some experiences of postpartum depression, the world and other people (and perhaps oneself too) are experienced as a threat not principally to the mother but to

---

[21] The questionnaire response I have quoted from contains 3100 words of testimony (not including background information), 21 references to a generic 'them', 'they', 'other people' or 'others', and no references at all to particular individuals or to differences between people. The author stated that she was depressed at the time of writing. She also described experiences of self-hate, self-loathing, guilt, and despair, along with a pronounced sense of the pointlessness of human existence.

her baby. How she relates to her baby is therefore quite different from how she relates to other people. The baby is experienced as utterly vulnerable and dependent upon her, a source of emotional and practical demands that present themselves as impossible to fulfil (Røseth, Binder, and Malt, 2011).[22] More generally, a parent might experience the majority of people as a source of threat, while her own children are experienced as demanding a kind of affective response and style of interaction that she is unable to offer them. So I concede that there is more to be said here. Even so, such experiences can be understood in the same general way—there is still a change in the overall structure of interpersonal experience, albeit one that might affect different kinds of interpersonal relation in different ways. The kinds of interpersonal experience that arise in existential forms of depression are all consistent with Sartre's view that our sense of others as persons has a bodily, felt phenomenology and is at the same time a sense of the possible. They also suggest that a fully rich experience of the personal approximates the kind of relation described by Løgstrup, insofar as anything that departs from it diminishes one's sense of the personal. Hence the interpersonal phenomenology of depression can be plausibly interpreted in terms of the view that a sense of others as persons consists primarily in an appreciation of the potential to enter into a kind of self-transformative relation with them, involving a balance of openness and vulnerability.

What I have described here are not simply different 'types' of existential depression; they also relate to each other in dynamic ways. Take the following description:

> #277. When I start to get depressed, I only filter through the negative messages from friends and family, so even the most benign comment can be perceived as an insult. As a result, they soon learn to step on egg shells around me, they become less affectionate because I'm less receptive to it and it generally compounds the situation. There have been a couple of exceptions to this, and they are the ones who have seen me through the worst of my depression. They are the ones who are there no matter what and are able to see that the negative reactions I have are not a reflection of how I feel about them, but rather a reflection of my inner state of self-loathing. It's a very hard thing to do to be able to step back and realize that someone who is depressed is projecting their own thoughts onto others, but in my opinion, it is one of the most amazing gifts that one can give to someone feeling that way.

---

[22] However, experiences of postpartum depression are as heterogeneous as depression experiences more generally. Beck (2002, p.462) surveys twenty qualitative studies of postpartum depression and remarks that 'postpartum depression can be likened to a chameleon. It takes on a different appearance depending on which specific mother is experiencing it'.

Remarks such as this indicate that how other people react to a depression experience has the potential to shape that experience, to exacerbate or alleviate it. The sense that others are hostile and uncaring can become a self-fulfilling prophecy. On the other hand, certain kinds of response might still be experienced as supportive. That others *appear* incapable of moving one in certain ways does not imply that they actually *are*. It is likely that different forms of depression experience are interpersonally permeable to varying degrees and in different ways.[23] The question therefore arises as to when, how, and to what extent interpersonal interactions of whatever kind might serve to reanimate the world and restore access to kinds of interpersonal possibility. To reiterate the conclusion of Chapter 5, phenomenological distinctions between forms of depression experience that would otherwise remain undifferentiated can help us to address such questions more clearly. Furthermore, as I will show in Chapter 9, an existential understanding of the varieties of depression experience can be integrated into an empathetic process.

---

[23] See also Aho and Guignon (2011) for a discussion of how therapy can involve a 'dialogical interplay' that opens up new possibilities for a person. A person is not, they say, an 'encapsulated center of experience', but intrinsically intersubjective, relational. They focus specifically on the role of changing linguistic self-interpretations. However, what they say is consistent with my emphasis on felt, bodily, self-affecting interaction. The two are closely associated and can shape each other.

Chapter 9

Depression and Empathy

I have suggested that an understanding of the existential changes involved in depression has the potential to inform psychiatric classification, diagnosis, and treatment. However, the project of distinguishing one or more 'types' of experience is distinct from that of understanding what a particular person is experiencing. The former seeks something generally applicable, while the latter attends to something specific: 'your experience', which is 'yours alone'. In this chapter, I offer an account of how phenomenological insights can be applied when engaging with someone's experience in its particularity, something that can proceed with or without categorizing it in terms of one or another psychiatric type. In other words, I am concerned with how phenomenology feeds into *empathy*. As we saw in Chapter 8, depressed people often feel that others do not or cannot empathize with them. By asking what exactly it is that they take to be lacking, we can better understand the nature of empathy. This then assists us in addressing the question of whether and how it is possible to empathize with depression, regardless of whether or not one's empathy is recognized as such.

Building on the account of interpersonal experience developed in Chapter 8, I argue that empathy is not—contrary to popular belief—a matter of 'simulating' another person's experience. It involves being open to varying degrees and kinds of interpersonal difference, rather than attempting to eliminate those differences by experiencing what the other person experiences in the same way that she does. Openness to phenomenological difference, of a kind that is inseparable from a distinctive kind of second-person attitude, is necessary for empathy and sufficient for some empathetic achievements. It can also serve as the starting point for a variably collaborative exploratory process that enables more sophisticated empathetic achievements. I further propose that adoption of a 'phenomenological stance' facilitates openness to kinds of experiential difference that would otherwise be misinterpreted or pass unnoticed, thus allowing empathy with existential forms of depression. Hence, although phenomenology is not to be identified with empathy (empathy is person-specific in a way that phenomenology need not be), its integration into a second-person attitude amounts to a distinctive form of empathy.

The aim of the chapter is not to prescribe a particular approach to therapy, and my account is quite consistent with what many therapists—of various different persuasions—are already doing. Nevertheless, there are potential implications for practice. Even though one might think that one is doing *p* when one is actually doing *q*, how one conceives of the nature and role of empathy in therapy is likely to have at least some influence on how one actually practices therapy. And any attempt to empathize with depression will be misguided to the extent that it takes first-person replication of the depressed person's experience as its goal.

The Nature of Empathy

A problem we face when trying to describe what it is to 'empathize' with depression is that that our subject matter is unclear—empathy is conceived of in a number of different ways. Empathy differs from both emotional contagion and sympathy, as it involves experiencing something of what another person experiences while recognizing that experience as hers. Emotional contagion involves experiencing the same thing as someone else but without attributing it to him, while sympathy is a response to someone else's experience rather than an experience of it. Given this initial characterization, it might seem obvious what empathy is. It is surely a matter of 'replication' or 'simulation'. You have a first-person experience that is to some degree isomorphic with that of another person, one that is somehow caused by his experience. Then you attribute an experience of that kind to him. Some have added that empathy further involves 'care' for the other person, which rules out counter-intuitive examples such as experiencing someone else's pain and then finding it hilariously funny (e.g. De Vignemont and Jacob, 2012).

Most recent philosophical discussions of empathy arise in relation to the debate between 'theory' and 'simulation' theories of interpersonal understanding (introduced in Chapter 8). Empathy is presumed to be a matter of simulation, and so attention focuses on the extent to which our understanding of others relies on this instead of (or alongside) application of a theory: how central is empathy/simulation to social cognition? Some simulation theorists simply identify 'simulation' with 'empathy', as though there were no alternative. For example, Goldman (2006, p.17) refers to the 'simulation (or empathy) theory', and Stueber (2006, p.4) similarly assumes that empathy is simulation. As noted in Chapter 8, a distinction is often drawn between explicit and implicit simulation, where the former involves applying conscious effort to replicate some aspect of another person's psychology, whereas the latter relies on non-conscious mechanisms and need not involve any awareness of the process.[1] So a distinction is similarly made between two kinds of empathy. We have what Stueber (2006, pp.20–21) calls 'basic empathy', where one perceives, for example, that someone is angry without knowingly simulating her emotional state. There is also what he calls 're-enactive empathy', where cognitive resources are consciously deployed to reconstruct the person's experience, enabling a more sophisticated appreciation of her mental life and behaviour. De Vignemont (2010) and Goldman (2011) draw much the same distinction, using the terms 'mirror empathy' or 'mirroring' and 'reconstructive empathy'.

However, this identification of empathy with simulation is questionable, and work in the phenomenological tradition by Scheler, Husserl, Stein, and others points to a different conception. As Zahavi (2010, p.291) puts it, empathy is instead construed as 'a basic, irreducible, form of intentionality that is directed towards the experiences of others'. In other words, 'empathizing' is comparable to 'perceiving', 'remembering', and 'believing'; it is a type of intentional state in its own right, a *second-person* experience of mental states that differs in kind from first-person experience. It is therefore a mistake to regard first-person access to experience as the sole mode of access. When we perceive the behaviour of others, we experience something of their experience *in* their behaviour. In doing so, we continue to encounter that experience *as theirs*, and thus in a different way to how we would if it were our own. Scheler (1954) advocates such a position, although he does not refer to the relevant accomplishment as 'empathy'. We also find it in Stein (1917/1989), whose account I will focus on here.

Stein uses the term 'empathy' to refer to all 'acts in which foreign experience is comprehended' (1989, p.6). She stresses that it is not a matter of having the same feeling as someone else and then attributing the feeling to him. From the outset, one experiences the feeling *as* his. There is a 'two-sidedness' to empathy: we have an experience of our own that 'announces' another experience as someone else's (p.19). Interestingly, Stein explicitly states that empathy is *never* a matter of simulating a mental state and then projecting it onto someone else. She acknowledges that we sometimes do this, but claims that we only resort to it when empathy fails. Suppose we were unable to experience a joyful person as joyful. We could still come to appreciate her joy via the indirect route of imaginatively putting

---

[1] Non-conscious or 'sub-personal' matching processes in the brain are, according to some accounts, ubiquitous. They occur whenever we perceive another person's behaviour and facilitate a quasi-perceptual appreciation of behaviour as expressive of experience. The discovery of so-called 'mirror neurons' is frequently cited as evidence. For further discussion of mirror neurons, see Ratcliffe (2007, Chapter 5).

ourselves in her position, experiencing joy ourselves and then attributing it to her. But then we never experience the joy as *her joy*. Instead, we experience *our own joy* and take her to be having an experience of the same type. What is missing is an experience of her joy, in its particularity. Stein is equally clear that empathy is not a 'feeling of oneness' or a matter of 'emotional contagion'. It essentially involves encountering someone else's experience *as theirs*, and thus maintains a distinction between self and other (pp. 14–23).

We might wonder how experience could be *perceived* in behaviour. For Stein, at least part of the answer is that experience and its expression are inextricable: 'Feeling in its pure essence is not something complete in itself. As it were, it is loaded with an energy which must be unloaded' (p.51). So, in perceiving the expression, you do perceive something of the feeling.[2] The term 'perception', as it is used here and also in the work of others who endorse this kind of approach, is perhaps unhelpful. Granted, there is an absence of conscious inference from observed behaviour—one simply *experiences* the behaviour as meaningful. However, whether this qualifies as 'perception', of the same kind as 'sensory perception', hinges on what we take sensory perceptual content to consist of. Phenomenological claims to the effect that we 'perceive' or 'directly perceive' experience in behaviour (e.g. Zahavi, 2010; 2011) would therefore benefit from engagement with debates in the philosophy of mind concerning the nature of perception and the kinds of content that specifically 'perceptual' experiences can have.

There is also a tension involved in taking empathy to be a *sui generis* form of intentionality and, at the same time, a kind of perception. If it is perceptual, then it is not a type of intentional state in its own right, and vice versa. Without further qualification, all the appeal to perception amounts to is the claim that empathy involves experiencing something of what someone else experiences without recourse to conscious inference from behavioural observation. And this is too permissive to be informative. I can 'perceive' that someone on a bicycle is 'heading somewhere', that she is engaged in goal-directed behaviour, and I can 'perceive' that someone is happy on the basis of a passing glance in the street. As these examples suggest, perceiving experience in behaviour need not amount to *second-person* experience. One can adopt a detached, third-person perspective towards someone and still 'see' something of her mental life. Indeed, all interpersonal encounters would seem to include some degree of 'empathy'.

A further problem for the view is a lack of clarity regarding the content of empathetic experience. Empathy at least involves recognizing another

---

[2] We find much the same view in Scheler (1954, pp.10–11).

person *as* a locus of experience and agency. This does not imply a more specific appreciation of *what* she experiences, but Stein maintains that it includes this as well (at least sometimes): we can experience another person as happy, sad, or scared. Even so, it is arguable that empathy, as conceived of by Stein, is restricted to a fairly shallow understanding of experience. Appealing to Scheler and Stein, Zahavi (2007, p.37) describes empathy as 'an ability to experience behaviour as expressive of mind'. But an emphasis on what we can experience in someone's behaviour, even when stripped of references to 'perception', seems to rule out more sophisticated empathetic achievements. There is much that we do not experience in this way. For example, we might experience someone as angry, but the content of our experience is less likely to include *what* she is angry about or *why* she is angry about it, unless the cause is a salient feature of her current environment and/or we draw upon prior knowledge in a way that is to be distinguished from our *experience* of her behaviour.

It might be argued that what some phenomenologists call 'empathy' can be identified with 'basic empathy', a perceptual or quasi-perceptual appreciation of others' experience that is enabled by sub-personal simulation. So there is nothing here that the simulationist has failed to accommodate. However, that *x* is involved in process *y* does not imply that *x* is responsible for those features of *y* that make *y* distinctive. Even if non-conscious matching processes are at play in empathy, appealing to them does not aid our understanding of what is most central to empathy as construed by Scheler, Stein, and Zahavi: experiencing someone else's experience *as* belonging to her. There is an important difference between empathy, conceived of as a type of attitude *towards* others, and a conception that appeals to the non-conscious replication of *x* generating a perceptual or perception-like experience of *x*. In my view, the central insight of phenomenological approaches is not that we 'perceive' someone else's experience in her behaviour but that empathy involves a distinctive kind of attitude towards another person, a kind of 'second-person experience'. This is more specific than the claim that we experience mental life in behaviour, something that applies to even the most fleeting of third-person encounters. The simulationist could respond that what makes certain 'second-person' experiences distinctive is the more sophisticated appreciation of experience that comes with them, something that arises when explicit simulation is brought into play. When we adopt a 'second-person stance' towards someone, we often think 'what is it like for you?' and use simulation to find out. But I will suggest that, as with the appeal to implicit simulation, this misses the point. Empathy is qualitatively different from any combination of simulation routines; its principal constituent is a distinctive kind of *attentiveness* towards another person, towards a 'you'.

I do not deny that we sometimes 'replicate' others' mental states in the first-person (consciously and perhaps non-consciously too, and with varying degrees of success) when trying to understand them. That would be phenomenologically implausible. It is often easier to empathize with someone when you have been through a similar experience yourself, as with experiences such as profound grief. Furthermore, an appreciation of what that person is experiencing can be enhanced by 'reliving'—to an extent—one's own past experiences, and also by imaginative exercises that draw on first-person experience. Although replication (conscious or otherwise) is not sufficient for the kind of engagement with someone else's experience that Stein describes, it can at least contribute to it. In fact, Stein (1989, p.6) is non-committal over *how* empathetic experience is generated; she is concerned instead with *what* it consists of. So her approach accommodates the possibility that some empathetic experiences are generated by cognitive processes, rather than in a 'perception-like' or 'quasi-perceptual' way, and therefore allows for empathetic experiences with more elaborate contents. Furthermore, I see no reason to rule out cognitive elaboration of an empathetic experience that leaves its second-person structure intact.

Hence, in response to the view that reconstructive or re-enactive empathy consists of explicit simulation, it can be argued that some 'reconstructions' are not adequately characterized in terms of first-person simulation followed by projection onto another person. They are embedded from the outset in a distinctive kind of attitude. So we seem to arrive at a 'hybrid' account of empathy, according to which people sometimes rely on explicit simulation, and perhaps implicit simulation too, but in the context of an attitude that is directed towards the other person.[3] Without that attitude, simulation does not amount to empathy, as the experience is not other-directed. However, I think this concedes too much to simulation. Some empathetic achievements are no doubt enabled, in part, by explicit simulation, and some may even be partly constituted by it. The distinction between enablement and constitution can be a difficult one to draw, and I will not attempt to do so here. But what

---

[3] Gordon (e.g. 1995, p.55) offers an account of what he calls 'radical simulation', which is fairly close to this. For Gordon, one does not imagine what one would do in someone else's situation; one imagines what *that person* would do, something that requires an experienced 'egocentric shift' to *her* perspective upon the world. However, Gordon construes this shift as a relocation of the first-person perspective from oneself to the other person, and I am concerned with something different: a second-person appreciation of her experience as hers, which does not require resignation of one's first-person perspective. Even if the kind of feat described by Gordon is possible (which I am doubtful of), it is not what I refer to as 'empathy'.

I will argue is that, even if explicit simulation is partly constitutive of empathy in a given instance, its role is a contingent one. Empathy, I will suggest, is a singular kind of cognitive achievement, and simulation is neither necessary nor sufficient for empathy. So, if we want to understand what distinguishes empathy as a *type* of cognitive achievement, we need to appeal to something else. By analogy, breeze blocks are partly constitutive of many houses, but their presence is neither a necessary nor a sufficient condition for something's being a house, and the subcategory 'houses with breeze blocks somewhere in their walls' is an arbitrary and uninformative one.

In what follows, I will suggest that a distinctive kind of 'openness' towards another person is both necessary and sufficient for empathy. It is quite different from explicit simulation, and involves an appreciation of phenomenological difference rather than the generation of similarity. An appeal to implicit simulation is similarly uninformative, given that the implicit generation of similarity does not explain the explicit appreciation of difference. Drawing on my account of the phenomenology of depression, I will suggest that empathy centrally involves a variant of something described in Chapter 8: a feeling of *being with* another person, of relating to her *as* a person. When we are in the company of others, a feeling of interpersonal connection often manifests itself primarily through how a shared situation is experienced, and need not involve our attending to their experiences. This is not always the case though. We are sometimes concerned with another person's experiences more so than our surroundings. So there is a distinction to be drawn between second-person experiences that are primarily 'world-oriented' and others that are primarily 'person-oriented' (the two being opposite ends of a spectrum). Central to empathy, I will argue, is an 'openness to phenomenological difference' that is integral to person-oriented second-person experience. Openness to difference can be sufficient for empathy and, in its absence, no amount of simulation will add up to empathy. Hence empathizing with an experience of depression need not involve simulating it. In fact, I will argue that it *cannot*.

Openness to Difference

My account of depression experiences points to a problem for the simulationist. In short, if empathy is essentially a matter of simulation, it is by definition impossible to empathize with some kinds of depression. In Chapter 8, we saw that depression often involves a sense that nobody else understands or cares: they do not or cannot empathize. An appreciation of being 'understood' by another person, at least in a certain way, is inextricable from an experience of interpersonal connection. So an all-enveloping loss of connection amounts to a feeling of not being understood by anyone. Some interpret their estrangement from others in terms of a lack of care. They cannot participate in those interpersonal relations that cultivate a feeling of being cared for, which leads to the conviction that they are not cared for. This loss of interpersonal connection also impairs the depressed person's ability to empathize with others, as is often acknowledged following recovery. This theme is prominent in Sally Brampton's memoir, which stresses throughout the need to connect with others, the inability to do so when depressed, and the profound isolation that results. She describes how her inability to be moved by others led inevitably to a degree of 'self-absorption'. For Brampton, this became most troubling when she was watching the events of 9.11 unfold on television:

> It was that lack of moral outrage and absence of any feeling that, more than anything else, convinced me that I had to do something to ease the terrible grip depression had on me. I was so lost in my own world that I had ceased to have compassion or feeling for any other. If the sight of bodies dropping from a burning building did not horrify me, that absence of feeling did. (2008, p.176)

What she describes is not just an absence of empathy. There is also a lack of sympathy, along with an inability to feel a range of other situationally appropriate emotions. Nevertheless, this 'absence of any feeling' does include—amongst other things—a substantially impaired ability to appreciate and engage with what others are experiencing. And here is the problem for similarity-based accounts of empathy: depression can involve a lack of empathy and, in such a case, duplicating what one is empathizing with would prevent one from empathizing with it. In order to grasp via isomorphism the profundity of the existential change that has occurred, one would need to lose access to certain kinds of possibility, including those needed for interpersonal connection. However, it is surely not impossible by definition to empathize with an experience that itself involves a lack of empathy.

In fact, it is arguable that simulationism similarly renders much of human experience impossible to empathize with. Goldie (2011b) observes that certain 'character' or 'personality' traits shape our experience in the ways they do partly because we are not reflectively aware of their influence, a point that also applies to many moods and existential feelings. If the empathizer explicitly recognizes their influence on another person's experience, she cannot then simulate the roles they play, as they can only play those roles when first-person insight is lacking. But, if she does not recognize them, she cannot feed them into a simulation process at all. So she cannot duplicate the other person's perspective by means of simulation. As Goldie acknowledges, we might be able to simulate how we would act in another person's situation, 'in his shoes'. However, to the extent that we are psychologically unable to take on board various moods and habitual dispositions, we are unable to transcend a first-person perspective and appreciate how it is for *him*.[4]

One might object that the failure of simulation in such cases should not be taken to imply that we do not empathize by simulating, just that we are sometimes not very good at it. However, that will not suffice. Simulation is constitutionally incapable of succeeding in cases like these, and so it would be rather odd if we all persisted in using it regardless. Furthermore, my point is that empathy *is* possible in cases where simulation is not possible, showing that simulation is not required for empathy. Of course, the simulationist need not insist that one has to model every aspect of another person's experience in order to empathize with it. Nevertheless, if one seeks to empathize with an experience that centrally involves an all-pervasive sense of interpersonal alienation, it is unclear how one could do so by simulating an experience that did not involve an all-pervasive sense of interpersonal alienation. And, if one could do that, it is unclear why simulation should be necessary at all, given that profound experiential differences are, by implication, bridged by something other than simulation.

Contrary to simulationist accounts, empathy can involve appreciating that one is *unable* to understand someone's experience in a first-person way. To illustrate this, let us consider what it is to recognize empathy on the part of another person, to *feel* empathized with. Appreciating that somebody has adopted a certain *attitude* towards one's experience can be sufficient. Central to this attitude is a kind of 'openness' to experiential difference. In the presence of an empathetic listener who is receptive to potential and actual phenomenological differences between self and other, a person may, as Havens (1986, p.24) puts it, 'light up in recognition of your sudden presence in their lives'; they 'feel found, and not in the sense of found out or criticized'. Pienkos and Sass (2012, p.32) note that an interviewer's acknowledgement of profound experiential differences, conveyed by the asking of certain kinds of question, can itself instil an appreciation of being understood: 'patients can feel quite moved in being asked about these experiences'. Halpern (2001, xii) similarly maintains that empathy in clinical

---

[4] Although Goldie describes his conclusion as 'anti-empathy', there is no conflict between his view and a conception of empathy that stresses the appreciation of difference rather than the creation of similarity.

contexts essentially involves 'genuine curiosity and openness to learning something new'; it is not so much a matter of undergoing a similar experience as 'acknowledging that you *don't* fully understand how the patient feels and are curious to learn more'. The point applies more specifically to empathizing with depression. For example, Kitanaka (2012, p.94) makes the following observations, with reference to psychiatrist-patient interactions in contemporary Japan:

> As patients revealed in my [...] interviews, a surprising number of them had had their worries dismissed by their families, even by other doctors. They thus found great relief in meeting someone who had even an inkling of what they were going through. Perhaps it was because of this that patients talked about the acknowledgement from a psychiatrist to be a defining, transformative moment. As one woman said to me: 'I knew, at that moment, that he understood, that I could entrust myself to him'. Establishing this moment of connection was, for doctors as well, important for ensuring diagnostic accuracy and therapeutic efficacy.

The 'inkling' she refers to does not consist of (i) being able to duplicate, to whatever extent, a patient's experience in the first-person and (ii) communicating the experience back to him so that he recognizes the phenomenological isomorphism between the two parties. Rather, it involves achieving a kind of second-person relationship, something that has more to do with asking certain questions, not asking others, and conducting oneself in a certain way. This can culture a feeling of connection, of being understood and somehow affirmed as a person. Granted, recognition of phenomenological difference implies at least some grasp of what another person does experience, but this can remain vague, ambiguous, indeterminate, without amounting to a failure of empathy. Where empathy (whether or not it is recognized as such by the other party) consists solely in the adoption of such an attitude, first-person replication of second-person experience has no role to play and the appeal to simulation is redundant.

I concede that depressed people will have difficulty imaginatively modelling the psychological attributes and/or behaviourally salient situations of others. If one lacks access to a kind of possibility, one will be unable to imagine experiences that incorporate that kind of possibility. It is therefore plausible to suggest that an ability to 'simulate' is impaired in depression, although not entirely absent. Furthermore, people who are not depressed will be unable to simulate what it is like to be depressed, given that they cannot shut off their own access to these same kinds of possibility. For the same reason, a depressed person will be better placed to simulate other depressed people, at least those with similar kinds of depression. But none of this relates to what sufferers claim is most lacking in their relations with others.

What is missing is an ability to 'connect', something that an experience of being understood depends upon. The problem centrally involves being unable to enter into certain kinds of relation with others, rather than being unable to model them or be modelled by them. Someone else is recognized as empathetic when she manages to foster at least some sense of interpersonal connection, the possibility of which might previously have been experienced as absent from the world.

It might be objected that registering the existence of interpersonal difference is too trivial to qualify as 'empathy'. Surely, appreciating that other people's experiences differ from one's own is such a banal achievement that it goes without saying? But a theme running throughout this book is that existential changes are often misinterpreted, with the result that the profundity of phenomenological difference between self and other is significantly underestimated. When you attempt to understand someone's experience but concede defeat, you at least recognize that there is a difference between the two of you, one that you have failed to fully comprehend. A more profound failure of empathy, however, is when you fail to recognize that there is a difference. Here, the possibility of empathizing with the other person's experience is not even entertained. In our everyday encounters with others, we of course appreciate that our own experiences differ from those of others in all manner of ways. Even so, we continue to take much for granted as shared. When you see someone running towards a bus waving, you experience something of her emotion, a sense of urgency and frustration (which you do not feel in quite the same way as you would if it were your own). But you experience this against a shared backdrop: it is *us* who co-inhabit a realm of interconnected artefact functions, norms, and social roles, a world that includes buses, bus stops, departure times, bus drivers, and so on. And you do not have to ascribe all of this to the other person by means of some psychological process. It is presupposed by your appreciation of psychological differences between self and other, a backdrop that is not 'yours' or 'mine' but 'ours'. So the phenomenological separation between self and other is incomplete. It is taken as given that both parties already find themselves in a common situation and, furthermore, a common world.

However, not all attempts to empathize can presuppose so much. For example, when empathizing with a young child, someone from a different culture, or someone with a very different set of interests and values, less can be assumed. If we know or suspect that another person has never seen buses before and has no grasp of the norms associated with them, we might, when engaging with her experience, bracket our more usual assumption that these are features of a *shared* world.[5] This is not to suggest that all instances of empathy are made more difficult, or made difficult to the same extent, by cultural differences. Much depends on the content of the experience with which we are trying to empathize. For example, when presented with a person covering her sobbing face with her hands, cultural differences might not interfere at all with the ability to appreciate her sadness (at least in some cases). When the content of the experience is not just 'B is sad' but 'B is sad about *p*', matters are more complicated. Some will find it harder than others to empathize with B's being sad about the fact that nobody ever visits his Facebook page. Empathizing with others thus involves suspending, to varying degrees, a background of norms, roles, artefact functions, self-interpretations, projects, values, and various other experiential contents. Phenomenologically speaking, this is not so much a matter of recognizing that other people do not have exactly the same internal psychological states as oneself (although recognition of differ-ence does *sometimes* take the form 'person B's mental life is unlike mine in respects *p, q*, and *r*'). Rather, the first step when engaging with difference is to stop presupposing aspects of what is more usually given as *our world*.

We do not take everyone to have exactly the same grasp of the social world, but it would be unusual to interpret another person without assuming at least some kind of shared socio-cultural backdrop. Let us suppose that we did though. Even then, the phenomenological separation of our own world from hers would not be complete. The interpreter would continue to assume that both parties find themselves *in the same world*, regardless of how dif-ferent the contents of that world might be for each of them. As discussed in Chapter 1, this sense of belonging to a shared world is seldom even recognized as a phenomenological achievement, let alone one that can vary in structure. However, it can be approached philosophically by adopting a 'phenomeno-logical stance', a broad methodological orientation common to the work of many phenomenologists. Hence, for an empathetic attitude to be open to

---

[5] When empathizing with someone from a very different background, we sometimes build up a positive understanding of the norms and so forth that she *does* subscribe to. Gallagher (2012) argues that empathy, here and more generally, is facilitated by 'shared narratives', which play a similar role to what I have referred to as a context of norms, roles, and artefact functions. When we try to empathize with someone who is not immersed in the same narrative context as ourselves, we need to get to know her narra-tives in order to appreciate something of her history, her situation, her life. This kind of understanding can be fostered through a dialogical, exploratory process, of a kind that I will go on to describe. See also Goldie (2000) for the view that empathy involves a nar-rative understanding of experience.

the possibility of 'existential difference' between self and other, it needs to incorporate a phenomenological stance. This amounts to a distinctive kind of empathy, which I have elsewhere called 'radical empathy'. It involves engaging with someone else's experiences, rather than one's own, while at the same time suspending the usual assumption that both parties share the same space of possibilities (Ratcliffe, 2012b).[6] In earlier chapters, I argued that recognizing *openness to kinds of possibility* as a phenomenological achievement enables us to explore changes in the structure of experience that would otherwise elude us. Although this kind of enquiry can be pursued in a second-person way, it can equally be carried out in the first-person. Someone prone to 'wobbles' in the sense of reality and belonging could use herself as an object of study and reveal something of the structure of experience by attending to its patterns of variation, while also drawing (successfully or unsuccessfully) on imagination. So my claim is not that phenomenology *must* amount to empathy, but that a phenomenological stance *can be* integrated into our attempts to engage with the experiences of others. And when one seeks to understand the experiences of particular individuals in this way, rather than phenomenological types, what we have is a form of empathy.

Empathy as Exploration

Openness to difference is sufficient for some empathetic achievements, but how do we account for other cases where there is a positive and sometimes elaborate understanding of experience? For instance, empathizing with someone's depression experience could involve some sense of the *kind* of experiential world she inhabits, as well as how she interprets her predicament. I suggest that openness to difference serves as the starting point for a dynamic, variably collaborative exploration of second-person experience. Hence the attempt to acquire a positive empathetic appreciation of depression could fail in two different ways: (1) the empathizer is not open to the relevant kinds of interpersonal difference; (2) an exploratory process, which involves some degree of mutual cooperation, breaks down or never gets going (perhaps because the other person does not *feel* empathized with).

This proposal is consistent with many accounts of 'clinical empathy', which emphasize an interpersonal process more so than an ability to simulate someone's experiences and then attribute them to her. Though something that could

---

6 Radical empathy therefore serves to challenge Heidegger's claim in *Being and Time* that 'only on the basis of Being-with does 'empathy' become possible' (1962, p.162). Radical empathy does not take for granted what Heidegger calls 'Being-in-the-world'; it involves grasping the possibility of variations in its structure.

be (but need not be) interpreted as 'simulation' often features in these accounts as well, it is not central. For instance, Havens (1986) construes empathy as a collaborative endeavour, one that can be obstructed in various ways by implicit and explicit strategies of non-cooperation.[7] He distinguishes several kinds of empathy: motor empathy, passive empathy (where a therapist waits to be affected by a client), cognitive empathy, affective empathy, and perceptual empathy. But all have a potential role to play in a unitary process. This does not involve replication of the other person's perspective but, Havens suggests, a self-affecting investigation of it: 'to find another, you must enter that person's world. The empathic visitor then discovers what he has taken for granted in his own world' (p.21). To *enter* someone's world is not to *become* it. Empathy, for Havens, involves a way of being 'with' the patient (p.27), which facilitates a kind of 'exploration' (p.67). It also requires an initial recognition of actual or potential differences between one's own 'world' and that of the patient, involving suspension of assumptions that are habitually made when interacting with people in many other circumstances.[8]

Other accounts similarly emphasize openness and exploration. For instance, Larson and Yao (2005) remark that, 'to cultivate an acute ability to empathize with others, one needs patience, curiosity, and willingness to subject one's own mind to the patient's world' (p.1100). This 'subjection' involves encountering an experiential world *as* someone else's and proceeding to explore it. Empathy is thus a 'psychological process', one that involves 'a collection of affective, cognitive, and behavioral mechanisms and outcomes in reaction to the observed experiences of another' (p.1102). As Halpern (2003, p.671) observes, the empathetic clinician's attention is directed principally at the patient and not 'unduly diverted to introspection'. Being 'empathetic' is not a matter of being able to perform a singular cognitive feat: first-person replication of someone else's experience. Instead, it is a *way* of approaching and interacting with another person. For Halpern (2001, xi), empathy is 'not an additional task but rather an adverb'; it is a style of conduct that involves proceeding with openness and curiosity. She adds that imagination has an important part to play (as it surely does in any complicated cognitive task), but its main role is not the first-person modelling of second-person

---

[7] There are also passages that *could* be interpreted in simulationist terms, but are equally compatible with a conception of empathy as second-person experience. For example, Havens (1986, p.16) refers to a 'capacity to participate in or experience another's sensations, feelings, thoughts, or movements', and talks of 'finding the other'.

[8] See Throop (2010; 2012) for a similar conception of empathy in the context of cultural anthropology. Throop maintains that empathy is a dialogical process, which is not an 'all or nothing affair' and does not require 'some set of homologous experiences shared between individuals' (2010, p.771).

experience. Rather, it contributes to a progressive appreciation of the patient's experience that involves coming to understand it as a cohesive whole: 'imagination work must be done to unify the details and nuances of the patient's life into an integrated affective experience' (Halpern, 2001, p.88). So, when empathy involves developing a positive conception of what someone experiences, its task is not that of understanding 'an experience' in isolation from the rest of the person's life. If one did replicate an isolated experience (whatever that might be; I am unsure how to individuate 'experiences' and I use the plural term in a noncommittal way) and attribute it to the other person, that would not amount to empathetic understanding. Empathy involves relating a person's experiences to her life, situating them against the backdrop of her hopes, aspirations, projects, commitments, concerns, loves, fears, successes, disappointments, and vulnerabilities. In cases of 'radical empathy', we can add to this an acknowledgement of the existential framework within which the person experiences things and interprets life events. In empathizing with an experience of depression, we might imagine various different transformations of the possibility space. The kind of existential change that the person has actually undergone could then be further clarified through an interpersonal, exploratory process.

Importantly, one empathizes not with an experience but with a person, something that involves second-person exploration of how her experiences fit into her life, rather than first-person replication of a current experience and its wider psychological context. To illustrate the *personal* focus of empathy and the fact that it is not captured by simulation, consider the following scenario: Persons A and B have both taken hallucinogenic drugs and are lying next to each other in a field. A says to B, 'This is amazing—are you seeing this?' and B replies 'Yes, it's fantastic'. In this case, A has much the same kind of experience as B and also attributes an experience of that kind to B, while recognizing his own experience as distinct from B's. However, what I have just described does not add up to empathy. One might respond on behalf of simulation that this is because A's experience is not caused by B's. But her appreciation of what B's experience consists of is indirectly caused by B's experience, given that it depends on B's communicating that experience to A. And to insist that the isomorphism between A and B must be caused in its entirety by B for empathy to occur would be too strict a criterion. It would preclude empathy in all those cases where one is already having an experience that is in any way similar to the target experience. Another response is to maintain that this is simple projection, and that empathy further requires imaginative modification of one's own experience before attribution. So let us add that B responds 'Yes, but I'm seeing pink cows, rather than butterflies'.

A then imaginatively modifies his own experiential contents from 'butterflies' to 'pink cows' and attributes the experience to B, after which he says 'Wow, this is great'. Again, A's experience of B seems somehow lacking as an example of empathy, but how? The answer is that both parties are attending to an experience, rather than to each other. It is the kind of experience they are both undergoing that interests them, and any curiosity about interpersonal differences is wholly symptomatic of their interest in the experience.

It has been suggested that empathizing with someone involves caring for her, in addition to simulating her experience (de Vignemont and Jacob, 2012). When one empathizes, one is concerned about another person, not about a kind of experience she is having, where *who* has the experience does not really matter. Perhaps this is what is missing from the above exchange? However, the type of 'care' we are looking for just *is* the second-person stance I have already described: a distinctive type of person-oriented attitude, involving openness to phenomenological difference. It is not an 'add-on' to a core process of simulation and is itself sufficient for empathy. Without it, an understanding of experience would not amount to empathy, even if it involved simulation, attribution, and care for the simulated party. Consider the fictional example of a doctor's receptionist who has the ability to reliably detect when someone is in despair by fleetingly entering an isomorphic state as the person walks past, and subsequently attributing it to him. She also feels concerned for these patients (she 'cares' about them) and so she alerts the doctor by pressing a button whenever she detects someone in despair. We can add that her ability is non-mysterious, involving a heightened but natural sensitivity to despair-specific gait, movement, and expression. Even so, this ability is not empathy, but some sort of idiosyncratic talent, quirk, or neat trick. The reason for this is that it does not involve the right kind of care, a way of being open to the other person that serves as the starting point for a certain style of relating.

Of course, empathy involves being open to the possibility of similarities too. One might suspend a similarity assumption in order to contemplate the possibility of difference, only to discover that the two parties are similar in that respect after all. But here too, empathy is not a matter of imposing one's own experience on someone else. One might recognize the possibility, or even the likelihood, that another person is experiencing something similar to what one currently experiences or experienced in the past. Nevertheless, where there is empathy, there is also a 'gap' between first-person and second-person experience. Simulation can contribute to a sense of what another person *might* be experiencing, but empathy demands restraint. Saying 'I know just how you feel' can lead the other person to conclude that you have not empathized, that you have failed to understand her, even if you are broadly right about what she feels. To engage with *her* experience, an attitude involving openness, curiosity, and reciprocity is needed. Imposing one's own experience on someone (even a modified version of it) without listening, without being open to alternatives, is a failure of empathy. First-person experience thus informs empathy, rather than serving as a substitute for it.

To further illustrate simulation's failure to capture the essentially personal nature of empathy, consider a case described by Minkowski (I am not sure what the diagnosis would be). He reports not that he failed to understand the patient but that he felt he understood him too well: 'I know all about him'; 'the psyche of the patient is too well understood' (1970, pp.177–8). This is not to be confused with his having a comprehensive understanding of the patient's world, as the *feeling* of understanding him 'too well' actually constitutes a sense of his being utterly different, somehow alien. According to Minkowski, what this person lacked was any sense of an open future in which he might actualize significant possibilities. The future appeared only in the guise of threat and he retreated into a closed, nostalgic world. This, Minkowski says, is something that could be *felt* while interacting with the patient:

> The individual, separated so brutally from becoming, can experience it only as a hostile force. And we, confronted by this psyche, flattened and reduced to a single dimension, have the impression, in listening to the patient speak, of being constrained to read in an open book, as if there were nothing behind the pages of that book. (1970, p.179)

The book is open because it is complete. The person is not oriented towards the future in any way, towards the possible. Instead, he wallows in the past, in what is already actualized. Rather than being a locus of possibilities and thus a potential influence on one's own world, he seems more like an object in one's world, oddly complete and therefore somehow diminished as a person. Minkoswki comes to empathize with the patient's predicament by attempting to engage with him as a person and feeling somehow impeded in his attempts to do so. This serves to reveal a profound phenomenological difference, of a kind that is then further clarified—something is missing from the patient's world, something inseparable from the ability to interact with others in a personal way. Minkowski's description of this experience stands in stark contrast to the view, common to both theory and simulation theories, that interpreting others (regardless of whether or not one does so by experiencing something of what they experience) involves solving an epistemic problem: one acquires knowledge about someone's psychology in order to predict or explain her behaviour. According to that view, if one somehow had the good fortune to know everything about the psychology of another person, it would make no difference to one's appreciation of her *as* a person. Minkowski's description suggests otherwise: not knowing everything about a person is integral to our sense of her as a person.

As I argued in Chapter 8, others are not merely experienced as objects within one's world. A sense of their *being* persons involves an appreciation of their potential to reshape one's world, to transform to varying degrees the possibilities it offers. Hence one cannot know everything about them, as they could not then open up new possibilities and would not be experienced as persons. The sense of uncertainty that is so central to our experience of others is not principally a matter of ignorance about the contents of their heads. A person is intrinsically unknowable in her entirety in a way that a rock is not, because a person is never fully inserted into one's own world and points to something beyond it.[9] It follows that imposing a simulation on someone amounts to a lack of empathy, rather than a successful empathetic achievement. Having a sense of phenomenological difference (of a kind that could never be comprehensively understood in a positive way) is inseparable from engaging with someone in a distinctively *personal* manner. And anything that did not include that openness could not amount to empathy, as empathy essentially involves personal engagement. Simulation without openness to difference would inevitably amount to a total failure of empathy; it could not be directed at another person without one's ceasing to experience her as a person at all.

I do not seek to challenge the intuitive view that empathy can be *aided* by similarities between people. To be more specific, it may be that depressed people are better able to understand the experiences of other depressed people. However, there are reasons to doubt that. Recognizing that another person is 'depressed like me' could involve typifying rather than empathizing, where one infers that both parties fall under the type 'depressed' and therefore have the same kinds of experience. There is also a risk of imposing one's own experience of depression on another person. Depression does not enhance the ability to engage with *someone else's* depression, to recognize the particularity of her experience. As I have argued, the potential for this kind of interaction is absent from the world of many depressed people. Nevertheless, a person's *past* experience of depression could feed into empathetic engagement with someone else's depression, giving her a clearer sense of what that person *might* be experiencing (including some appreciation that profound experiential disturbances may be involved, of a kind that others are often oblivious to). Matters are complicated by the heterogeneity of depression. Although

---

[9] We find similar themes in Levinas (1961/1969).

one's own experience is potentially informative, it cannot be assumed with any confidence that the other person's 'depression experience' is similar in kind. Openness to existential difference therefore remains the starting point for an exploratory process, through which a more refined understanding of second-person experience may then be developed. Imagining how one would feel or remembering how one did feel in similar circumstances can inform that task. But an over-emphasis on simulation eclipses something that is central to all empathetic achievements: attentiveness to actual and potential degrees and kinds of phenomenological difference. Even so, having experienced profound existential changes oneself could serve to cultivate an empathetic openness to existential differences more generally, and thus a greater sensitivity to various forms of suffering that are more usually misinterpreted.

Empathy does not arise solely in face-to-face interactions, and the second-person openness I have described can also feature in engagement with written narratives, whether autobiographical or fictional. So, although I stated that phenomenology is insufficient for empathy and that understanding *types* of experience should not be confused with empathizing, the attitude I have sought to adopt towards individual testimonies does qualify as one of empathy. However, more sophisticated empathetic achievements usually involve an interpersonal process, which facilitates clarification, disambiguation, correction, and elaboration of an initial understanding of experience. There are exceptions to this though, such as when one already knows another person well, and is better placed to situate her experience in the context of her life. It is also important to note that empathetic understanding need not be a one-sided attempt by A to understand B. There are varying degrees of 'mutual empathy', where A and B empathize with each other in the course of interactions that involve feelings of mutual relatedness on the part of both. The process is more one-sided when it comes to depression, given that depression experiences generally involve a felt inability to engage in precisely such processes. Whether an empathetic process is achieved depends, amongst other things, on whether and to what extent the potential for interpersonal connection really is blocked, rather than just experienced as blocked.

It has been pointed out that clinical empathy is a form of 'professional interaction' (Mercer and Reynolds, 2002, p.10). So it might be objected that what I have described in this chapter is a skill acquired through exposure and training, rather than a wider-ranging ability of the kind that simulationists are concerned with. But I do not take this to be problematic, as the point applies equally to empathy in other contexts. Empathy invariably draws on skills that people acquire to varying degrees and in a range of ways. And the kind of second-person phenomenological stance that I have described is a case in point. However, it can be added that 'radical empathy' is not dependent upon specifically *philosophical* training. Whereas phenomenological research involves employing a stance, as well as describing that stance and what it reveals, radical empathy requires only the former. It is possible to adopt a phenomenological stance without being able to characterize the achievement as such. In other words, one can engage in this kind of empathy without being able to offer an explicit account of exactly what one has come to appreciate or how one has done so. For example, one first-person account of depression (which I also quoted in Chapter 6) describes the experience as one of having lost 'life itself', a 'habitable earth'. What has been lost, the author says, is 'something that people don't even know is', which is why 'it's so hard to explain' (Hornstein, 2009, pp.2012–13). This is something he seeks to communicate to others, implying an appreciation that 'how we find ourselves in the world' can be altered in profound but seldom recognized ways. This kind of appreciation, although bereft of theoretical baggage, could equally be integrated into an empathetic project. So radical empathy may well be uncommon, but it is not tied to a form of philosophical enquiry; it is something that arises in our relations with others, in clinical settings and more widely.[10]

---

[10] Regardless of whether or not one is able to describe the relevant achievement, radical empathy can also involve varying degrees of effort. One might set out to empathize with a person and draw on various imaginative resources in order to do so. In contrast, it could simply 'happen', to some extent at least, without prior intention or effort.

Chapter 10

The Nature of Depression

I have argued that the phenomenology of depression is heterogeneous, in a way that is obscured by superficial similarities in symptom descriptions. Despite the substantial differences between existential and non-existential changes in experience, categories such as 'major depression' do not distinguish them. There are also several different kinds of existential depression. So, in addition to the variation explicitly acknowledged by the DSM, there is considerable further variation that goes unnoticed. Furthermore, first-person descriptions of depression convey different aspects of a unitary phenomenological change rather than separate 'symptoms'. The same shift in *how one finds oneself in the world* can be expressed in terms of the body, the world, hope, guilt, agency, time, interpersonal relations, and/or certain kinds of belief. For instance, a 'loss of all hope' also amounts to a sense that significant change and meaningful action are impossible, as well as a blurring of the distinction between past, present, and future, and an inability to 'connect' with other people. All existential depression experiences can be located somewhere within a malleable possibility space, and involve subtly different shifts in the kinds of possibility one is open to. This approach, I have suggested, can facilitate a deeper, more detailed, and more discriminating understanding of the phenomenology of depression, allowing us to distinguish forms of experience that might otherwise be regarded as much the same.[1] I have not offered any specific proposals regarding how depression experiences ought to be classified, diagnosed, or treated. Rather, I have offered an interpretative framework, as well as a number of phenomenological distinctions, which together have the potential to inform research, classification, diagnosis, and treatment.

Where do these conclusions leave the concept of 'depression'? In this chapter, I bring the discussion to a close by addressing four interrelated issues. First of all, I further consider the implications of my various claims for the categories 'depression' and 'major depression'. I propose that they are best construed as

---

[1] By 'deeper', I mean that phenomenology can enable an appreciation of something that I addressed in Chapter 5: the way in which 'existential changes' are more profound than 'intentional changes'.

'ideal types' that can play a methodological role in certain areas of enquiry and practice. Then I turn to the question of whether and how a distinction might be drawn between experiences of depression and experiential disturbances that are more typical of the early stages of schizophrenia. Despite the heterogeneity of depression, I show that there are qualitative differences to be discerned between all of the depression experiences described here and at least some of those existential changes more usually associated with schizophrenia diagnoses. I also offer some thoughts on the relationship between depression and depersonalization. Following this, I ask whether and why depression experiences should be deemed 'pathological' or otherwise. Although various criteria for making the distinction prove problematic, I suggest that it can often be drawn in practice by relying on pragmatic considerations. Finally, I address the question of whether or not depression is what we might call 'epistemically pathological': does it invariably supply a misleading view of things or is there some truth to the world of depression? I focus more specifically on an especially profound form of existential despair, which manifests itself as a revelation about the unavoidable structure of all human life. This can be construed as an intellectual position of sorts, one with a built-in feeling of certainty. I conclude that the epistemic allure of existential despair is symptomatic of a contingent loneliness, rather than an inevitable human condition.

What is 'Depression'?

As noted in Chapter 9, it is possible to empathize with an experience of depression without classifying it. Empathy involves engaging with the *particularity* of someone's experience and can operate without the mediation of psychiatric typification. However, classification is needed in other contexts, such as that of diagnosis. What, then, are the implications of my discussion for the diagnostic categories 'depression' and 'major depression'? A category need not have 'natural kind' status in order for its retention to be defensible. In other words, it does not have to be an accurate or uniquely accurate reflection of how the world really divides up. For certain purposes, its utility may be justification enough. Historical entrenchment is also a consideration. The fact that category x is already in widespread and habitual use gives it a pragmatic edge over a newly proposed category y. Even though y might be preferable according to some criteria, the cost of switching from x to y, the time and effort involved, might offset any potential benefits. It is clear that 'depression' and 'major depression' accommodate a range of different kinds of experience. There are currently no additional non-phenomenological criteria that we might appeal to in order to unite them. Furthermore, it is unlikely that any such criteria are forthcoming. For instance, as we saw in Chapter 3, the aetiology of depression is most likely diverse as well. So I will not address the various metaphysical conceptions of 'natural kind' that 'depression' could, in principle conform to, as it does not approximate even the more permissive ones.[2]

I suggest instead that we construe 'depression' in terms of what Jaspers (1963), drawing on the work of Max Weber, calls an 'ideal type'. In a more recent discussion, from which I take my lead, Schwartz and Wiggins (1987a, b) construe ideal types in psychiatry in a way that involves no metaphysical commitment and credits them only with a methodological role. They are starting points from which to navigate, and the types one works with are partly a reflection of one's values and goals. In the context of mental health, the values are those of 'promoting health and ameliorating mental illness', and the goals are to facilitate informative generalizations and engage with individual patients. So an ideal type does not have a 'truth value'; it is to be evaluated solely in terms of its 'heuristic value' (1987a, pp.280–85). Where the categories 'depression' and 'major depression' are concerned, I think this is the most we can commit to with any confidence. They serve as initial orientations, which constrain attention and focus enquiry. Where an ideal type *p* is reliably associated with the presence of *a, b, c,* or *d,* it can be informative even where *a, b, c,* and *d* have little in common, as it still gives us an initial sense of what we might expect to find. By starting with broad categories that impose at least some order on an object of investigation, we gain the focus needed for enquiry to get off the ground. This non-committal approach does not imply that 'depression' serves our purposes any better than various other types that we might conceive of.[3]

---

[2] For a good discussion of natural kinds and psychiatric classification, see Cooper (2005). My conception of depression is, however, compatible with Ian Hacking's influential account of 'human kinds', where a human kind is a way of classifying people that itself influences their thought and behaviour, along with that of others, thus shaping and reshaping the kind in question. See, for example, Hacking (1995). There is no tension between this and my view that 'depression' also operates as an 'ideal type'.

[3] See Sass and Pienkos (2013, a, b) for a recent defence of an 'ideal types' approach along similar lines. See also Ghaemi (2007, p.124), who warns that, although ideal types such as 'depression' and 'mania' have their uses, they should not be reified. That, he says, would risk obscuring 'the more complex texture of the actual experience of mixed states'. For a different conception of ideal types in psychiatry, see Murphy (2009, pp.114–115), who proposes moving away from a syndrome-based approach and attempting to identify disease entities that are 'abstracted away from individual variation'. Idealization, he maintains, is needed if we are to identify 'robust processes' that may be masked by superficial diversity. I do not wish to dismiss such an approach, only to suggest that it is not applicable to the categories 'depression' and 'major depression' as they currently stand, given the considerable (and non-superficial) heterogeneity that they encompass. However, these categories could at least serve as initial foci for the kind of approach Murphy advocates.

Even if depression is an 'ideal type', in this sense of the term, it is arguable that the category would benefit from further refinement. Many experiences of 'depression' involve existential changes, but others do not. Symptom checklists are insensitive to differences between loss of existential hope and loss of hopes, loss of practical significance and loss of life projects, and so forth. To serve as a more effective focus for research and practice, the label 'depression' could be restricted to cases that involve existential changes. It is not informative to lump these together with non-existential changes that are superficially similar but structurally quite different. Provisional classification of an experience as one of 'depression' would thus amount to the acknowledgement that some existential change is likely to be involved, a change that is likely to be of type *a*, *b*, *c*, or *d*, rather than *p*, *q*, *r*, or *s*. The same can be said of 'major depression'. This is more specific than just 'depression', as it includes an indication of severity, but it likewise accommodates considerable variety, much of which is not explicitly acknowledged. One could then proceed from these initial characterizations to a more nuanced appreciation of depression experiences, a task that would involve discriminating various subcategories of existential depression.

Restricting the scope of 'depression' to its existential forms also serves to distinguish it more clearly from some somatic illness experiences. Where those experiences do not involve existential changes, they can be discounted as instances of 'depression'. Even so, this does not dispense with all of the concerns raised in Chapter 3. Where a somatic illness experience does involve an existential change, of a kind that could equally be associated with a depression diagnosis, there is no principled way of distinguishing the two. Appealing to aetiology is ineffective, as depression is already aetiologically diverse and it is not clear why several different aetiologies should be admitted and others excluded. One approach is simply to exclude all those predicaments that are reliably caused by known disease processes. The ideal type 'depression' would then amount to this: 'broad family of existential predicaments; aetiology unknown'. It would operate as a temporary placeholder, the aim being to surpass it by identifying associated disease processes and removing them from the category 'depression' until nothing is left. An alternative option would be to widen the scope of 'depression' to include existential changes that are currently excluded on the basis of their being attributable to other medical conditions.

An 'ideal type' view of depression is complicated by the likelihood of discrepancies between theory and practice. As Schwartz and Wiggins (1987b) point out, diagnosis is a practical skill, which can involve a quasi-perceptual ability to assign a patient to a category. What a skilful clinician is *actually* sensitive to need not map onto the explicit contents of diagnostic manuals. Hence clinicians are most likely attuned to some (perhaps many) of the distinctions drawn here, even though certain literature is not. Schwartz and Wiggins add that a degree of practical skill is also needed to use diagnostic criteria competently, skill that is acquired and refined through interaction with patients rather than exposure to concepts. This is probably right—much of the relevant expertise will not be articulated, at least not in the form of diagnostic criteria and superficial symptoms descriptions. Nevertheless, skill acquisition is surely shaped by conceptual knowledge as well. And it is unlikely that cursory and simplistic descriptions of depression experience fail to impede, in any way, the development of skilful discrimination. So it is plausible to suggest that a better conceptual grasp of depression has implications for practice. It can be added than many depression diagnoses are not made by psychiatrists but by general practitioners, who are more reliant on explicit guidance.

In addressing the more specific kinds of existential change associated with the labels 'depression' and 'major depression', phenomenological enquiry proceeds beyond these initial orienting categories to describe something that has *phenomenological reality*. There is a fact of the matter concerning (i) the types of possibility that human experience does and does not incorporate and (ii) the types of existential change it is and is not susceptible to. And this is something we are able to investigate. If it turns out that possibility type p can be lost while possibility type q remains, it is clear that our experience respects a distinction between them. However, if loss of p invariably entails loss of q, with no time lag, there may well be a dependence of intelligibility or even a relationship of identity (where the same kind of possibility is described in two different ways). The kind of phenomenological work needed to draw such distinctions is not easy, but it is possible. And the outcome of enquiry is a contestable account of how human experience is structured, rather than something that is to be assessed solely in terms of its methodological utility or other pragmatic merits. The distinctions made in this book are not rigid and categorical; they allow for alterations of the possibility space that lie somewhere between the kinds of existential change I have described. But this is not to concede that 'anything goes'. Because existential changes are unitary in structure, there are numerous constraints on the forms that experience can take. For instance, it is not possible to have temporal experience p, which is ordinarily associated with loss of hope q, instead associated with loss of hope r, where r is qualitatively different and less profound than q.

Reflecting on his own experience, Shenk (2001, p.245) states that the concept 'depression' is 'cobbled together of so many different parts, causes, experiences, and affects as to render the word ineffectual and perhaps even noxious to a full, true narrative'. I am not entirely unsympathetic to that view and, even if 'depression' is tightened up to include only those cases that involve existential changes, an ideal type conception—of the kind that I have advocated here—does not imply any commitment to its retention.[4] However, discarding the term or even aspiring to do so would be premature. Although I have distinguished several different kinds of depression experience, the distinctions I have drawn can also be integrated into a more dynamic construal of depression. Different kinds of experience may well feature in a single, structured, longer-term process. By analogy, two musical notes may sound quite different as well as separate from each other when heard in isolation, but can also be integrated into many different and equally cohesive melodies. Here is one of many scenarios we might explore: The person first feels exhausted and increasingly unable to do things. She feels unsupported by others, gradually loses trust in the world and then experiences a growing sense of non-localized dread. This exacerbates the feeling of inability so that everything now appears utterly impossible, after which feelings of irrevocable worthlessness and guilt take hold. It should be re-emphasized that self-narrative also has a role to play in shaping and regulating how an experience unfolds. So there are temporal patterns to discern, involving relations of causation and also intelligibility. Any causal story we tell must respect constraints on intelligibility. One cannot lose all sense of practical significance while one's experience of time remains intact, and one cannot experience profound existential guilt while still feeling enticed to act in the usual way by one's surroundings.

Thus, what I have tried to do in this book is provide a starting point for a form of enquiry that brings phenomenology into dialogue with psychiatry, therapy, and empirical research. It is not my intention to dictate where that enquiry should lead us. So far as finer-grained diagnostic categories are concerned, it is not at all clear where we ought to end up, partly because the issue hinges on what we want those categories to do for us, and partly because diagnostic categories are not motivated exclusively by phenomenological concerns. Even so, phenomenological research can at least

---

[4] The problem that Shenk draws attention to is not specific to current classifications of depression. It is arguably something that has always dogged historically changing conceptions of melancholia and depression. For example, Radden (2009, p. 61) observes that, at the time Burton was writing (in the early seventeenth century), 'not only does "melancholy" seem to have been extended to cover a broader spectrum of mental abnormalities than those that would today be classified as clinical depression. In addition, melancholy traits were represented as ranging from despair and the black moods described by poets to wit, wisdom, and inspiration. And, finally, "melancholy" refers as much to a passing or long-term attribute of a normal person as to a mental disturbance. To our contemporary minds, the concept of melancholy at that period is at first so broad as to be almost meaningless'.

inform debates over classification. Take, for instance, the contested distinction between so-called 'endogenous', 'reactive', and 'neurotic' subtypes of depression, a distinction that has been drawn in a number of different ways.[5] It is based partly on aetiological considerations, but appeals are also made to phenomenological differences, the emphasis being on endogenous depression's distinctiveness.[6] An interpretative framework of the kind formulated here can be used to further address and clarify the nature of any proposed phenomenological differences. In the process, it can also facilitate better focused investigations of aetiology. A distinctive phenomenological type is surely more likely to be associated with a distinctive causal process than a category of depression that fails to differentiate a range of profoundly different experiences.[7]

Another issue to consider is that of whether and how the kinds of existential change described here are culturally variable. The DSM acknowledges cultural differences in how depression is experienced and expressed: 'Culture can influence the experience and communication of symptoms of depression' (DSM-IV-TR, p.353). More specifically, it is noted that depression is sometimes couched in somatic terms that are themselves culturally variable, with 'nerves' and 'headaches' often featuring in Latino and Mediterranean cultures, 'imbalance', weakness, and tiredness in Chinese and Asian cultures,

---

[5] See Klein, Shankman, and McFarland (2006) for a survey and discussion.

[6] One way of distinguishing the three forms of depression aetiologically is as follows: endogenous depression arises without an appropriate or proportionate environmental cause, while reactive depression is both proportionate and appropriate to some cause, and neurotic depression involves responding to a situation in a way that may be appropriate but is still disproportionate. However, 'reactive' is sometimes identified with 'neurotic'.

[7] The most detailed phenomenological account of endogenous or melancholic depression is that of Tellenbach (1980, 1982). He associates it with a distinctive personality type, the 'typus melancholicus', which he describes as follows: 'Its decisive characteristic consists of *being-pinned-down* to orderliness, high demands to individual production, a painful concern with avoiding guilt [...] and lastly an inclination towards a sympathetic, even symbiotic mode of communication' (1982, p.192). In this book, I have offered an account of the possibility space within which depression experiences more generally are to be located, compared, and contrasted. The kind of 'melancholia' that Tellenbach describes can be placed within that space. However, more nuanced distinctions between different types of existential change (involving different ways of experiencing the body, agency, time, guilt, despair, and other people) also offer the potential to further clarify, refine, and disambiguate his account. For instance, it is not clear whether 'melancholia' encompasses loss of enticing possibilities, loss of significant possibilities, a combination of the two, or all three kinds of experience.

problems of the 'heart' in Middle Eastern cultures, and so forth.[8] I indicated in Chapter 3 that claims about the extent of cultural difference are mitigated by the recognition that depression is invariably a 'bodily' experience, but this is compatible with the view that bodily experiences are shaped by 'cultural systems of meaning' (Kirmayer, 2008, p.319). I also acknowledged in Chapter 5 that depression experiences are influenced by how they are conceptualized, expressed, and narrated. I do not conceive of existential feeling as a layer of experience that is impervious to the influence of interpretative and communicative practices, some of which are to be understood at the level of culture. My account therefore allows for considerable variation, of a kind that is not itself to be interpreted in existential terms. Ways of experiencing the world that involve access to the same kinds of possibility can differ in other respects.[9] Furthermore, I do not want to discount the possibility that some kinds of existential feeling are more or less prevalent in certain cultures. Culture has a substantial influence on how depression is experienced and interpreted, and may also dispose people to some kinds of existential change and not others.

However, I do not think there are grounds for the more radical view that certain *kinds of possibility* are only accessible within certain cultures (where 'kind of possibility' is understood in terms of the content-independent level of description adopted in Chapter 2). Indeed, it is unclear what positive evidence there could be for such a view, as its proponent would have to acknowledge types of possibility that he was constitutionally incapable of finding intelligible. The possibility space I have described amounts to *the having of an experiential world*. It is presupposed by the ability to encounter entities as 'present', experience others as persons, have goals, inhabit time, have a sense of agency, and adopt beliefs. Granted, it can vary in structure, often quite profoundly. And my own *description* of it is no doubt lacking in certain respects, some of which may be symptomatic of social and cultural as well as individual limitations. But what I am attempting to describe (in contrast to how I have actually described it) is a malleable structure within which all the existential variants of human experience are to be located.

---

[8] DSM-5 (p.352) contains a shorter statement about 'cultural differences in the expression of major depressive disorder'. See, for example, Radden (2009) for further discussion of depression and culture, and Kirmayer (2001) for an account of how culture influences the ways in which experience is shaped, expressed, categorized, and regulated.

[9] For example, Kitanaka (2012) describes, at length, historically shifting conceptions of depression in Japanese culture. Despite the considerable diversity that arises due to changing interpretative practices, all of the phenomena she describes could be construed in terms of the malleable possibility space charted here.

Insofar as my account is found lacking, it requires correction, refinement, or elaboration (a process that can itself be informed by engagement with cultural difference) rather than restriction to a particular culture and/or historical period.

Depression, Schizophrenia, and Depersonalization

I have suggested that some somatic illness experiences are phenomenologically indistinguishable from some 'depression' experiences. But what about forms of experience associated with other psychiatric illness categories? For instance, it is plausible to suggest that schizophrenia involves existential changes. Phenomenological accounts of schizophrenia offered by Sass (e.g. 1992, 2004, 2007) and Sass and Parnas (2007) emphasize a loss of practical engagement and a profound shift in the sense of reality, along with pervasive disconnection from the world and other people. They further suggest that delusional experiences with specific contents are symptomatic of this more enveloping transformation in one's sense of self, world, and other people.[10] If something along these lines is right, how might we distinguish the types of existential feeling that arise in depression from those that arise in schizophrenia? In addressing this question, I do not wish to imply that the category 'schizophrenia' is unproblematic. Indeed, many of the concerns I have raised about 'depression' may apply equally to 'schizophrenia'. However, this does not prevent us from considering whether and how certain existential changes that tend to be associated with the label 'schizophrenia' differ from those described here.

It is well established that depression and anxiety diagnoses often precede schizophrenia diagnoses (e.g. Broome et al., 2005). So it might be argued that the two have much in common phenomenologically. Perhaps schizophrenia involves an existential change of much the same kind, but one that is more extreme? Association does not imply similarity, even where there is a close causal relationship; one form of experience could dispose a person towards another, quite different form of experience. But it could be added that those cases where a schizophrenia diagnosis is made in conjunction with a depression diagnosis show that the two cannot be clearly distinguished. One might object, though, that the existence of 'in between' cases poses no more of a problem for the distinction between schizophrenia and depression than the existence of moderate drinkers poses a problem for that between alcoholism

---

[10] Stanghellini (2004) similarly suggests that schizophrenia involves a global change in a person's relationship with the world and with other people.

and life-long abstinence. However, the success of this analogy hinges on depression and schizophrenia experiences being distinct 'poles', akin to alcoholism and abstinence. And we should at least be open to the possibility that phenomenological differences between the two—however pronounced they may seem—are only superficial and serve to obscure underlying existential changes that are similar in kind.[11] Nevertheless, I suggest that there is a qualitative difference between depression experiences that involve *diminution* or *erosion* of what some have called the 'minimal self' (see Chapter 6) and a *disruption* or *fragmentation* of self that is more typical of schizophrenia. This difference can be conceived of in terms of the anticipation-fulfilment dynamic described in Chapter 2. To show how, I will focus on the 'delusional atmosphere' that often precedes the onset of schizophrenic psychosis. This is more difficult to distinguish from depression than full-blown schizophrenia, given that characteristic delusions are absent. Furthermore, the phenomenological change it involves is elusive and hard to describe. Consider Jaspers' well known description:

> Patients feel uncanny and that there is something suspicious afoot. Everything gets a *new meaning*. The environment is somehow different—not to a gross degree—perception is unaltered in itself but there is some change which envelops everything with a subtle, pervasive and strangely uncertain light. A living-room which formerly was felt as neutral or friendly now becomes dominated by some indefinable atmosphere. Something seems in the air which the patient cannot account for, a distrustful, uncomfortable, uncanny tension invades him. (Jaspers, 1963, p.98)

This differs from the static world of depression, in that everything appears somehow novel, surprising. In the face of an enduring, all-enveloping feeling of anomaly, a confident style of anticipation is replaced by a growing sense of everything as unpredictable. Expectation takes the form 'I don't know what is coming next'. This is compatible with continuing to feel surprised by what does come next. Although the person expects things to be somehow different, what is anticipated is indeterminate, and the more determinate ways in which things then appear are not anticipated. By analogy, even if you enter a room with a vague anticipation that its contents will be somehow out of the ordinary, you can still be surprised by what you actually find. The experience thus differs from forms of anxious anticipation described in earlier

---

[11] The broad categorical distinction between depression and schizophrenia has also been challenged on other grounds. For instance, Van Os (2009) proposes that psychosis in depression, mania, and schizophrenia should instead be construed in terms of the single, broader category 'salience dysregulation syndrome'.

chapters. Whereas anxiety is a mode of anticipation, delusional atmosphere also involves a sense that something is already happening:

> Superficially this state of mood is similar to anxiety, but its internal structure is different. In a state of anxiety anything can happen, whereas in delusional moods something strange, enigmatic and incomprehensible is already happening. (Lopez-Ibor, 1982, p.147)

How, though, do things look anomalous? As with other kinds of existential change, the experience is not to be construed in terms of their seeming to have physical properties that they previously lacked, or vice versa. Instead, there is a shift in the kinds of possibility that are experienced. I have suggested that existential changes in depression can involve failing to anticipate possibilities of type p or anticipating them but encountering a world from which they are absent. What Jaspers describes is different. Entities have an unanticipated significance or a kind of significance that differs from what was anticipated: one anticipates p but experiences q, or one fails to anticipate p and experiences p. Furthermore, the kinds of significant possibility that they do offer are dissociated from their physical properties. Ordinarily, a hammer appears threatening when someone is waving it at you due to its potential to cause harm, and practically significant in relation to a project due to its nail-hitting potential. These kinds of significance are consistent with its properties and, in the latter case, with habitual use. Delusional atmosphere involves experiencing possibilities in a less structured way. A comfortable sofa may look somehow menacing, thus conflicting with the prior expectation that it will appear as something 'for sitting on' and perhaps also 'entice' one to sit. So it looks somehow wrong, strange and unfamiliar. This might fascinate or terrify, depending on what kind of anomalous significance it possesses. While existential depression involves impoverishment of the anticipation-fulfilment dynamic due to the consist *loss* of certain kinds of possibility from experience, delusional atmosphere involves a pervasive mismatch between kinds of anticipated and experienced significance. This amounts to a fragmentation of experience, a loss of the confident interplay of anticipation and fulfilment that more usually operates as a backdrop to experiences of uncertainty, doubt, and anomaly. We can distinguish privation from fragmentation in this way, while also allowing that they can occur together. A person might lack access to certain kinds of possibility, while the anticipation-fulfilment structure breaks down in relation to others. In addition, fragmentation may come in varying degrees and different forms, where the forms are to be distinguished in terms of the kinds of possibility affected.

Schizophrenia can therefore involve an erosion of practical significance that differs from what I have described in relation to depression. The world lacks a coherence that is required for the intelligibility of sustained purposive activity.[12] A breakdown of the dynamic, structured unfolding of practically salient possibilities constitutes a sense of being unable to practically engage with the world. However, when objects cease to invite activity, perceptual curiosity may be retained. The world still draws one in perceptually—it appears somehow anomalous, bewildering, fascinating. As there is a diminished sense of agency, involving loss of practical solicitation from the world, things no longer appear significant in relation to one's own potential activities. Instead, a seemingly autonomous significance emanates from them (Lopez-Ibor, 1982). Other people may appear different too. Insofar as they fail to offer kinds of possibility that are integral to distinctively *interpersonal* experience, they will look somehow impersonal, curiously mechanical, or artificial. With a loss of the interpersonal from experience, the line between 'my world' and a 'shared world' (in which my perspective is just one amongst many) becomes blurred, resulting in a quasi-solipsistic, voyeuristic predicament of the kind described in detail by Sass (1992, 1994).

Fuchs (2005) proposes a further way of distinguishing between experiences of schizophrenia and depression: the 'corporealization' typical of depression is to be contrasted with schizophrenic 'disembodiment'. Though this distinction is complicated by the range of bodily experiences associated with depression, it is consistent with the emphasis on a disengaged, spectatorial form of experience in schizophrenia. If the significant possibilities offered by one's surroundings are disrupted, they will no longer correspond to bodily capacities in a structured way, and so experience will no longer be shaped by a coherent sense of one's body. Hence the passive fascination that I have described could equally be construed as a pervasive feeling of detachment from one's body. In summary, then, I think that a very general (and admittedly rough) distinction can be drawn between different disturbances of the anticipation-fulfilment structure. Existential depression experiences involve privation, whereas schizophrenia is often associated with disruption. Various

---

[12] This is consistent with the view that schizophrenia involves 'aberrant salience' (see e.g. Kapur, 2003; Kapur, Mizrahi and Li, 2005). It thus points to the potential for mutually illuminating interactions between phenomenology, neurobiology, and pharmacology. For instance, phenomenological analysis enables us to distinguish different kinds of 'salience' and 'aberrance', by clarifying the various kinds of significant and enticing possibility that could be at play in any given case.

different combinations of privation and disruption are possible, which themselves amount to unitary existential feelings. Hence a clear line should not be drawn between 'schizophrenic' and 'depressive' forms of experience.[13]

More problematic is the distinction between depersonalization and depression. Depersonalization can arise in conjunction with both depression and schizophrenia, but 'depersonalization syndrome' or 'depersonalization-derealization' is also increasingly acknowledged as a condition in its own right (Medford et al, 2005; Simeon and Abugel, 2006; Colombetti and Ratcliffe, 2012). It is characterized by a feeling of being somehow detached from one's body and from the world. The world seems 'unreal', while one's body is experienced as strange or bereft of feeling. Medford et al. (2005, p.93) describe the symptoms as follows:

> ...some patients report feeling 'like a robot', 'different from everyone else' and 'separate from myself' [...]. Others describe feeling 'half-asleep' or 'as if my head is full of cotton wool', with associated difficulties in concentration. External reality may also be strangely altered: it may appear somehow artificial—as if 'painted, not natural', or 'two-dimensional' or 'as if everyone is acting out a role on stage, and I'm just a spectator'. Even though the world does not necessarily look unreal, it is nevertheless experienced as 'less interesting and less alive than formerly'. A reduction in, or complete absence of, bodily feelings is often described ('as if I were a phantom body', 'my hands seem not to belong to me'), as are reduced intensity in the experience of thirst, hunger and physical pain. Another frequent theme is a reduction or loss of emotional responses: 'my emotions are gone, nothing affects me', 'I am unable to have any emotions, everything is detached from me'.

Some but not all depression experiences involve depersonalization: the person feels curiously detached from other people and from the world more

---

[13] See also Sass and Pienkos (2013a, b) for a discussion of phenomenological similarities and differences between depression and schizophrenia. Sass and Pienkos (2013a) suggest that phenomenological changes in melancholic depression, which involve fatigue and loss of vitality, are generally less profound than those that occur in schizophrenia, where there is disturbance of a minimal or core experience of self and—with it—the sense of being part of a world. However, they also acknowledge that the differences are often unclear. I have suggested that existential changes in depression do concern this core experience of self, but that there is a distinction to be drawn between fragmentation and partial loss of the anticipation-fulfilment structure. My approach is thus consistent with the view that changes in self-experience associated with schizophrenia diagnoses tend to be more profound than those associated with depression diagnoses: fragmentation can involve a more pronounced existential shift than partial loss. However, Sass and Pienkos add that the disturbance in melancholia 'may occur more at the level of narrative identity' (2013a, p.118). I have argued that, in existential forms of depression, disruptions of self-narrative are symptomatic of changes in existential feeling, something that is presupposed by narrative and inseparable from a core sense of self.

generally, and she goes about her business mechanically rather than being drawn in by things.[14] I have suggested that such experiences be interpreted in terms of a loss of 'enticing possibilities', which leaves one feeling distant and disengaged. However, other kinds of depression experience are also associated with the theme of detachment. As discussed in Chapter 4, profound forms of existential hopelessness can involve feeling driven to act, but in a way that is quite different from responding to enticing possibilities that are embedded in significant projects:

> #117. I have stood on an edge of a pavement and felt like stepping out in front of a car. You do not feel this is your true self that is making this choice. It is as though a black fog has descended and you are trapped within a black sea of treacle being dragged to a bottomless pit. The deeper you go the blacker it gets and the more of your 'self' is lost.

Descriptions of feeling detached from one's actions are to be interpreted with caution. That action and choice are experienced differently when they cease to emanate from a 'true self' does not imply that this 'true self' is currently present in the guise of a detached spectator. A salient sense of something's absence from experience is quite different from a sense of its continuing but dislocated presence. In the above passage, detachment of a 'true self' from action is also described in terms a profoundly diminished sense of self—something has been 'lost'. The distance is more plausibly construed in temporal than spatial terms: one currently experiences the felt absence of something that used to be there. Hence some depression experiences involve a sense of 'dislocation' from things that is consistent with descriptions of depersonalization, while others involve something subtly but profoundly different—a sense of having lost something. If the latter are also to be characterized as involving a kind of 'depersonalization', then it is a very different kind of depersonalization. The schizophrenia experience described earlier involves a further form of 'depersonalization': a voyeuristic sense of detachment from one's body and one's surroundings that arises due to fragmentation of the anticipation-fulfilment structure. All three types of experience are to be conceived of in terms of unitary existential changes, rather than experiences of depression or schizophrenia *plus* something else. Once the existential change is described, there is no additional 'experience of depersonalization' to account for.

What about when depersonalization arises without depression or schizophrenia? Depersonalization is a 'syndrome', rather than a singular 'symptom' (Sierra et al, 2005). The case for its existence is based almost entirely on

---

[14] See Gaebler et al. (2013) for the view that depersonalized depression is a distinctive subtype.

first-person reports of experience, in the absence of detailed phenomenological analyses. So, as with depression, it is likely to include a range of different existential changes that people are inclined to describe in similar ways. In the light of the phenomenological distinctions I have drawn with respect to depression, it is not at all clear whether or how feeling 'half-asleep' is similar to feeling 'separate' from oneself or 'like a robot', or whether a world 'less interesting and alive' is anything like a world that looks 'artificial'. But this is not to deny that there are similarities between depersonalization experiences in depression and some of those that arise in other circumstances. As noted by Medford et al. (2005, p.95), 'healthy individuals exposed to life-threatening danger almost always report at least some features of depersonalization'. So we might expect something like this to happen when someone experiences a pronounced, all-enveloping dread, of a kind that crystallizes into the conviction that she is about to die. Again, though, it should not be concluded from this that the experience is one of depression *plus* depersonalization. When depression is 'added' to depersonalization or vice versa, there is a transition from one kind of existential feeling to another. The resultant experience differs from depersonalization in other contexts, as it is also shaped by the absence of certain kinds of possibility from experience. Simeon and Abugel (2006, p,72) observe that depersonalization is not always an unpleasant experience; sometimes 'the dissociation is a safe, comforting place for them to retreat, which shields them from being overwhelmed and envelops them in a state of nothingness'. However, the possibility of retreating to a 'safe, comforting place', whatever that might amount to, is absent from the world of depression.

Depression and Pathology

What, if anything, makes a depression experience 'pathological'? In addressing this question, I will use the term 'pathological' in a loose way, to mean simply that depression involves something going 'wrong' according to one or another criterion. Phenomenological descriptions can help us to better appreciate what depression experiences consist of, but they do not contain normative judgments to the effect that a *way of finding oneself in the world* is somehow pathological. Do they provide us with grounds for making these judgments though? I have referred throughout to *losses* of possibility and to what is *lacking* from the world of depression, indicating both privation of experience and experience of privation. However, as noted in Chapter 2, talk of 'loss' and 'addition' of possibility types is a convenient shorthand for capturing what are in fact *changes* in the structure of experience. The same change might be described in terms of the loss of p or the addition of q. In any

DEPRESSION AND PATHOLOGY | 265

case, loss, or even experienced loss, of something from experience does not imply wrongness. Loss of intense pain is not a matter of something having gone wrong, and neither is the feeling of absence experienced when a cast is removed after a broken bone has healed.

We could add that depression involves suffering. However, whether or not suffering is deemed 'pathological' depends on the circumstances. For instance, although intense grief involves great suffering, many would insist that it is often a healthy reaction to circumstances. A further criterion to consider is 'proportionality'. According to Horwitz and Wakefield (2007), all of the DSM depression symptoms can be normal, healthy reactions to life events. They are properly regarded as pathological only when disproportionate to their causes, and it is then that depression should be diagnosed, but removal of a proportionality criterion from the DSM classification scheme has resulted in a failure to distinguish depression from 'normal sadness', and thus to a proliferation of depression diagnoses. There are several problems with Horwitz and Wakefield's approach. First of all, depression is not simply a matter of intense 'sadness'. I have argued that existential changes are quite different from non-existential changes that are often described in superficially similar ways. So the possibility of drawing a distinction on phenomenological grounds (in addition to or instead of appealing to 'proportionality') should not be discounted. Furthermore, it is not clear how we go about determining whether a reaction is or is not proportionate in intensity (or appropriate in kind). Somebody who is devastated by the death of a pet goldfish could be reacting proportionately and appropriately, given an idiosyncratic set of cares and concerns that prioritized the goldfish's well-being over everything else. To label this reaction disproportionate, we would have to regard the value system in which it is embedded as inappropriate. When attempting to devise criteria on which to base such judgments, there would be a significant risk of sliding into ideologically dubious generalizations about which kinds of value system are and are not appropriate in the context of a human life. Of course, there may be other cases where a reaction is excessive in relation to the values one does have. Perhaps the person was indifferent to the goldfish until it died. But this presents us with an epistemological problem: it is difficult to distinguish a disproportionate reaction from an alternative scenario where 'I didn't realize how much that goldfish meant to me until it died'.

A further epistemological problem is that causal links between depressions and life events are hard to establish. The depressed person may interpret life events through a depressed mood and, in the process, mistakenly posit causes in the guise of unpleasant events. Even if her depression then seems proportionate to a cause, it may not be if the wrong cause has been identified.

Depression can also expose a person to unpleasant life events. For instance, a marriage breakdown could be partly attributable to depression. So cause and effect are difficult to disentangle (Maj, 2011). It is also plausible to suggest that a reaction can be both appropriate and proportionate to circumstances but—at the same time—obviously pathological. If somebody puts me in a boxing ring with Rocky Balboa, from which I am dragged shortly afterwards bruised and bleeding, there is obviously something wrong with me, something that requires urgent medical attention. I need not have a 'bruising disorder', one that causes me to have an over-reaction to Balboa's punches, in order to have a serious pathological condition.[15]

Nevertheless, perhaps the distinction can be drawn in a more specifically biological way, where disproportionate reactions are to be construed in terms of aberrant biological processes.[16] We do not have a comprehensive account of the various causal processes that culminate in depression experiences. However, we can still assign the status 'pathological' by appealing to the likelihood of something having gone biologically wrong or 'malfunctioned' (where 'malfunction' is construed in evolutionary terms, as a biological structure's having failed to perform a task that it was selected to perform). It can be added that the malfunction in question is a 'harmful' one (Horwitz and Wakefield, 2007). As we saw in Chapter 2, many depression experiences are much like illness experiences. Indeed, some (but certainly not all) are likely to be wholly or partly attributable to the same inflammatory processes. Nevertheless, disease *symptoms* are not themselves pathological. What is pathological is the disease process that causes them. And we have a choice between two conceptions of 'depression': (i) depression consists of one or more as yet unidentified pathological processes, to be detected by identifying characteristic symptoms; (ii) depression just *is* a 'syndrome' or cluster of symptoms (Radden, 2009, pp.79–80).

Depression 'symptoms', I have argued, include a range of different existential changes, as well as other kinds of experience. If a causal conception of

---

[15] Wilkinson (2000) makes this point with regard to grief, which he argues could be proportionate, appropriate, and understandable in the circumstances, while still warranting medical treatment. Grief, he suggests, might be considered analogous to a burn in this respect.

[16] There is much controversy over whether depression should be a 'medical' or a 'moral' concern (see, for example, Graham, 1990; Hansen, 2004; Martin, 1999). Although I have described the 'existential' structure of depression, this emphasis does not preclude a complementary biological approach. An existential conception of depression can inform biological enquiry, and vice versa. For example, Ghaemi (2013, p.64), drawing on Jaspers, advocates what he calls a 'biological existentialism'.

depression and its symptoms is adopted, then it is unclear why depression experiences should *themselves* be pathological: if y depends causally on x, where x is pathological, it does not follow that y is pathological. Of course, y could still serve to signal the presence of a disease process. But that position is mortgaged on there being pathological processes associated with *all* kinds of depression experience, a view that seems implausible given the degree of heterogeneity I have described. A less committal position, maintaining that at least *some* depression experiences arise due to disease processes, faces the problem that we are not yet in a position to determine which do and which do not. Distinguishing the various different kinds of experience that 'depression' encompasses is an important step in addressing that problem.

This is not to suggest that all of the relevant phenomenological work must be done before other forms of enquiry can get off the ground. Just as phenomenological considerations can inform scientific studies, empirical findings can assist in phenomenological research (as discussed in Chapters 3 and 6). Nevertheless, the empirical study of depression cannot proceed in ignorance of the relevant phenomenology. A singular account of the aetiology of phenomenon p will not be forthcoming when p includes but fails to distinguish q, r, and s, where q, r, and s are quite different from each other. Enquiry will lack focus, and the conflation of q, r, and s will result in conflicting findings and confusion. If we rely on cursory and superficial symptom descriptions, rather than on more discriminating phenomenological analyses of depression, this is exactly what we will face. The point applies equally to all of the different evolutionary, genetic, developmental, and neurobiological stories that might be told about depression. Insofar as we lack a clear conception of what it is that we seek to account for, the various competing or seemingly competing hypotheses cannot be satisfactorily assessed.[17]

If depression is instead identified with its symptoms, it is unclear what criteria we should appeal to in order to assign pathological status. What we are left with, I suggest, are various pragmatic criteria. These might well lead to judgments of pathology that turn out to be consistent with the deliverances of more specifically biological approaches, but there could equally be conflict. In short, one evaluates the effects that depression has on a person's life. This does not give us rigid criteria and admits of considerable vagueness. There is also the risk of being guided by various questionable presuppositions. Even so, pragmatic criteria can be quite sufficient in practice, at least in more severe cases (and many

---

[17] See, for example, some of the essays in Pariante et al eds. (2009) and Gotlib and Hammen eds. (2009) for discussions of the evolutionary basis, genetics, and developmental psychopathology of depression.

milder forms of depression will be excluded from my account on the basis that they do not involve existential changes). If a person won't get out of bed, won't eat, can't face other people, can't perform mundane tasks, aches all over, experiences all-pervasive dread, and wants to die, there is clearly something 'wrong'. She is unable to do what she ordinarily does, and she is suffering.[18]

One might object that there are also benefits to having depression. People can and often do gain something from it. They may adjust their projects, priorities, goals, and attitudes towards others, in ways that they and/or others regard as an improvement. And they may come to be grateful for something they previously took for granted. But this observation is consistent with the view that, overall, depression is a bad thing to have. People make similar life changes having endured conditions that clearly are pathological, including serious illness and injury. It can be added that *types* of depression experience are not reliably associated with *types* of benefit, indicating a tenuous connection at best, and that many plausibly involve no benefit at all. However, matters are less clear when we turn to the question of whether or not depression has specifically *epistemic* benefits. The potential benefits of having experienced depression certainly include that of learning something from it. For instance, I have suggested that having undergone a profound existential change can serve to culture recognition of the fact that *finding oneself in the world* is a phenomenological achievement, one that is fragile and changeable. But I am concerned with something different: the epistemic credentials of depression experiences themselves. Does *being depressed* facilitate recognition of certain truths that one would otherwise be unlikely or unable to appreciate? Alternatively, does depression present one with a view of the world that is distorted or misleading (a view that may itself contribute to depression's detrimental effect on one's well-being)?

Epistemic benefit is to be distinguished from pragmatic benefit, given the possibility of acquiring true beliefs that are emotionally devastating and detrimental to one's well-being.[19] Even so, pragmatic and epistemic considerations are closely related, and how we respond to a depression experience

---

[18] What I am suggesting here is consistent with the more detailed account of values-based practice offered by Jackson and Fulford (1997, 2002) and Fulford (e.g. 1994, 2004).

[19] For much the same reason, epistemic and biological 'wrongness' can also come apart. It is often pointed out that certain false beliefs (including evaluative beliefs) could be biologically advantageous, while access to certain truths could put one at a biological disadvantage. For example, the belief 'I am invincible in battle' conceivably enhances fighting ability in a way that increases the likelihood of survival. Hence, even if we concede that a form of experience and the kinds of belief it disposes one towards are undesirable in a biological sense, we need not give up on the view that it is revelatory.

will reflect—amongst other things—how we regard its epistemic credentials. 'Treating' a predicament that centrally involves an accurate but disruptive evaluation of a person's life is more problematic than treating one that involves a false and similarly disruptive evaluation. By analogy, p's grief over the death of q, in a case where q has indeed died, warrants a different response to r's phenomenologically indistinguishable grief over the death of s, where s has not died and r is somehow unable to register the fact. Now, a *way of finding oneself in the world* does not in itself amount to an intellectual position that can be regarded as right or wrong, reliable or unreliable, appropriate or inappropriate, well informed or poorly informed. However, some kinds of depression experience do incorporate a contestable 'view of the world', one that is not always easy to dismiss. In order to address the question of whether or not such experiences are symptomatic of what we might call 'epistemic pathology', I will focus more specifically upon a distinctive kind of 'existential despair', as described by Tolstoy.[20]

The Truth or Otherwise of Existential Despair

In *A Confession*, Tolstoy recounts an experience of suicidal despair that would nowadays be classified as one of major or severe depression. At one point, he conveys it in terms of an 'Eastern fable, told long ago'. A traveller runs from a beast and seeks refuge in a well. At the bottom of the well is a dragon, and so the traveller is unable to climb out or climb down. He clings to a twig growing from the side of the well, which two mice—one black and the other white—chew at in turn. As the traveller awaits his inevitable fate, he consoles himself by licking drops of honey from leaves that grow on the twig, the taste of which distracts him from his plight. Tolstoy's problem was that the honey stopped tasting sweet:

> So I too clung to the twig of life, knowing that the dragon of death was inevitably awaiting me, ready to tear me to pieces; and I could not understand why I had fallen into such torment. I tried to lick the honey which formerly consoled me; but the honey no longer gave me pleasure, and the white and black mice of day and night gnawed at the branch by which I hung. I saw the dragon clearly, and the honey no longer tasted sweet. I only saw the unescapable dragon and the mice, and I could not tear my gaze from them. And this is not a fable, but the real unanswerable truth intelligible to all. (Tolstoy, 2005, p.18)[21]

---

[20] See Graham (1990) for the view that depression can, in some circumstances at least, be appropriate or justified. However, he states that his claims apply only to 'intentional' forms of depression. These are to be contrasted with the existential forms I have focused on here.

[21] If one replaces the word 'honey' with 'alcohol', what Tolstoy describes is remarkably similar to what some alcoholism memoirs describe. For example, it conforms to most of

This description makes salient the sense of revelation and certainty that is integral to Tolstoy's despair. It presents itself as the 'real unanswerable truth', and as something that was always lurking in the background but formerly eclipsed by distractions. Once those distractions are swept away, he can no longer hide from a way of being that offers only futility and then extinction.[22] There is some similarity here with more mundane experiences of losing ourselves in something in order to take our minds off something else. One might spend an evening with friends and feel temporary relief from the pain of bereavement, or go to the cinema to forget about an impending job interview. But what Tolstoy describes is more profound—one flees not from some contingent circumstance but from the structure of human life.

It is important to distinguish the kind of despair Tolstoy describes from other predicaments associated with depression diagnoses, which might also be labelled as 'hopelessness' or 'despair'. Tolstoy's despair involves an especially profound loss of existential hope (of a kind described in Chapter 4). It is not specific to him; it relates to all human life. And it is not just that he takes all human life to be without value. He cannot even contemplate the possibility of its being otherwise, and the experience has a *feeling* of irrevocable certainty to it. The capacity to take pleasure in anything, to be drawn in by situations, or to engage in meaningful activity is altogether absent. As a result, there is no source of distraction from the well. But this does not suffice to characterize the experience fully. Why does all human activity appear but a futile distraction? A heightened and/or altered awareness of mortality seems to be largely responsible, and Tolstoy couches existential despair in terms of a negative response to the question 'is there any meaning in my life that the inevitable death awaiting me does not destroy?' (2005, p.21). There is more to it than this, however. In addition to the poignant awareness of life as finite and meaningless, it involves—in Tolstoy's case, at least—an unpleasant feeling of

---

the 43 first-person accounts in the Alcoholics Anonymous *Big Book*. The person's sense of significant possibilities contracts until all that appears enticing and significant in a positive way is the next drink. Everything else is to be endured, with alcohol offering consolation and temporary relief. But the source of consolation itself becomes a source of suffering. Life then takes the form of a journey into increasing wretchedness, upon which the person feels compelled to travel due to the absence of any other kinds of enticing or significant possibility.

[22] We find similar themes in some of Heidegger's works, where it is claimed that certain mood changes involve the 'awakening' of a mood that was already there, rather than the replacement of one mood by another: 'Whatever is sleeping' is in a peculiar way absent and yet there. When we awaken an attunement [*Stimmung*], this means that it is already there. At the same time, it expresses the fact that in a certain way it is *not* there' (Heidegger, 1995, p.60).

urgency (which corresponds to an experience of bodily agitation described in Chapter 7). There is a felt need to act for the sake of some end, which is rendered insatiable by the ever-present sense of mortality and all-embracing futility:

> Had I been like a man living in a wood from which he knows there is no exit, I could have lived; but I was like one lost in a wood who, horrified at having lost his way, rushes about, wishing to find the road. (Tolstoy, 2005, p.19)

So the experience is something like this: a heightened sense of mortality comes to light when the capacity for effortless, pleasurable immersion in activity is blocked, and this renders worthwhile activity unintelligible. An agitated need to achieve something lingers on, with no possible outlet. Why, though, should an appreciation of mortality be incompatible with purposive activity? The answer, it seems, is that a sense of any activity's being worthwhile tacitly depends on the possibility of its infinite teleological development. This is incompatible with the extinction of every human accomplishment, something one accepts as inevitable in properly grasping the nature of mortality. There is a felt realization that everything we do will ultimately leave no trace upon the universe. The association between mortality and futility can be further illuminated by drawing attention to the theme of evil. This is more prominent in some of William James's works, especially *Varieties of Religious Experience* (in a well-known chapter entitled 'The Sick Soul' where James quotes and discusses Tolstoy's *A Confession* at length). James describes an intense awareness of human mortality and the inevitability of suffering, which develops into an experience of the world as fundamentally evil, a place in which we can never be safe or feel at home. Our projects crumble, given that they rest upon a hope or faith in the goodness of life that reveals itself as utterly unfounded:

> The fact that we *can* die, that we *can* be ill at all, is what perplexes us; the fact that we now for a moment live and are well is irrelevant to that perplexity. We need a life not correlated with death, a health not liable to illness, a kind of good that will not perish, a good in fact that flies beyond the Goods of nature. (James, 1902, p.140)

For those James calls 'sick souls', the feeling of evil is ever-present: 'the evil aspects of our life are of its very essence, and [...] the world's meaning most comes home to us when we lay them most to heart' (James, 1902, p.131). The theme is present in Tolstoy's account too when, for instance, he recalls witnessing an execution in Paris some years earlier and feeling that the horror of the guillotine could never be reconciled with a fundamentally good world that accommodates worthwhile human activity.

How might one respond to such an experience? Tolstoy's existential journey ends with religious conversion. He comes to recognize that what first struck him as a truth about all human life was actually more parochial and concerned the privileged, parasitic social elite to which he belonged. He distances himself from that way of life to discover the faith of the peasants. Tolstoy is clear that there is no purely intellectual solution to be found, as existential despair sweeps away the ground on which all intellectual endeavours rest. What he discovers is a new way of living, more so than a new way of thinking. However, his 'solution' is unsatisfying for several reasons. The view of Tolstoy's pre-conversion life that he presents in *A Confession* is one-sided and uncharitable. Furthermore, after his conversion, he was inconsistent and conflicted in many respects, and he was consumed until his death by an exceptionally unhappy and destructive marriage. As one biographer remarks, 'once one is alerted to the danger signals, *A Confession*, precisely because of its artless sincerity, is revealed as a transparent piece of self-deception: transparent, that is, to everyone except the author' (Wilson, 2001, p.312). Regardless of such concerns, Tolstoy's solution is historically specific and does not offer clear guidance to us now. Who, for us, are analogous to his 'simple laboring folk'? With so many cultures and attitudes to sample, it is not at all clear where to look for practical wisdom. In any case, the epistemological question I want to address is somewhat different. I am not concerned so much with potential first-person responses but with what form a third-person response to the view that 'this is what human life consists of' should take. In refusing to accept the deliverances of existential despair, what grounds do I have for believing that I am not simply impervious to the truth? If existential despair of this kind is symptomatic of epistemic pathology, what criteria can we appeal to in order to determine that?

One approach is to address the more general question of how depression affects the capacity for evaluative judgment, and then regard existential despair accordingly. Does depression render the relevant cognitive processes more or less reliable? According to so-called 'depressive realism' (mentioned briefly in Chapter 2), it fosters more accurate evaluations, at least in relation to matters such as one's social status, abilities, and degree of culpability for undesirable outcomes (Alloy and Abramson, 1988). The general idea was nicely expressed much earlier by Freud:

> If [...] he describes himself as a petty, egoistic, insincere and dependent person, who has only ever striven to conceal the weakness of his nature, he may as far as we know have come quite close to self-knowledge, and we can only wonder why one must become ill in order to have access to such truth. (Freud, 2005, p.206)

However, it would be implausible to suggest that depressive realism supports the case for existential despair. Proponents of depressive realism concede that depression not only corrects certain biases; it also renders the person more susceptible to others (Alloy and Abramson, 1988, p.243). Furthermore, the evidence for depressive realism is questionable in several respects. It is not always clear that there is an objective standard for comparison to support claims about the appropriateness or otherwise of an evaluation; the design of some studies has been called into question; the experimental results are amenable to several interpretations; and almost as many findings are inconsistent with it as are consistent with it (Ackermann and DeRubeis, 1991).[23] At best, depressive realism seems to be a fragile phenomenon that shows up only under certain conditions. Crucially, much of the empirical support for it involves subjects who are not severely depressed, and the effect diminishes and disappears as severity increases (Ghaemi, 2007). So, if we assume that what Tolstoy describes is generally associated with more severe forms of depression, the depressive realism findings are inapplicable.

Does the evidence instead favour the view that severe depression is associated with unreliable evaluative judgments? It is plausible to suggest that all stages of intellectual enquiry are motivated and guided by emotions of various kinds, such as curiosity, doubt, wonder, surprise, and satisfaction (e.g. Hookway, 2002; Thagard, 2002; Morton, 2010). Given that depression lessens or even extinguishes the capacity for some of these, it surely interferes with belief-forming processes, especially where value judgments are concerned. Elliott (1999, pp.93–97) therefore raises the concern that, although a person's reasoning may appear intact when she is depressed, her decision-making ability can still be impaired. Her access to cares and concerns that would more usually shape decision-making is impeded by an inability to feel:

> To put the matter simply, if a person is depressed, he may be *aware* that a protocol carries risks, but simply not *care* about those risks. [...] When a person is caught in the grip of depression, his values, beliefs, desires and dispositions are dramatically different from when he is healthy. In some cases, they are so different that we might ask whether his decisions are truly his.

Hence it is arguable that existential despair, which arises from an inability to experience certain feelings and a consequent loss of access to values, is a deceptive, impoverished evaluation of human life. However, that view is also problematic. Our epistemic capacities are surely to some degree heterogeneous, a point that may well apply more specifically to our evaluative tendencies. The capacities needed to appreciate the irrevocable futility of all human life could be quite different from those needed to make other types of value

---

[23] Allan, Siegel, and Hannah (2007) attribute the phenomenon not to an enhanced capacity for certain kinds of evaluative judgment but to the simple fact that depressives are 'nay-sayers', who have to be more confident about something before endorsing it.

judgment. Furthermore, an overarching evaluation of all human activity as irrevocably futile would most likely have a detrimental effect on cognitive ability more generally. So it is not enough to make a case for impaired evaluation in some other context and then appeal to guilt by association. A disturbing and accurate evaluation of human life could be precisely what impedes one's ability to evaluate in that other context. It would be comparable to grief in this respect: an experience of profound grief can involve an accurate evaluation of loss, while interfering with thought and activity more generally.

A more promising approach is to maintain that existential despair is epistemically pathological because, like depression more generally, it involves losing kinds of possibility that play an essential epistemic role (regardless of whether or not it is also describable in terms of the 'addition' of other kinds of possibility). The way the despairing person evaluates her predicament (and that of others too) is symptomatic of her inability to contemplate alternatives. In order to competently evaluate a state of affairs as p rather than q, one must be able to first comprehend the possibility of q and then rule it out. If an ability to even entertain the possibility of q were lost, then one's commitment to p would reflect incapacity rather than p's relative plausibility. As we have seen, feelings of certainty that arise in depression are often deceptive. For instance, the belief that recovery is impossible stems from an inability to contemplate something that is not only possible but probable. We can understand both the content of the evaluation and the associated sense of unwavering conviction in the same way: inability to contemplate alternatives leads to a pared-down evaluation of the world that presents itself as certain. If access to alternatives were restored, it would again reveal itself as a contingent evaluation, and not a very enticing one either.[24] Consider the analogy with dreaming, which likewise involves an epistemic asymmetry: we might not be aware that we are dreaming while we are dreaming, but we can usually make the distinction with confidence once awake, when the limitations of the dream-world become readily apparent. Existential despair, we might suggest, is akin to the dream-world, in that it is oblivious to its shortcomings. Those who are not stuck in it have access to kinds of possibility that reveal its certainties as misguided.

Unfortunately, matters are not so clear. What applies to depression arguably applies more generally: feelings restrict the options for belief. When beliefs amount to mere intellectual play, commitment to p rather than q might not demand a feeling of certainty. But those convictions that matter to us most,

---

[24] See also Meynen (2011) for a discussion of how the inability to experience possibilities affects decision-making in depression.

that regulate our activities and our aspirations, are not a matter of putting ticks next to propositions. Confidence comes as we cease to *feel* the pull of significant alternatives. This applies to our most cherished intellectual commitments, as well as many religious beliefs. Similarly in depression, one not only believes that p; one becomes increasingly unable to appreciate how anyone could possibly believe otherwise, as nothing else feels salient. So, why is existential despair to be singled out as intellectually dubious, rather than all those evaluative beliefs that are held with strong conviction? A difference is that other cases involve an inability to contemplate *token* possibilities rather than *types* of possibility. One retains access to the various ways in which things could be significant; it just happens that alternative q is not experienced as significant in some or all of these ways. Hence the ability to evaluate is not deficient; one does not form the belief that q doesn't matter because one is incapable of taking anything to matter. Depression and, more specifically, existential despair are therefore special cases.

However, let us briefly return to Heidegger's discussion of the phenomenological role of anxiety in *Being and Time*. He describes the 'mood' of anxiety as amounting to a total loss of practical significance from the experienced world. It is not that one no longer finds p, q, or r practically significant. Rather, one's ability to find anything practically significant is absent, temporarily at least. Even so, Heidegger regards this as potentially revelatory. Ordinarily, he claims, we lose ourselves in the everyday, public world in ways that eclipse the underlying structure of human existence. By sweeping away the capacity to find things practically significant, a capacity upon which the disposition to misinterpret ourselves depends, anxiety gives us phenomenological access to something that would otherwise be obscured. If something like this is at all plausible (in this or any other case we manage to cook up), it could be that loss of possibility in depression does not always cultivate illusion. Some such experiences may free us from something that hides the truth. In order to reveal what is obscured, access has to be suspended.[25]

We can respond by observing that, when people recover from depression, they regain access to possibilities, the effect of which is to reveal the contingency of what they previously took as certain. Despair loses its allure and is revealed as a symptom of privation. Furthermore, even if we cannot show conclusively that despair is mistaken (as there is no objective measure

---

[25] Another example of the association between loss of possibility and revelation is the 'dark night of the soul', as described by St John of the Cross (Kavanaugh, ed. 1987). In order to find God, he maintains, one must first endure a purification process that culminates in complete loss of the intelligibility of hope, the 'dark night of the spirit'.

for comparison), other factual and evaluative beliefs, such as 'recovery from depression is impossible' and 'things cannot get better', are clearly false. We know that recovery is possible and that a belief to the contrary is symptomatic of an inability to contemplate alternatives. Existential despair has the same structure, and is thus plausibly regarded in the same way, as a symptom of contingent limitation rather than a source of revelation. So the comparison with Heideggerian anxiety does not apply. Even if Heidegger is right about the kind of existential change he describes, his account does not concern *all* such changes, and this one is different in structure.

However, there is a problem. For some people, recovery from depression is not accompanied by rejection of the evaluation of human life that it embodied. Instead, a sense of revelation remains. Existential feelings, I have argued, comprise a sense of the possible, and this can include a sense of their own contingency, their susceptibility to change. Once one has left the world of depression, the place one returns to can be imbued with a new kind of contingency. One recognizes the fragility of a way of belonging to the world that was previously taken for granted. And this contingency can involve the appreciation that one might re-enter a place where something that now seems distant will again appear with the force of revelation. Many of those who have suffered from depression describe their recovery in terms of regaining something they were previously deprived of. But for some, although despair becomes less salient with the return of possibilities, it continues to lurk in the background like a preying monster, with a feeling of undeniable truth still attached to it:

> #154. I do not have that 'switch', that 'normal' function, and those like me (other people that are affected by mental illness) are able to see past the 'programmed' normality that the majority of humans have and realize that there is no point to the world, there is nothing to look forward to, humans simply exist to perpetuate themselves. [...] This 'explanation' of how the world works doesn't go completely when I come out of a depression, the thoughts are still there, they are just lighter and further away...

Depression is often (perhaps even always) the route via which one arrives at existential despair, but a sense of futility can outlast the depression. Ghaemi (2007, p.126) thus raises the concern that some treatments may tackle depression while leaving a person in 'existential despair'. We should concede, then, that despair cannot be attributed solely to an inability to contemplate alternatives; it can persist in some form after that ability has returned and still 'feel like truth'. James (1889, pp.327–330) describes how we move between various 'sub-universes' in our day to day lives, including the world of sense, the world of science, the supernatural world, and the world of madness. One of these we select as our 'world of *ultimate* realities'. For most of us, this is the world of sense, but others place the flag of truth in the supernatural realm or in scientifically described reality. Something along these lines applies to existential feeling. Our existential feelings wobble in subtle ways, but most of us retain a sense that some ways of finding ourselves in the world are better grounded in 'how things are' than others. The detachment of jet lag, for instance, is experienced *as* something that dislodges one from the world, from a place where thoughts are more reliably formed. How, then, do we respond to someone who continues to place the flag of truth in the world of existential despair? What grounds are there for rejecting the view that he subscribes to a legitimate or even uniquely appropriate evaluation of human life?

Rather than challenging existential despair on the basis that it is the product of unreliable cognitive processes or an impoverished possibility space, we might take issue with the plausibility of its content. A simple objection to existential despair, considered as an intellectual position, is that awareness of mortality just does not need to be associated with existential catastrophe. I can be well aware that I and everyone else will suffer and die, without all of my projects becoming unintelligible or the universe taking on an air of evil. However, it is arguable that both the content of the position and the attitude of acceptance are partly constituted by existential feeling, and that neither can be *fully* appreciated without having (or having had) the required feeling. Some feelings may, as Wynn (2005, p.9) remarks, 'offer our only mode of access to certain values'. Thus, when the association between mortality and futility is casually dismissed, this could be due to confusion between the content of existential despair and some other content that is superficially similar but subtly different.[26] So, even if our own thoughts about death and the worth of human action do not add up to existential despair, we can still ask whether those who do suffer from it might have stumbled upon a truth that we have the good fortune of being unable to access.

Even if those of us who have not glimpsed existential despair cannot rule out its being an accurate appraisal of human life, we can at least insist that we ourselves have no reason to be intellectually troubled by it. Just as one cannot fully appreciate its content and pull without experiencing the requisite feelings, so too those in existential despair lack full experiential access to non-despairing ways of being in the world (whether or not they are depressed). Neither party can be, or ought to be, intellectually swayed by the

---

[26] This is consistent with Tolstoy's well-known contrast in his short novel *The Death of Ivan Ilych* between two different ways of believing that one will die. The protagonist comes to understand that he will die, in a felt way that differs from conceding propositionally that all people die, that he is a person, and that he will therefore die.

other, and we end up with a stalemate of conflicting feelings. Having established a stalemate, we could then argue on pragmatic grounds for the superiority of a non-despairing stance: choosing despair over hope is a lose-lose bet (Garrett, 1994). However, it is debatable whether and to what extent there could be a choice over despair; it has an affective allure that plausibly cannot be over-ridden by any amount of cold calculation. A similar concern applies to Cooper's (2002) view that despair is to be alleviated by nurturing a sense of the world as fundamentally mysterious. When stuck in Tolstoy's well, one is unable to contemplate the possibility of the world's being mysterious in an ultimately good or even indeterminate way. The only sense of mystery one is able to cultivate involves a sense of inchoate evil, which may linger on even after one has recovered from depression. So the stalemate persists. Even supposing the relevant feelings could be re-trained, there is the worry that success would involve steering someone away from a sound evaluation of human life and towards a more bearable illusion. One cannot simply entertain existential despair and decide, on pragmatic or other grounds, to reject it, as it has an epistemic allure; it *feels* right. One would have to try to escape it, to forget it, to trick oneself. And there is also the concern that existential despair eventually gets the upper hand anyway. James (1902, p.140) points out how we at least *glimpse* something like Tolstoy's well when we are injured, fatigued, or sick:

> ...so with most of us: a little cooling down of animal excitability and instinct, a little loss of animal toughness, a little irritable weakness and descent of the pain-threshold, will bring the worm at the core of our usual springs of delight into full view, and turn us into melancholy metaphysicians.

Hence it is arguably something that we are untroubled by only if we have not yet had the kinds of experience that serve to reveal it. To be free of the pull of despair is to be ignorant of something, and only for a time. If that view could be made convincing, it would leave us with a case for despair rather than a stalemate.

I will bring my discussion to a close by briefly outlining a different approach. What if, instead of trying to challenge existential despair, we accept it but seek to mitigate it? Upon recovery from depression, certain kinds of significant possibility become accessible again. And the loss of these possibilities is debilitating regardless of any relationship it might have to despair. In the absence of depression, the person is at least capable of immersing herself in activities again, and of enjoying herself. Of course, it might be suggested that this just amounts to a revitalized capacity for distraction, a taste for honey. However, it is not at all clear why all activities should be incompatible with a heightened appreciation of mortality and finitude. Consider activities such as building a sandcastle with one's children or spending the day gardening. One knows, from the outset, that the sandcastle will soon be washed away without a trace, that many of the plants one handles with such care will die as winter approaches, that the fruits of such activities are short-lived. It is doubtful that the majority of sandcastle builders and gardeners fall prey to the illusion that things are otherwise, but their projects do not strike them as futile, incoherent, or unintelligible. The point applies equally to all of those intellectual and practical activities that are driven by curiosity, fascination, aesthetic feelings, and perhaps a wide range of other modes of 'enticement'. In short, much of what we preoccupy ourselves with does not tacitly rest on a conception of life teleology that is inconsistent with our mortality.

In response, one might object that a constant, felt awareness of one's unavoidable demise disrupts these activities too. However, there is a distinction between disruption attributable to the realization that one will die and disruption caused by repeated occurrences of beliefs that happen to have the content 'I will die'. If I experienced incessant intrusive beliefs with the content 'Durham Cathedral is bigger than York Minster', they would no doubt disrupt my concentration. But their content is incidental, and my life when I am not thinking 'Durham Cathedral is bigger than York Minster' is not in conflict with that belief content. So the disruptive effect of a psychological state does not have to be primarily due to its content. The point applies to 'death' beliefs too. What is disruptive is the intrusiveness of the occurrent thought that one will die, not acceptance of the fact that one will die, even if it is acknowledged that full recognition of mortality can indeed be distressing and that death beliefs are therefore more disruptive than cathedral beliefs. It is thus arguable that a substantial proportion of our activities are untarnished by the acceptance of existential despair, at least when despair is considered separately from a loss of possibilities that is symptomatic of severe depression and not just despair, a loss that *does* amount to privation of epistemic ability. Only certain kinds of project, with a distinctive kind of motivational structure, present themselves as incompatible with mortality. And it is difficult to determine exactly which projects are vulnerable, as the evaluative framework that threatens them involves feeling and cannot be fully appreciated without the required feelings.

This response can be supplemented by another line of argument. James (1889, p.333) suggests that the allure of a broad conception of reality is symptomatic of the extent to which it relates to one's life: 'Whatever things have intimate and continuous connexion with my life are things of whose reality I cannot doubt. Whatever things fail to establish this connexion are things which are practically no better for me than if they existed not at all'. Existential despair, one might retort, is not 'related' to the structure of a life. It entails the unintelligibility of any meaningful way of finding oneself in the world and is opposed to any system of life projects, preferences, commitments, cares, and concerns. But the point can be rephrased: existential despair *feels right* in the context of a certain kind of life. What kind of life though? Implicit in many accounts of despair is a curiously individualistic way of construing life projects: what is of worth in *my* life; can the worth of *my* projects withstand *my* mortality? I have suggested that an all-enveloping sense of alienation from other people is absolutely central to experiences of depression in general. People who look back on their depression often remark on the extent to which they were lonely, self-absorbed, cut off from others. And others who 'recover' from depression may continue to feel socially isolated, something that is likely to involve an enduring preoccupation with *one's own life*.

It is by no means clear why all *interpersonal* cares, concerns, and commitments should be rendered futile in the light of one's mortality, everyone's mortality, or even by a conviction that the world is fundamentally evil. The point is nicely illustrated by the 2011 film *Melancholia*, directed by Lars von Trier. Two sisters, Claire and Justine, are confronted with the prospect of Earth's imminent and unavoidable destruction by the approaching planet Melancholia. What kinds of activity are appropriate or even meaningful while the annihilation of humanity and anything it might have accomplished fast approaches? Justine, who has been suffering from severe depression, tells her sister that life on Earth is evil and that she somehow *knows* there is no life anywhere else. As the film progresses, her depression lifts and she starts to wash and eat again, but her appraisal of human life does not falter. Indeed, it is made concrete for the viewer in the guise of the planet's approach. Even so, as the end nears, she chooses to be with her nephew, to comfort him— she builds a 'shelter' with him, a 'magic cave'. Nothing renders that kind of concern unintelligible to her. At the same time, she dismisses as absurd her sister's suggestion that they await the end of the world with a glass of wine on the terrace—they might as well meet on the toilet; there is no meaningful difference between the two scenarios.

The evaluation of human life contained in Tolstoy's well is not obviously a barrier to interpersonal concern, other than when it is accompanied by an inability to connect with others that is attributable to loss of access to certain kinds of possibility. The questions 'What is the point in my doing *x*; what will I achieve by it?' and 'What is the point in caring for my children?' address different kinds of concern. Whereas the former can be a legitimate request for justification, one that is sometimes met with a negative answer, the latter is different. The question is somehow poorly formed. That kind of care more usually goes without saying and even asking a question like this points to one's lacking something: access to a type of concern that does not require legitimation through reference to one or another forward-looking project. Both types of concern can be affected by loss of possibilities in depression, but any lingering sense of revelation one might have regarding one's projects does not automatically extend to the kind of care one has for one's children or, indeed, for people more generally. And, to the extent that one's projects are structured by interpersonal concerns, they are similarly insulated from existential despair. So, although it could well be that certain projects are existentially incoherent in structure—tacitly premised on a drive towards ever-greater achievements of whatever kind, without a *felt* recognition of their impermanence—it would be a mistake to generalize from these to all kinds of project.

Of course, there is a lot more to be said, but these reflections at least point towards the conclusion that existential despair, of the kind that I have described here, is something that only some kinds of project and some kinds of human life are susceptible to, those shaped by a contingent form of self-absorption that also amounts to a way of relating to others. There is a profound sense of social isolation and loneliness at the heart of many depression experiences, which does not always disappear completely when depression is no longer diagnosed. A person's actual interpersonal circumstances may not change much, and feelings of rejection, alienation, abandonment, and disconnection may still predominate in her relations with others. As well as nice-tasting honey, what is absent from Tolstoy's well is the possibility of certain kinds of interpersonal connection and concern. When the despair outlasts the depression, it is symptomatic of a more subtle existential privation in the interpersonal domain, rather than the universal, irrevocable structure of human life.

Appendix

Details of Depression Questionnaire Respondents

The table below contains the following information for all Depression Questionnaire respondents quoted in this book:

1. Questionnaire number
2. Gender: (M)ale; (F)emale; (O)ther
3. Age at the time of response (2011)
4. Year of first depression diagnosis
5. Diagnosis, as stated by respondent
6. Other psychiatric diagnoses, as stated by respondent
7. Currently depressed: (Y)es; (N)o

The numbers in column 1 correspond to the numbers that appear with each quotation.

1	2	3	4	5	6	7
8	O	55	2008	Moderate depression	Gender dysphoria	Y
14	F	28	2000	Major depression	Anxiety	Y
15	F	34	2005	Severe depression	Borderline personality disorder	Y
16	F	16	2010	Severe depression with hypermanic [sic] traits		Y
17	F	25	2009	Major depression		N
20	F	35	1999	Depression	Bipolar II disorder	N
21	F	24	2001	Depression		N
22	F	23	2007	Major depression		N
23	F	24	2009	Major depression		Y
24	F	19	2009	Major depression		N
26	F	43	2008	Bipolar disorder	Borderline personality disorder	Y

1	2	3	4	5	6	7
28	M	37	2011	Clinical depression		Y
30	M	17	2010	Clinical depression	Severe anxiety disorder	Y
34	F	39	1996	Depression	Anxiety disorder; borderline personality disorder	N
37	F	40	1999	Post-natal depression; depression		N
38	F	35	2009	Depression		N
41	F	36	2010	Major depression		Y
45	F	20	2006	Depression	Borderline personality disorder; eating disorder	Y
49	F	22	2005	Mild depression	Anxiety	N
51	F	18	2006	Depression	Attention Deficit disorder; Posttraumatic stress disorder	Y
53	F	17	2008	Mild depression	Generalized anxiety disorder	N
54	F	38	1999	Major depression	Complex posttraumatic stress disorder, with related psychosis	Y
61	F	35	1993	Clinical depression		N
65	F	33	2009	Depression		Y
66	F	50	1983	Reactive depression and anxiety		Y
75	F	26	2004	Major depression	Eating disorder	N
84	F	58	1982	Depression		Y
85	F	31	2009	Severe depression		Y
88	F	31	2009	Severe depression		Y
97	F	30	2000	Major depression and anxiety		Y
98	F	44	2001	Multiple diagnoses, including bipolar disorder	Borderline personality disorder	Y
106	F	45	1985	Severe depression		Y
107	F	21	2009	Depression		Y
110	F	48	1997	Depression	Panic attacks; anxiety disorder	N
112	F	32	2010	Severe depression		Y

1	2	3	4	5	6	7
117	F	49	1997	Depression		N
124	F	20	2008	Depression	Anxiety disorder; anorexia; bulimia; social phobia	Y
129	M	37	1991	Depression	Drug-induced psychosis	Y
130	F	21	2005	Cyclic dysthymia with major depressive disorder		Y
133	F	21		No diagnosis		Y
134	F	37	1988	Depression	Agoraphobia; social phobia; generalized anxiety disorder	Y
137	F	65	1964	Major depression		N
138	F	18	2009	Depression; emotional dysregulation	Borderline personality disorder; anxiety; body dysmorphic disorder	Y
143	M	54	2006	Depression	Affect disorder	Y
147	F	22	2009	Depression		Y
150	F	37	1993	Clinical depression	Brief period of psychosis	Y
153	F	63	1967	Unspecified depression	Compulsive hoarding	N
154	?	50	2000	Bipolar disorder with prominent depressive episodes		N
155	M	50s	1996	Chronic depression		Y
158	F	20	2009	Clinical depression	Borderline personality disorder	Y
161	F	30		No diagnosis		Y
166	F	28	2006	Depression		Y
168	F	40	1996	Depression		Y
171	F	33	1987	Depression; dysthymia	Attention deficit disorder; social anxiety; generalized anxiety	Y
179	F	40	1996	Depression	Posttraumatic stress disorder; anorexia nervosa	N
180	M	30	2004	Depression; severe depression		Y

1	2	3	4	5	6	7
186	F	54	1985	Postnatal depression; depression; severe anxiety and depression; severe depression		Y
189	F	24	2001	Major depression		Y
199	F	34	2011	Depression	Obsessions; posttraumatic stress disorder	Y
200	F	35	2011	Major depression		Y
224	F	30	2010	Depression and anxiety	Acute transient psychotic episode	N
228	F	33	2009	Depression and anxiety		Y
231	M	49	1985	Clinical depression; dysthymia		Y
240	F	21	2005	Depression with psychotic features	Anxiety; social phobia	?
266	F	41	2010	Severe clinical treatment resistant depression	Personality disorder	Y
271	F	26	2001	Chronic depression	Generalized anxiety disorder; posttraumatic stress disorder	Y
277	F	25	2003	Major depressive disorder	Generalized anxiety disorder; borderline personality disorder	N
280	F	23	2003	Recurrent depressive disorder	Schizophrenia; bipolar disorder; psychosis; personality disorders; anxiety disorders; obsessive compulsive disorder	Y
282	M	42	2000	Major depression		Y
311	F	26	2011	Depression and anxiety		Y
312	F	31	1995	Clinical depression		Y
324	F	17		No diagnosis		Y
325	F	23	2010	Major depression	Anxiety; panic attacks	Y
326	F	34		No diagnosis		?
334	F	19	2007	Major depression		N
343	F	34	1995	Major depression	Possible bipolar disorder or cyclothymia	Y

1	2	3	4	5	6	7
347	M	47	1990	Bipolar disorder		N
352	M	55	2009	Depression		Y
357	M	43	2007	Endogenous depression	Anxiety; social phobia	Y
367	F	20	2005	Depression		N
370	F	17	2010	Major depressive episode	Anorexia nervosa	Y

References

Abramson, L. Y., Metalsky, G. I., and Alloy, L. B. 1989. Hopelessness Depression: a Theory-Based Subtype of Depression. *Psychological Review 96*: 358–372.

Abramson, L. Y., Seligman, M. E. P., and Teasdale, J. D. 1978. Learned Helplessness in Humans: Critique and Reformulation. *Journal of Abnormal Psychology 87*: 49–74.

Ackermann, R. and DeRubeis, R. J. 1991. Is Depressive Realism Real? *Clinical Psychology Review 11*: 565–584.

Aho, K. and Guignon, C. 2011. Medicalized Psychiatry and the Talking Cure: a Hermeneutic Intervention. *Human Studies 34*: 293–308.

Alcoholics Anonymous. 2001. *The Big Book.* (Fourth Edition.) New York City: Alcoholics Anonymous World Services, Inc.

Allan, L. G., Siegel, S. and Hannah, S. 2007. The Sad Truth about Depressive Realism. *The Quarterly Journal of Experimental Psychology 60*: 482–495.

Alloy, L. B. ed. 1988. *Cognitive Processes in Depression.* New York: The Guilford Press.

Alloy, L. B. and Abramson, L. Y. 1988. Depressive Realism: Four Theoretical Perspectives. In Alloy, L. B. ed. *Cognitive Processes in Depression.* New York: Guildford Press: 223–265.

Alloy, L.B., Abramson, L.Y., Whitehouse, W.G., Hogan, M.E., Panzarella, C. and Rose, D.T. 2006. Prospective Incidence of First Onsets and Recurrences of Depression in Individuals at High and Low Cognitive Risk of Depression. *Journal of Abnormal Psychology 115*: 145–156.

Alvarez, A. 2002. *The Savage God: A Study of Suicide.* London: Bloomsbury.

American Psychiatric Association. 2000. *Diagnostic and Statistical Manual of Mental Disorders* (Fourth Edition, Text Revision). Washington, DC: American Psychiatric Association.

American Psychiatric Association. 2013. *Diagnostic and Statistical Manual of Mental Disorders* (Fifth Edition). Washington DC: American Psychiatric Association.

Améry, J. 1999. *At the Mind's Limits: Contemplations by a Survivor on Auschwitz and its Realities* (Trans. Rosenfeld, S. and Rosenfeld, S. P.). London: Granta Books.

Baier, A. 1986. Trust and Antitrust. *Ethics 96*: 231–260.

Bayne, T. and Levy, N. 2006. The Feeling of Doing: Deconstructing the Phenomenology of Agency. In Sebanz, N. and Prinz, W. eds. *Disorders of Volition.* Cambridge MA: MIT Press: 49–68.

Bayne, T. and Montagu, M. eds. 2011. *Cognitive Phenomenology.* Oxford: Oxford University Press.

Beck, A. T. 1967. *Depression: Clinical, Experimental and Theoretical Aspects.* New York: Harper and Row.

Beck, A. T., Weissman, A., Lester, D. and Trexler, L. 1974. The Measurement of Pessimism: The Hopelessness Scale. *Journal of Consulting and Clinical Psychology 42*: 861–865.

Beck, C. T. 2002. Postpartum Depression: a Metasynthesis. *Qualitative Health Research* 12: 453–472.

Beilke, D. 2008. The Language of Madness: Representing Bipolar Disorder in Kay Redfield Jamison's *An Unquiet Mind* and Kate Millett's *The Loony Bin Trip*. In Clark, H. ed. *Depression and Narrative: Telling the Dark*. New York: State University of New York Press: 29–39.

Bennett, C. 2002. The Varieties of Retributive Experience. *Philosophical Quarterly* 52: 145–163.

Benson, O., Gibson, S. and Brand, S, 2013. The Experience of Agency in the Feeling of Being Suicidal. *Journal of Consciousness Studies 20* (7–8): 56–79.

Benzon, K. 2008. A Dark Web: Depression, Writing and the Internet. In Clark, H. ed. *Depression and Narrative: Telling the Dark*. New York: State University of New York Press: 145–156.

Berg, J. H. van den. 1952. The Human Body and the Significance of Human Movement: A Phenomenological Study. *Philosophy and Phenomenological Research* 13: 159–183.

Berg, J. H. van den. 1966. *The Psychology of the Sickbed*. Pittsburgh: Duquesne University Press.

Berg, J. H. van den. 1972. *A Different Existence: Principles of Phenomenological Psychopathology*. Pittsburgh: Duquesne University Press.

Bernstein, J. M. 2011. Trust: On the Real but Almost Always Unnoticed, Ever-changing Foundation of Ethical Life. *Metaphilosophy 42*: 395–416.

Berridge, K. C. 2007. The Debate over Dopamine's Role in Reward: The Case for Incentive Salience. *Psychopharmacology 191*: 391–431.

Binswanger, L. 1964. On the Manic Mode of Being-in-the-world. In Straus, E. ed. *Phenomenology: Pure and Applied*. Pittsburgh: Duquesne University Press: 127–141.

Binswanger, L. 1975. *Being-in-the-world: Selected Papers of Ludwig Binswanger*. (Trans. Needleman, J.). London: Souvenir Books.

Blackburn, S. 1998. *Ruling Passions*. Oxford: Oxford University Press.

Blattner, W. 2006. *Heidegger's Being and Time*. London: Continuum.

Bovens, L. 1999. The Value of Hope. *Philosophy and Phenomenological Research* 59: 667–681.

Brampton, S. 2008. *Shoot the Damn Dog: A Memoir of Depression*. London: Bloomsbury.

Brison, S.J. 2002. *Aftermath: Violence and the Remaking of a Self*. Princeton: Princeton University Press.

Broome, M. R. 2005. Suffering and the Eternal Recurrence of the Same: the Neuroscience, Psychopathology, and Philosophy of Time. *Philosophy, Psychiatry & Psychology 12*: 187–194.

Broome, M. R., Woolley, J. B., Tabraham, P., Johns, L. C., Bramon, E., Murray, G. K., Pariante, C., McGuire, P. K. and Murray, R. M. 2005. What Causes the Onset of Psychosis? *Schizophrenia Research 79*: 23–34.

Bruner, J. 1990. *Acts of Meaning*. Cambridge MA: Harvard University Press.

Burnard, P. 2006. Sisyphus Happy: the Experience of Depression. *Journal of Psychiatric and Mental Health Nursing 13*: 242–246.

Callahan, C. M. and Berrios, G. E. 2005. *Reinventing Depression: a History of the Treatment of Depression in Primary Care* 1940–2004. Oxford: Oxford University Press.

Campbell, S. 1997. *Interpreting the Personal: Expression and the Formation of Feelings.* Ithaca: Cornell University Press.

Capuron, L. and Miller, A.H. 2011. Immune System to Brain Signaling: Neuropsycho-pharmacological Implications. *Pharmacology and Therapeutics 130*: 226–238.

Carel, H. 2008. *Illness: The Cry of the Flesh.* Stocksfield: Acumen.

Cataldi, S. 1993. *Emotion, Depth and Flesh: A Study of Sensitive Space.* Albany: State University of New York Press.

Clarke, D. M. and Kissane, D. W. 2002. Demoralization: its Phenomenology and Importance. *Australian and New Zealand Journal of Psychiatry 36*: 733–742.

Cole, J. 2004. *Still Lives: Narratives of Spinal Cord Injury.* Cambridge MA: MIT Press.

Colombetti. G. 2005. Appraising Valence. *Journal of Consciousness Studies 12* (8–10): 103–126.

Colombetti, G. 2009. What Language does to Feelings. *Journal of Consciousness Studies 16*: 4–26.

Colombetti, G. 2011. Varieties of Pre-reflective Self-awareness: Foreground and Background Bodily Feelings in Emotion Experience. *Inquiry 54*:293–313.

Colombetti, G. and Ratcliffe, M. 2012. Bodily Feeling in Depersonalisation: a Phenomenological Account. *Emotion Review 4*: 145–150.

Colombetti, G. and Torrance, S. 2009. Emotion and Ethics: An Inter(en)active Approach. *Phenomenology and the Cognitive Sciences 8*: 505–526.

Cooper, D. E. 2002. *The Measure of Things: Humanism, Humility and Mystery.* Oxford: Clarendon Press.

Cooper, R. 2005. *Classifying Madness: A Philosophical Examination of the Diagnostic and Statistical Manual of Mental Disorders.* Dordrecht: Springer.

Csordas, T. 2013. Inferring Immediacy in Adolescent Accounts of Depression. *Journal of Consciousness Studies 20* (7–8): 239–253.

Davies, M. and Stone, T. eds. 1995a. *Mental Simulation: Evaluations and Applications.* Oxford: Blackwell

Davies, M. and Stone, T. eds. 1995b. *Folk Psychology: The Theory of Mind Debate.* Oxford: Blackwell.

De Jaegher, H. and Di Paolo, E. 2007. Participatory Sense-Making: An Enactive Approach to Social Cognition. *Phenomenology and the Cognitive Sciences 6*: 485–507.

De Sousa, R. 1990. *The Rationality of Emotion.* Cambridge MA: MIT Press.

De Vignemont, F. 2010. Knowing Other People's Mental States as if they were One's Own. In Gallagher, S. and Schmicking, D. eds. *Handbook of Phenomenology and Cognitive Science.* Dordrecht: Springer.

De Vignemont, F. and Jacob, P. 2012. What is it Like to Feel Another's Pain? *Philosophy of Science 79*: 295–316.

Debus, D. 2007. Being Emotional about the Past: On the Nature and Role of Past-Directed Emotions. *Noûs 41*: 758–779.

Deonna, J. A. 2006. Emotion, Perception and Perspective. *Dialectica 60*: 29–46.

Dreyfus, H. L. 1991. *Being-in-the-World: A Commentary on Heidegger's Being and Time Division 1*. Cambridge MA: MIT Press.

Ehrenberg, A. 2010. *The Weariness of the Self: Diagnosing the History of Depression in the Contemporary Age*. Montreal: McGill—Queen's University Press.

Elliott, C. 1999. *A Philosophical Disease: Bioethics, Culture and Identity*. London: Routledge.

Elster, J. 1999. *Alchemies of the Mind: Rationality and the Emotions*. Cambridge: Cambridge University Press.

Emmons, K. 2008. Narrating the Emotional Woman: Uptake and Gender in Discourses on Depression. In Clark, H. ed. *Depression and Narrative: Telling the Dark*. New York: State University of New York Press: 111–125.

Flanagan, O. 2013. Identity and Addiction: What Alcoholic Memoirs Teach. In Fulford, K.W.M., Davies, M., Gipps, R.G.T., Graham, G., Sadler, J.Z., Stanghellini, G. and Thornton, T. eds. *The Oxford Handbook of Philosophy and Psychiatry*. Oxford: Oxford University Press: 865–888.

Foulds, A. 2009. *The Quickening Maze*. London: Jonathan Cape.

Frankl, V. 1973. *Psychotherapy and Existentialism: Selected Papers on Logotherapy*. London: Penguin Books.

Freud, S. 1919/2003. *The Uncanny*. London: Penguin.

Freud, S. 1917/2005. Mourning and Melancholia. In *On Murder, Mourning and Melancholia* (Trans. Whiteside, S.). London: Penguin: 201–218.

Fuchs, T. 2001. Melancholia as a Desynchronization: Towards a Psychopathology of Interpersonal Time. *Psychopathology 34*: 179–186.

Fuchs, T. 2003. The Phenomenology of Shame, Guilt and the Body in Body Dysmorphic Disorder and Depression. *Journal of Phenomenological Psychology 33*: 223–243.

Fuchs, T. 2005. Corporealized and Disembodied Minds: A Phenomenological View of the Body in Melancholia and Schizophrenia. *Philosophy, Psychiatry & Psychology 12*: 95–107.

Fuchs, T. 2007. Fragmented Selves: Temporality and Identity in Borderline Personality Disorder. *Psychopathology 40*: 379–387.

Fuchs, T. 2013a. Depression, Intercorporeality and Interaffectivity. *Journal of Consciousness Studies 20* (7–8): 219–238.

Fuchs, T. 2013b. Temporality and Psychopathology. *Phenomenology and the Cognitive Sciences 12*: 75–104.

Fulford, K. W. M. 1994. Value, Illness and Failure of Action. In Graham, G. and Stephens, G. L. eds. *Philosophical Psychopathology*. Cambridge MA: MIT Press: 205–233.

Fulford, K. L. M. 2004. Facts/Values: Ten Principles of Values-based Medicine. In Radden, J. ed. *The Philosophy of Psychiatry: A Companion*. Oxford: Oxford University Press: 205–234.

Gaebler, M., Lamke, J-P, Daniels, J.K. and Walter, H. 2013. Phenomenal Depth: a Common Phenomenological Dimension in Depression and Depersonalization. *Journal of Consciousness Studies 20* (7–8): 269–291.

Gallagher, S. 2000. Philosophical Conceptions of the Self: Implications for Cognitive Science. *Trends in Cognitive Sciences 4*: 14–21.

Gallagher, S. 2001 The Practice of Mind: Theory, Simulation, or Interaction? *Journal of Consciousness Studies 8* (5–7): 83–107.

Gallagher, S. 2005. *How the Body Shapes the Mind.* Oxford: Oxford University Press.

Gallagher, S. 2006. Where's the Action? Epiphenomenalism and the Problem of Free Will. In Banks, W., Pockett, S. and Gallagher. S. eds. *Does Consciousness Cause Behavior? An Investigation of the Nature of Volition.* Cambridge MA: MIT Press: 109–124.

Gallagher, S. 2008. Intersubjectivity in Perception. *Continental Philosophy Review 41:* 163–178.

Gallagher, S. 2009. Two Problems of Intersubjectivity. *Journal of Consciousness Studies 16* (6–8): 289–308.

Gallagher, S. 2012. Empathy, Simulation and Narrative. *Science in Context 25:* 355–381.

Gallagher, S. and Zahavi, D. 2008. *The Phenomenological Mind.* London: Routledge.

Garner, A. and Hardcastle, V. G. 2004. Neurobiological Models: An Unnecessary Divide—Neural Models in Psychiatry. In Radden, J. ed. *The Philosophy of Psychiatry: A Companion.* Oxford: Oxford University Press.

Garrett, R. 1994. The Problem of Despair. In Graham, G. and Stephens, G. L. eds. *Philosophical Psychopathology.* Cambridge MA: MIT Press.

Gerrans, P. and Scherer, K. 2013. Wired for Despair: the Neurochemistry of Emotion and the Phenomenology of Depression. *Journal of Consciousness Studies 20* (7–8): 254–268.

Ghaemi, S. N. 2007. Feeling and Time: the Phenomenology of Mood Disorders, Depressive Realism, and Existential Psychotherapy. *Schizophrenia Bulletin 33:* 122–130.

Ghaemi, S.N. 2008. Why Antidepressants are not Antidepressants: Step-BD, STAR*D, and the Return of Neurotic Depression. *Bipolar Disorders 10:* 957–968.

Ghaemi, N. 2013. *On Depression: Drugs, Diagnosis, and Despair in the Modern World.* Baltimore: John Hopkins University Press.

Ghatavi, K., Nicolson, R., MacDonald, C., Osher, S. and Levitt, A. 2002. Defining Guilt in Depression: A Comparison of Subjects with Major Depression, Chronic Medical Illness and Healthy Controls. *Journal of Affective Disorders 68:* 307–315.

Gibson. J. J. 1979. *The Ecological Approach to Visual Perception.* Hillsdale, New Jersey: Lawrence Erlbaum Associates.

Glas, G. 2003. A Conceptual History of Anxiety and Depression. In Boer, J. A. den and Sitsen, A. eds. *Handbook of Anxiety and Depression.* (Second Edition.) New York: Marcel Dekker: 1–47.

Goldie, P. 2000. *The Emotions: A Philosophical Exploration.* Oxford: Clarendon Press.

Goldie, P. 2007. Seeing what is the Kind Thing to Do: Perception and Emotion in Morality. *Dialectica 61:* 347–361.

Goldie, P. 2009. Getting Feeling into Emotional Experience in the Right Way. *Emotion Review 1:* 232–239.

Goldie, P. 2011a. Grief: a Narrative Account. *Ratio XXIV:* 119–137.

Goldie, P. 2011b. Anti-Empathy. In Coplan, A. and Goldie, P. eds. *Empathy: Philosophical and Psychological Perspectives.* Oxford: Oxford University Press: 302–317.

Goldman, A. 2006. *Simulating Minds: The Philosophy, Psychology, and Neuroscience of Mindreading.* Oxford: Oxford University Press.

Goldman, A. 2011. Two Routes to Empathy: Insights from Cognitive Neuroscience. In Coplan, A. and Goldie, P. eds. *Empathy: Philosophical and Psychological Perspectives*. Oxford: Oxford University Press: 31–44.

Good, B. J. 1994. *Medicine, Rationality and Experience: an Anthropological Perspective*. Cambridge: Cambridge University Press.

Gordon, R. 1995. Folk Psychology as Simulation. In Davies, M. and Stone, T. eds. *Mental Simulation*. Oxford: Blackwell: 60–73.

Gotlib, I.H. and Hammen, C.L. eds. 2009. *Handbook of Depression*. (Second Edition). London: The Guilford Press.

Graham, G. 1990. Melancholic Epistemology. *Synthese 82*: 399–422.

Grahek, N. 2007. *Feeling Pain and Being in Pain* (second edition). Cambridge MA: MIT Press.

Haaga, D. A. F. and Beck, A. T. 1995. Perspectives on Depressive Realism: Implications for Cognitive Theory of Depression. *Behaviour Research and Therapy 33*: 41–48.

Hacking, I. 1995. The Looping Effects of Human Kinds. In Sperber, D., Premack, D. and Premack, A.J. eds. 1995. *Causal Cognition: a Multi-Disciplinary Debate*. Oxford: Clarendon Press: 351–383.

Halpern, J. 2001. *From Detached Concern to Empathy*. Oxford: Oxford University Press.

Halpern, J. 2003. What is Clinical Empathy? *Journal of General Internal Medicine 18*: 670–674.

Hansen, J. 2004. Affectivity: Depression and Mania. In Radden, J. ed. *The Philosophy of Psychiatry: a Companion*. Oxford: Oxford University Press: 36–53.

Harrison, N.A., Brydon, L., Walker, C., Gray, M.A., Steptoe, A. and Critchley, H.D. 2009. Inflammation causes Mood Changes through Alterations in Subgenual Cingulate Activity and Mesolimbic Connectivity. *Biological Psychiatry 66*: 407–414.

Haugeland, J. 2000. Truth and Finitude: Heidegger's Transcendental Existentialism. In Wrathall, M. and Malpas, J. eds. *Heidegger, Authenticity, and Modernity: Essays in Honor of Hubert L. Dreyfus*: Volume 1. Cambridge MA: MIT Press: 43–77.

Havens, L. 1986. *Making Contact: Uses of Language in Psychotherapy*. Cambridge MA: Harvard University Press.

Hawley, K. and MacPherson, F. eds. 2011. *The Admissible Contents of Experience*. Oxford: Wiley-Blackwell.

Healy, D. 1993. Dysphoria. In Costello, C. G. ed. *Symptoms of Depression*. New York: John Wiley & Sons, Inc: 23–42.

Heidegger, M. 1927/1962. *Being and Time* (Trans. Macquarrie, J. and Robinson, E.). Oxford: Blackwell.

Heidegger, M. 1927/1996. *Being and Time* (Trans. Stambaugh, J.). New York: State University of New York Press.

Heidegger, M. 1983/1995. *The Fundamental Concepts of Metaphysics*. (Trans. McNeill, W. and Walker, N.). Bloomington: Indiana University Press.

Heidegger, M. 2001. *Zollikon Seminars: Protocols—Conversations—Letters* (ed. Boss, M.; Trans. Mayr, F. and Askay, R.). Evanston: Northwestern University Press.

Hobson, R. P. 1993. *Autism and the Development of Mind*. Hove: Erlbaum.

Hobson, R. P. 2002. *The Cradle of Thought*. London: Macmillan.

Hobson, R. P. 2010. Is Jealousy a Complex Emotion? In Hart, S.L. and Legerstee, M. eds. *Handbook of Jealousy: Theory, Research, and Multidisciplinary Approaches.* Oxford: Blackwell: 293–311.

Hohwy, J. 2007. The Sense of Self in the Phenomenology of Agency and Perception. *Psyche 13*(1).

Holton, R. 2009. Determinism, Self-Efficacy, and the Phenomenology of Free Will. *Inquiry 52*: 412–428.

Hookway, C. 2002. Emotions and Epistemic Evaluations. In Carruthers, P., Stich, S. and Siegal, M. eds. *The Cognitive Basis of Science.* Cambridge: Cambridge University Press: 251–262.

Horne, O. and Csipke, E. 2009. From Feeling too Little and too Much, to Feeling More and Less? A Non-Paradoxical Theory of the Functions of Self-Harm. *Qualitative Health Research 19*: 655–667.

Hornstein, G. A. 2009. *Agnes's Jacket: A Psychologist's Search for the Meanings of Madness.* New York: Rodale.

Horwitz, A. V. and Wakefield, J. C. 2007. *The Loss of Sadness: How Psychiatry transformed Normal Sorrow into Depressive Disorder.* Oxford: Oxford University Press.

Hull, J. 1990. *Touching the Rock: An Experience of Blindness.* New York: Pantheon Books.

Husserl, E. 1931/1960. *Cartesian Meditations: An Introduction to Phenomenology* (Trans. Cairns, D.). The Hague: Martinus Nijhoff.

Husserl, E. 1954/1970a. *The Crisis of European Sciences and Transcendental Phenomenology* (Trans. Carr, D.). Evanston: Northwestern University Press.

Husserl, E. 1954/1970b. The Vienna Lecture. In his *The Crisis of European Sciences and Transcendental Phenomenology.* (Trans. Carr, D.). Evanston: Northwestern University Press: 269–299.

Husserl, E. 1948/1973. *Experience and Judgment.* Trans. Churchill, J. S. and Ameriks, K. London: Routledge.

Husserl, E. 1952/1989. *Ideas Pertaining to a Pure Phenomenology and to a Phenomenological Philosophy: Second Book* (Trans. Rojcewicz, R. and Schuwer, A.). Dordrecht: Kluwer.

Husserl, E. 1991. *On the Phenomenology of the Consciousness of Internal Time* (1893–1917). (Trans. Brough, J. B.). Dordrecht: Kluwer.

Husserl, E. 2001. *Analyses concerning Passive and Active Synthesis: Lectures on Transcendental Logic* (Trans. Steinbock, A. J.). Dordrecht: Kluwer.

Hutto, D. D. 2008. *Folk Psychological Narratives: The Sociocultural Basis of Understanding Reasons.* Cambridge MA: MIT Press.

Jackson, M. C. and Fulford, K. W. M. 1997. Spiritual Experience and Psychopathology. *Philosophy, Psychiatry & Psychology 4*: 42–65.

Jackson, M. C. and Fulford, K. W. M. 2002. Psychosis Good and Bad: Values-Based Practice and the Distinction between Pathological and Nonpathological Forms of Psychotic Experience. *Philosophy, Psychiatry & Psychology 9*: 387–394.

Jacobsen, J. C., Maytal, G. and Stern, T. A. 2007. Demoralization in Medical Practice. *Primary Care Companion to the Journal of Clinical Psychiatry 9*: 139–143.

James, W. 1889. The Psychology of Belief. *Mind 14*: 321–352.

James, W. 1890. *The Principles of Psychology. Volume II.* New York: Holt.

James, W. 1902. *The Varieties of Religious Experience*. New York: Longmans, Green and Co.

Jaspers, K. 1963. *General Psychopathology*. (Trans. Hoenig, J. and Hamilton, M. W.). Manchester: Manchester University Press.

Jones, K. 2004. Trust and Terror. In Des Autels, P. and Walker, M. U. eds. *Moral Psychology: Feminist Ethics and Social Theory*. Lanham, Maryland: Rowman and Littlefield: 3–18.

Kane, S. 2000. *4.48 Psychosis*. London: Methuen.

Kangas, I. 2001. Making Sense of Depression: Perceptions of Melancholia in Lay Narratives. *Health 5*: 76–92.

Kapur, S. 2003. Psychosis as a State of Aberrant Salience: a Framework linking Biology, Phenomenology, and Pharmacology in Schizophrenia. *American Journal of Psychiatry 160*: 13–23.

Kapur, S., Mizrahi, R. and Li, M. 2005. From Dopamine to Salience to Psychosis—linking Biology, Pharmacology and Phenomenology of Psychosis. *Schizophrenia Research 79*: 59-

Karp, D. 1996. *Speaking of Sadness: Depression, Disconnection, and the Meanings of Illness*. Oxford: Oxford University Press.

Kavanaugh, K. ed. 1987. *John of the Cross: Selected Writings*. New York: Paulist Press.

Kaysen, S. 2001. One Cheer for Melancholy. In Casey, N. ed. *Unholy Ghost: Writers on Depression*. New York: William Morrow: 38–43.

Kendell, R.E. 2001. The Distinction between Mental and Physical Illness. *British Journal of Psychiatry 178*: 490–493.

Kierkegaard, S. 1849/1989. *The Sickness unto Death* (Trans. Hannay, A.). London: Penguin.

Kirmayer, L. J. 2001. Cultural Variations in the Clinical Presentation of Depression and Anxiety: Implications for Diagnosis and Treatment. *Journal of Clinical Psychiatry 62* (Supplement 13): 22–28.

Kirmayer, L. J. 2008. Culture and the Metaphoric Mediation of Pain. *Transcultural Psychiatry 45*: 318–338.

Kirsch, I. 2009. *The Emperor's New Drugs: Exploding the Antidepressant Myth*. London: The Bodley Head.

Kissane, D. W. and Clarke, D. M. (2001). Demoralization Syndrome—a Relevant Psychiatric Diagnosis for Palliative Care. *Journal of Palliative Care, 17*, 12–21.

Kitanaka, J. 2012. Depression in Japan: Psychiatric Cures for a Society in Distress. *Princeton: Princeton University Press*.

Klass, D., Silverman, P. R. and Nickman, S. L. eds. 1996. *Continuing Bonds: New Understandings of Grief*. London: Routledge.

Klein, D. N., Shankman, S. A. and McFarland, B. 2006. Classification of Mood Disorders. In Stein, D. J., Kupfer, D. J. and Schatzberg, A. D. eds. *The American Psychiatric Publishing Textbook of Mood Disorders*. Arlington, VA: American Psychiatric Publishing, Inc.

Kleinman, A. 1988. *Rethinking Psychiatry: From Cultural Category to Personal Experience*. New York: The Free Press.

Kraepelin, E. 1921. *Manic-Depressive Insanity and Paranoia* (Trans. Barclay, R.M.). Edinburgh: E. & S. Livingstone.

Krishnadas, R. and Cavanagh, J. 2012. Depression: an Inflammatory Illness? *Journal of Neurology, Neurosurgery and Psychiatry 83*: 495–502.

Laing, R. D. 1960. *The Divided Self: A Study of Sanity and Madness*. London: Tavistock Publications.

Larson, E.B. and Yao, X. 2005. Clinical Empathy as Emotional Labor in the Patient-Physician Relationship. *Journal of the American Medical Association 293*: 1100–1106.

Law, I. 2009. Motivation, Depression and Character. In Broome, M. R. and Bortolotti, L. eds. *Psychiatry as Cognitive Neuroscience: Philosophical Perspectives*. Oxford: Oxford University Press: 351–364.

Lear, J. 2006. *Radical Hope: Ethics in the Face of Cultural Devastation*. Cambridge MA: Harvard University Press.

Leder, D. 1990. *The Absent Body*. Chicago: University of Chicago Press.

Legrand, D. and Ravn, S. 2009. Perceiving Subjectivity in Bodily Movement: the Case of Dancers. *Phenomenology and the Cognitive Sciences 8*: 389–408.

Levinas, E. 1961/1969. *Totality and Infinity* (Trans. Lingis, A.). Pittsburgh: Duquesne University Press.

Lewis, C.S. 1966. *A Grief Observed*. London: Faber & Faber.

Lewis, G. 2006. *Sunbathing in the Rain: A Cheerful Book about Depression*. London: Harper Perennial.

Libet, B. 2004. *Mind Time: The Temporal Factor in Consciousness*. Cambridge MA: Harvard University Press.

Løgstrup, K. E. 1956/1997. *The Ethical Demand*. Notre Dame: University of Notre Dame Press.

Lopez-Ibor, J. 1982. Delusional Perception and Delusional Mood: a Phenomenological and Existential Analysis. In A.J.J. Koning and F.A. Jenner eds. *Phenomenology and Psychiatry*. London: Academic Press: 135–152.

Lott, T. 1996. *The Scent of Dried Roses*. London: Viking.

Lowe, E. J. 1996. *Subjects of Experience*. Cambridge: Cambridge University Press.

Lowe, E. J. 2008. *Personal Agency: The Metaphysics of Mind and Action*. Oxford: Oxford University Press.

Lysaker, P. H., Johannesen, J. K., and Lysaker, J. T. 2005. Schizophrenia and the Experience of Intersubjectivity as Threat. *Phenomenology and the Cognitive Sciences 4*: 335–352.

MacPherson, F. ed. 2011. *The Senses: Classic and Contemporary Philosophical Perspectives*. Oxford: Oxford University Press.

Madary, M. 2013. Anticipation and Variation in Visual Content. *Philosophical Studies 165*: 335–347.

Maj, M. 2011. When does Depression become a Mental Disorder? *British Journal of Psychiatry 199*: 85–86.

Martin, A. M. 2010. Hopes and Dreams. *Philosophy and Phenomenological Research LXXXIII*: 148–173.

Martin, M. W. 1999. Depression, Illness, Insight and Identity. *Philosophy, Psychiatry & Psychology* 6: 271–286.

Mayberg, H.S. 2003. Modulating Dysfunctional Limbic-Cortical Circuits in Depression: Towards Development of Brain-Based Algorithms for Diagnosis and Optimised Treatment. *British Medical Bulletin* 65: 193–207.

Mayberg, H.S., Liotti, M, Branna, S.K., McGinnis, S., Mahurin, R.K., Jerabek, P.A., Silva, J.A., Tekell, J.L., Martin, C.C., Lancaster, J.L. and Fox, P.T. 1999. Reciprocal Limbic-Cortical Function and Negative Mood: Converging PET Findings in Depression and Normal Sadness. *American Journal of Psychiatry 156*: 675–682.

Mayberg, H.S., Lozano, A.M., Voon, V., McNeely, H.E., Seminowicz, D., Hamani, C., Schwalb, J.M. and Kennedy, S.H. 2005. Deep Brain Stimulation for Treatment-Resistant Depression. *Neuron 45*: 651–660.

McGeer, V. 2004. The Art of Good Hope. *The Annals of the American Academy of Political and Social Science* 592: 100–127.

McGeer, V. 2008. Trust, Hope and Empowerment. *Australasian Journal of Philosophy* 86: 237–254.

Medford, N., Sierra, M., Baker, D. and David, A. S. 2005. Understanding and Treating Depersonalisation Disorder. *Advances in Psychiatric Treatment* 11: 92–100.

Meirav, A. 2009. The Nature of Hope. *Ratio XXII*: 216–233.

Mercer, S. W. and Reynolds, W. J. 2002. Empathy and Quality of Care. *British Journal of General Practice 52* (Quality Supplement): S9–S12.

Merleau-Ponty, M. 1945/1962. *Phenomenology of Perception* (Trans. Smith, C.). London: Routledge.

Merleau-Ponty, M. 1964. *The Primacy of Perception. And Other Essays on Phenomenological Psychology, and Philosophy of Art, History and Politics.* (Edited with Introduction by Edie, J. M.). Evanston: Northwestern University Press.

Merleau-Ponty, M. 1968. *The Visible and the Invisible* (Trans. Lingis, A.). Evanston: Northwestern University Press.

Meynen, G. 2011. Depression, Possibilities and Competence: a Phenomenological Perspective. *Theoretical Medicine and Bioethics 32*: 181–193.

Mill, J. S. 1873. *Autobiography.* London: Longmans, Green, Reader & Dyer.

Miller, A. H., Maletic, V. and Raison, C. L. 2009. Inflammation and its Discontents: the Role of Cytokines in the Pathophysiology of Major Depression. *Biological Psychiatry* 65: 732–41.

Minkowski, E. 1958. Findings in a Case of Schizophrenic Depression. (Trans. Blis, B. In May, R., Angel, E. and Ellenberger, H. eds.). *Existence.* New York: Simon and Schuster:127–138.

Minkowski, E. 1970. *Lived Time: Phenomenological and Psychopathological Studies* (Trans. Metzel, N.). Evanston: Northwestern University Press.

Mittal, V., Brown, W.A. and Shorter, E. 2009. Are Patients with Depression at Heightened Risk of Suicide as they Begin to Recover? *Psychiatric Services* 60: 384–386.

Morton, A. 2010. Epistemic Emotions. In Goldie, P. ed. *The Oxford Handbook of Philosophy of Emotion.* Oxford: Oxford University Press: 385–399.

Moyal-Sharrock, D. 2005. *Understanding Wittgenstein's On Certainty.* Basingstoke: Palgrave Macmillan.

Müller, N., Schwarz, M.J., Dehning, S., Douhe, A., Cerovecki, A., Goldstein-Müller, B., Spellmann, I., Hetzel, G., Maino, K., Kleindienst, N., Möller, H.-J., Arolt, V. and Riedel, M. 2006. The Cyclooxygenase-2 Inhibitor Celecoxib has Therapeutic Effects in Major Depression: Results of a Double-Blind, Randomized, Placebo Controlled, Add-on Pilot Study to Roboxetine. *Molecular Psychiatry 11*: 680–684.

Murphy, D. 2009. Psychiatry and the Concept of Disease as Pathology. In Broome, M. and Bortolotii, L. eds. *Psychiatry as Cognitive Neuroscience.* Oxford: Oxford University Press: 103–117.

National Collaborating Centre for Mental Health. 2010. *Depression in Adults with a Chronic Physical Health Problem: The NICE Guideline on Treatment and Management.* London: RCPsych Publications.

Nichols, S. 2004. The Folk Psychology of Free Will: Fits and Starts. *Mind & Language 19*: 473–502.

Nietzsche, F. 2003. *Beyond Good and Evil* (Trans. Hollingdale, R.J.). London: Penguin Books.

Noë, A. 2004. *Action in Perception.* Cambridge MA: MIT Press.

Nolen-Hoeksema, S. 1990. *Sex Differences in Depression.* Stanford: Stanford University Press.

Northoff, G. 2008. Are our Emotional Feelings Relational? A Neurophilosophical Investigation of the James-Lange Theory. *Phenomenology and the Cognitive Sciences 7*: 501–527.

O'Callaghan, C. 2011. Lessons from beyond Vision (Sounds and Audition). *Philosophical Studies 153*: 143–160.

O'Callaghan, C. 2012. Perception and Multimodality. In Margolis, E., Samuels, R. and Stich, S. eds. *Oxford Handbook to Philosophy and Cognitive Science.* Oxford: Oxford University Press: 92–117.

Panskepp, J. 1999. The Periconscious Substrates of Consciousness: Affective States and the Evolutionary Origins of the Self. In Gallagher, S. and Shear, J. eds. *Models of the Self.* Exeter: Imprint Academic: 113–130.

Pariante, C.M., Nesse, R.M., Nutt, D. and Wolpert, L. eds. 2009. *Understanding Depression: a Translational Approach.* Oxford: Oxford University Press.

Parker, M. 2004. Medicalizing Meaning: Demoralization Syndrome and the Desire to Die. *Australian and New Zealand Journal of Psychiatry 38*: 765–773.

Pettit, P. 2004. Hope and its Place in Mind. *The Annals of the American Academy of Political and Social Science 592*: 152–165.

Pienkos, E. and Sass, L.A. 2012. Empathy and Otherness: Humanistic and Phenomenological Approaches to Psychotherapy of Severe Mental Illness. *Pragmatic Case Studies in Psychotherapy 8*: 25–35.

Pies, R. 2013. From Context to Phenomenology in Grief and Depression. *Psychiatric Annals 43*: 286–290.

Plath, S. 1966. *The Bell Jar.* London: Faber & Faber.

Pugmire, D. 2005. *Sound Sentiments: Integrity in the Emotions.* Oxford: Oxford University Press.

Radden, J. 2000. Introduction: From Melancholic States to Clinical Depression. In Radden, J. ed. *The Nature of Melancholy: from Aristotle to Kristeva*. Oxford: Oxford University Press: 3–51.

Radden, J. 2009. *Moody Minds Distempered: Essays on Melancholy and Depression*. Oxford: Oxford University Press.

Raison, C.L., Capuron, L. and Miller, A.H. 2006. Cytokines Sing the Blues: Inflammation and the Pathogenesis of Depression. *Trends in Immunology* 27: 24–31.

Ratcliffe, M. 2005. The Feeling of Being. *Journal of Consciousness Studies* 12 (8–10): 43–60.

Ratcliffe, M. 2007. *Rethinking Commonsense Psychology: A Critique of Folk Psychology, Theory of Mind and Simulation*. Basingstoke: Palgrave Macmillan.

Ratcliffe, M. 2008. *Feelings of Being: Phenomenology, Psychiatry and the Sense of Reality*. Oxford: Oxford University Press.

Ratcliffe, M. 2009a. Understanding Existential Changes in Psychiatric Illness: the Indispensability of Phenomenology. In Broome, M. and Bortolotti, L. eds. *Psychiatry as Cognitive Neuroscience*. Oxford: Oxford University Press: 223–244.

Ratcliffe, M. 2009b. There are no Folk Psychological Narratives. *Journal of Consciousness Studies 16/6–8*: 379–406.

Ratcliffe, M. 2010a. Depression, Guilt and Emotional Depth. *Inquiry 53*: 602–626.

Ratcliffe, M. 2010b. The Phenomenology of Mood and the Meaning of Life. In Goldie, P. ed. *Oxford Handbook of Philosophy of Emotion*. Oxford: Oxford University Press: 349–371.

Ratcliffe, M. 2012a. Varieties of Temporal Experience in Depression. *Journal of Medicine and Philosophy 37*: 114–138.

Ratcliffe, M. 2012b. Phenomenology as a Form of Empathy. *Inquiry 55*: 473–495.

Ratcliffe, M. 2012c. What is Touch? *Australasian Journal of Philosophy 90*: 413–432.

Ratcliffe, M. 2013a. Depression and the Phenomenology of Free Will. In Fulford, K.W.M., Davies, M., Gipps, R.G.T., Graham, G., Sadler, J.Z., Stanghellini, G. and Thornton, T. eds. *The Oxford Handbook of Philosophy and Psychiatry*. Oxford: Oxford University Press: 574–591. <http://ukcatalogue.oup.com/product/9780199579563.do>

Ratcliffe, M. 2013b. What is it to Lose Hope? *Phenomenology and the Cognitive Sciences* 4: 597–614.

Ratcliffe, 2013c. Phenomenology, Naturalism and the Sense of Reality. *Royal Institute of Philosophy Supplement 72*: 67–88.

Ratcliffe, M. 2013d. Why Mood Matters. In Wrathall, M. ed. *Cambridge Companion to Being and Time*. Cambridge: Cambridge University Press: 157–176.

Ratcliffe, M. 2013e. Delusional Atmosphere and the Sense of Unreality. In Stanghellini, G. and Fuchs, T. eds. *One Century of Karl Jaspers' General Psychopathology*. Oxford: Oxford University Press: 229–244.

Ratcliffe, M. 2013f. Some Husserlian Reflections on the Contents of Experience. In Haug, M.C. ed. *Philosophical Methodology: the Armchair or the Laboratory?* London: Routledge: 353–378.

Ratcliffe, M. 2014a The Structure of Interpersonal Experience, In Moran, D. and Jensen, R. *The Phenomenology of Embodied Experience*. Dordrecht: Springer: 221–238.

Ratcliffe, M. 2014b. Evaluating Existential Despair. In Roeser, S. and Todd, C. *Emotion and Value*. Oxford: Oxford University Press: 229–246. <http://ukcatalogue.oup.com/product/9780199686094.do.>

Ratcliffe, M. and Broome, M. 2012. Existential Phenomenology, Psychiatric Illness and the Death of Possibilities. In Crowell, S. ed. *Cambridge Companion to Existentialism*. Cambridge: Cambridge University Press: 361–382.

Ratcliffe, M., Broome, M., Smith, B. and Bowden, H. 2013. A Bad Case of the Flu? The Comparative Phenomenology of Depression and Somatic Illness. *Journal of Consciousness Studies* 20(7–8): 198–218.

Read, J. and Reynolds, J. eds. 1996. *Speaking our Minds: An Anthology*. Basingstoke: Palgrave Macmillan.

Reddy, V. 2008. *How Infants Know Minds*. Cambridge MA: MIT Press.

Rhodes, J. and Gipps, R. G. T. 2008. Delusions, Certainty and the Background. *Philosophy, Psychiatry & Psychology* 15: 295–310.

Rhodes, J. and Smith, J. A. 2010. 'The Top of My Head Came Off': An Interpretative Phenomenological Analysis of the Experience of Depression. *Counselling Psychology Quarterly* 23: 399–409.

Riley, D. 2012. *Time Lived, Without Its Flow*. London: Capsule Editions.

Roberts, J. R. 2001. Mental Illness, Motivation and Moral Commitment. *Philosophical Quarterly* 51: 41–59.

Roberts, R. C. 2003. *Emotions: an Essay in Aid of Moral Psychology*. Cambridge: Cambridge University Press.

Røseth, I., Binder, P-E. and Malt, U. F. 2011. Two Ways of Living through Postpartum Depression. *Journal of Philosophical Psychology* 42: 174–194.

Rowe, D. 1978. *The Experience of Depression*. Chichester: John Wiley & Sons.

Sartre, J. P. 1943/1989. *Being and Nothingness*. (Trans. Barnes, H. E.). London: Routledge.

Sartre, J. P. 1939/1994. *Sketch for a Theory of the Emotions*. (Trans. Mairet, P.). London: Routledge.

Sass, L. A. 1992. *Madness and Modernism: Insanity in the Light of Modern Art, Literature and Thought*. New York: Basic Books.

Sass, L. A. 1994. *The Paradoxes of Delusion: Wittgenstein, Schreber, and the Schizophrenic Mind*. Ithaca: Cornell University Press.

Sass, L. A. 2003. 'Negative Symptoms', Schizophrenia, and the Self. *International Journal of Psychology and Psychological Therapy* 3: 153–180.

Sass, L. A. 2004. Affectivity in Schizophrenia: A Phenomenological View. In Zahavi, D. ed. *Hidden Resources: Classical Perspectives on Subjectivity*. Exeter: Imprint Academic: 127–147.

Sass, L. A. 2007. Commentary on Maxine Sheets-Johnstone's 'Schizophrenia and the Comet's Tail of Nature'. Time, Trauma and Schizophrenia. *Philoctetes* 1: 35–41.

Sass, L. A. and Parnas, J. 2007. Explaining Schizophrenia: The Relevance of Phenomenology. In Chung, M. C., Fulford, K. W. M. and Graham, G. eds. *Reconceiving Schizophrenia*. Oxford: Oxford University Press: 63–95.

Sass, L.A. and Pienkos, E. 2013a. Varieties of Self-Experience: A Comparative Phenomenology of Melancholia, Mania and Schizophrenia, Part I. *Journal of Consciousness Studies* 20 (7–8): 103–130.

Sass, L.A. and Pienkos, E. 2013b. Space, Time and Atmosphere: A Comparative Phenomenology of Melancholia, Mania and Schizophrenia, Part II. *Journal of Consciousness Studies 20* (7–8): 131–152.

Saury, J-M. 2009. The Phenomenology of Negation. *Phenomenology and the Cognitive Sciences 8*: 245–260.

Scarry, E. 1985. *The Body in Pain: the Making and Unmaking of the World.* Oxford: Oxford University Press.

Scheler, M. 1954. *The Nature of Sympathy* (Trans. Heath, P.). London: Routledge.

Schutz, A. 1967. *The Phenomenology of the Social World* (Trans. Walsh, G. and Lehnert, F.). Evanston: Northwestern University Press.

Schwartz, M.A. and Wiggins, O.P. 1987a. Diagnosis and Ideal Types: a Contribution to Psychiatric Classification. *Comprehensive Psychiatry 28*: 277–291.

Schwartz, M.A. and Wiggins, O.P. 1987b. Typifications: the First Step for Clinical Diagnosis in Psychiatry. *The Journal of Nervous and Mental Disease 175*: 65–77.

Searle, J. R. 1983. *Intentionality: An Essay in the Philosophy of Mind.* Cambridge: Cambridge University Press.

Sebald, W. G. 2002. *The Rings of Saturn.* (Trans. Hulse, M.). London: Vintage.

Sechehaye, M. 1970. *Autobiography of a Schizophrenic Girl.* New York: Signet.

Seligman, M. E. P., Abramson, L. Y., Semmel, A. and von Baeyer, C. 1979. Depressive Attributional Style. *Journal of Abnormal Psychology 88*: 242–247.

Shaw, F. 1997. *Out of Me: The Story of a Postnatal Breakdown.* London: Penguin.

Sheets-Johnstone, M. 2009. *The Corporeal Turn: an Interdisciplinary Reader.* Exeter: Imprint Academic.

Shenk, J. W. 2001. A Melancholy of Mine Own. In Casey, N. ed. *Unholy Ghost: Writers on Depression.* New York: William Morrow: 242–255.

Shorter, E. and Tyrer, P. 2003. Separation of Anxiety and Depressive Disorders: Blind Alley in Psychopharmacology and Classification of Disease. *British Medical Journal 327*: 158–160.

Shriver, L. 2006. *Double Fault.* London: Serpent's Tail.

Sierra, M., Baker, D., Medford, N. and David, A.S. 2005. Unpacking the Depersonalization Syndrome: an Exploratory Factor Analysis on the Cambridge Depersonalization Scale. *Psychological Medicine 35*: 1523–1532.

Simeon, D. and Abugel, J. 2006. *Feeling Unreal: Depersonalization Disorder and the Loss of the Self.* Oxford: Oxford University Press.

Slaby, J. 2008. Affective Intentionality and the Feeling Body. *Phenomenology and the Cognitive Sciences 7*: 429–444.

Slaby, J. 2012. Affective Self-construal and the Sense of Ability. *Emotion Review 4*: 151–156.

Slaby, J. and Stephan, A. 2008. Affective Intentionality and Self-Consciousness. *Consciousness and Cognition 17*: 506–513.

Smith, A. 1759/2000. *The Theory of Moral Sentiments.* New York: Prometheus Books.

Smith, B. 1999. The Abyss: Exploring Depression through a Narrative of the Self. *Qualitative Inquiry 5*: 264–279.

Solomon, A. 2001. *The Noonday Demon.* London: Chatto and Windus.

Solomon, R.C. 1993. *The Passions: Emotions and the Meaning of Life* (revised edition). Cambridge: Hackett.

Solomon, R. C. ed. 2004. *Thinking about Feeling: Contemporary Philosophers on Emotions*. Oxford: Oxford University Press.

Speer, A. 1975/2010. *Spandau: the Secret Diaries*. New York: Ishi Press.

Stanghellini, G. 2004. *Disembodied Spirits and Deanimated Bodies: The Psychopathology of Common Sense*. Oxford: Oxford University Press.

Stanghellini, G. and Rosfort, R. 2013. Borderline Depression: a Desperate Vitality. *Journal of Consciousness Studies* 20 (7–8): 153–177

Stein, E. 1917/1989. *On the Problem of Empathy*. (Trans. Stein, W.). Washington, D.C.: ICS Publications.

Steinbock, A. 2007. The Phenomenology of Despair. *International Journal of Philosophical Studies* 15: 435–451.

Steinke, D. 2001. Poodle Bed. In Casey, N. ed. *Unholy Ghost: Writers on Depression*. New York: William Morrow: 60–66.

Stephan, A. 2012. Emotions, Existential Feelings, and their Regulation. *Emotion Review* 4:157–162.

Stern, D. 1985. *The Interpersonal World of the Infant*. New York: Basic Books.

Stern, D. 2010. *Forms of Vitality: Exploring Dynamic Experience in Psychology, the Arts, Psychotherapy and Development*. Oxford: Oxford University Press.

Stocker, M. 2007. Shame, Guilt and Pathological Guilt. In Thomas, A. ed. *Bernard Williams*. Cambridge: Cambridge University Press: 135–154.

Stocker, M. and Hegeman, E. 1996. *Valuing Emotions*. Cambridge: Cambridge University Press.

Stolorow, R. D. 2007. *Trauma and Human Existence: Autobiographical, Psychoanalytic and Philosophical Reflections*. New York: Routledge.

Stolorow, R. D. 2011. *World, Affectivity, Trauma: Heidegger and Post-Cartesian Psychoanalysis*. London: Routledge.

Stompe, T., Ortwein-Swoboda, G., Chaudhry, H. R., Friedmann, A., Wenza, T. and Schanda, H. 2001. Guilt and Depression: A Cross-Cultural Comparative Study. *Psychopathology* 34: 289–298.

Strasser, S. 1977. *Phenomenology of Feeling: An Essay on the Phenomena of the Heart*. Pittsburgh: Duquesne University Press.

Straus, E. W. 1947. Disorders of Personal Time in Depressive States. *Southern Medical Journal* 40: 254–259.

Strawson, P. F. 1959. *Individuals: An Essay in Descriptive Metaphysics*. London: Methuen.

Stueber, K. 2006. *Rediscovering Empathy: Agency, Folk Psychology and the Human Sciences*. Cambridge MA: MIT Press.

Styron, W. 2001. *Darkness Visible*. London: Vintage.

Svenaeus, F. 2013. Depression and the Self: Bodily Resonance and Attuned Being-in-the-World. *Journal of Consciousness Studies* 20 (7–8): 15–32.

Tellenbach, H. 1980. *Melancholy: History of the Problem, Endogeneity, Typology, Pathogenesis, Clinical Considerations*. Pittsburgh: Duquesne University Press.

Tellenbach, H. 1982. Melancholy as Endocosmogenic Psychosis. In De Koning, A.J.J. and Jenner, F.A. eds. *Phenomenology and Psychiatry*. London: Academic Press: 187–200.

Teroni, F. 2007. Emotions and Formal Objects. *Dialectica* 61: 395–415.

Thagard, P. 2002. The Passionate Scientist: Emotion in Scientific Cognition. In Carruthers, P., Stich, S. and Siegal, M. eds. *The Cognitive Basis of Science.* Cambridge: Cambridge University Press: 235–250.

Thompson. T. 1995. *The Beast: A Reckoning with Depression.* New York: Putnam.

Thompson, E. 2007. *Mind in Life: Biology, Phenomenology, and the Sciences of Mind.* Cambridge MA: Harvard University Press.

Throop, J.C. 2010. Latitudes of Loss: On the Vicissitudes of Empathy. *American Ethologist* 37: 771–782.

Throop, J.C. 2012. On the Varieties of Empathic Experience: Tactility, Mental Opacity and Pain in Yap. *Medical Anthropology Quarterly* 26: 408–430.

Tolstoy. L. 1882/2005. *A Confession.* (Trans. Maude, A. Mineola, N.Y.): Dover Publications Inc.

Toombs, S. K. 1990. The Temporality of Illness: Four Levels of Experience. *Theoretical Medicine and Bioethics* 11: 227–241.

Toombs, S. K. 2001. The Role of Empathy in Clinical Practice. *Journal of Consciousness Studies* 8 (5–7): 247–258.

Trevarthen, C. 1993. The Self born in Intersubjectivity: The Psychology of an Infant Communicating. In Neisser, U. ed. *The Perceived Self: Ecological and Interpersonal Sources of Self-Knowledge.* Cambridge: Cambridge University Press: 121–173.

Tronick, E. Z. el. 1998. Dyadically Expanded States of Consciousness and the Process of Therapeutic Change. *Infant Mental Health Journal* 19: 290–299.

Undurraga, J. and Baldessarini, R.J. 2012. Randomized, Placebo-Controlled Trials of Antidepressants for Acute Major Depression: Thirty-Year Meta-Analytic Review. *Neuropsychopharmacology* 37: 851–864.

Ussher, J. M. 2010. Are we Medicalizing Women's Misery? A Critical Review of Women's Higher Rates of Reported Depression. *Feminism and Psychology* 20: 9–35.

Van Os, J. 2009. A Salience Dysregulation Syndrome. *British Journal of Psychiatry* 194: 101–103.

Varga, S. 2014. Cognition, Representations and Embodied Emotions: Investigating Cognitive Theory. *Erkenntnis* 79: 165–190.

Verster, J.C. 2008. The Alcohol Hangover—a Puzzling Phenomenon. *Alcohol & Alcoholism* 43: 124–126.

Vogeley, K. and Kupke, C. 2007. Disturbances of Time Consciousness from a Phenomenological and a Neuroscientific Perspective. *Schizophrenia Bulletin* 33: 157–165.

Webb, D. 2007. Modes of Hoping. *History of the Human Sciences* 20: 65–83.

Weiner, S. 2003. Unity of Agency and Volition: Some Personal Reflections. *Philosophy, Psychiatry & Psychology* 10: 369–372.

Westphal, M. 1984. *God, Guilt and Death: An Existential Phenomenology of Religion.* Bloomington: Indiana University Press.

Whybrow, P. C. 1997. *A Mood Apart.* London: Picador.

Wilkinson, S. 2000. Is 'Normal Grief' a Mental Disorder? *Philosophical Quarterly* 50: 289–304.

Wilson, A.N. 2001. *Tolstoy: a Biography.* New York: W.W. Norton & Company.

Wittgenstein, L. 1975. *On Certainty.* (Trans. Paul, D. and Anscombe, G.E.M.). Oxford: Blackwell.

Wolpert, L. 1999. *Malignant Sadness: The Anatomy of Depression.* London: Faber & Faber.

Woolf, V. 1930/2002. *On Being Ill.* Ashfield MA: Paris Press.

World Health Organization 1992. *The ICD-10 Classification of Mental and Behavioural Disorders: Clinical Descriptions and Diagnostic Guidelines.* Geneva: World Health Organization.

Wurtzel, E. 1996. *Prozac Nation: Young and Depressed in America.* London: Quartet Books.

Wyllie, M. 2005. Lived Time and Psychopathology. *Philosophy, Psychiatry & Psychology* 12: 173–185.

Wynn, M. 2005. *Emotional Experience and Religious Understanding: Integrating Perception, Conception and Feeling.* Cambridge: Cambridge University Press.

Wynn, M. 2012. Renewing the Senses. *International Journal for Philosophy of Religion* 72: 211–226.

Young, I. M. 2005. *On Female Bodily Experience: 'Throwing like a Girl' and Other Essays.* Oxford: Oxford University Press.

Zahavi, D. 2005. *Subjectivity and Selfhood.* Cambridge MA: MIT Press.

Zahavi, D. 2007. Expression and Empathy. In Hutto, D.D. and Ratcliffe, M. eds. *Folk Psychology Re-assessed.* Dordrecht: Springer: 25–40.

Zahavi, D. 2010. Empathy, Embodiment and Interpersonal Understanding: From Lipps to Schutz. *Inquiry 53*: 285–306.

Zahavi, D. 2011. Empathy and Direct Social Perception: a Phenomenological Proposal. *Review of Philosophy and Psychology 2*: 541–558.

Author Index

Note: References to footnotes are indicated by the suffix 'n' followed by the note number, for example, 115n7.

Subject Index

Note: References to footnotes are indicated by the suffix 'n' followed by the note number, for example, 91n22.

endogenous depression 256
energy, lack of 76
enticing possibilities 45–6, 52, 59, 179–80
    loss of 166–8, 182, 186–7, 225–6, 263
episodic memories 139–40
epistemic benefits of depression 268
estrangement 9–10, 15, 202–3, 236–7, 280
    and guilt 143
    and interpersonal experience 218–19, 224,
        226–7
    and loss of hope 112
    and loss of possibilities 71
evaluative judgement, capacity for 272–5
exhaustion 76
existential changes 2–3, 6, 8, 14–15, 250
    and altered sense of reality 19
    awareness of 36–7
    benefits of 268
    in bereavement 199
    cultural variability of 256–7
    in depression questionnaire 27–8
    and depression diagnosis 253
    and depths of feeling 130–1
    and phenomenological stance 22
    and possibilities 71
    in schizophrenia 258–62
    variants of 98
    see also temporal experience
existential despair 94
    as an accurate appraisal of life 277–8
    and awareness of mortality 277
    and capacity for evaluative
        judgement 272–4
    as distinct from depression 276–7
    and interpersonal experience 280–1
    mitigation of 278–9
    and pathology 274–7
    Tolstoy's account of 269–72
existential feelings 2, 33, 36–7, 51, 83
    and bodily dispositions 61
    'felt' character of 41, 59–64
    influence of self-narrative on 149–51
    influence on narrative capacity 151–4
    interpersonal variation in 39n7
    linguistic expression of 146–51
        difficulties with 39, 41
        in literature 37–9
        and reference to causes 40
        and use of metaphor 39–40
    and moods 58
    and possibilities 41–55, 64
    regulation of 151n15, 154
    relationship to cognitive approaches 73–4
    relationship to other aspects of
        experience 150
    role in religious and metaphysical
        doctrines 148–9
    role of bodily dispositions in 59–64

in schizophrenia 39n6, 41
unity of 63
see also existential despair; existential
    guilt; existential hope
existential guilt
    causes of 153–4
    compared to intentional guilt 138–43
    depths of 143
    and diminished agency 170–1
        and temporal experience 174
        experience of the past 192–3
    types of 144–5
existential hope 103–5
    and life events 105–7
    loss of 110–14
        aspiring hope 117–19
        demoralization 119–22
        diagnostic implications 115
        sense of loss 115–16
        and suicide risk 114–15
    radical hope 106–10
explicit simulation 208
explicit time 177
    changes in experience of 191

F
faith, comparison with existential
    hope 109n4
falling, sense of 60
false beliefs, value of 268n19
fatigue 94, 170
fear 112–13
    in Heidegger 56–7
    in Sartre 161
feelings 35–6
    loss of 237
    see also bodily feelings; existential feelings
fragmentation of experience 259, 260
free will 157
    and phenomenology of agency 158–60
    reality of 172–3
freedom 171–2
    loss of 171–2
    phenomenology of
        and bodily limitations 162–3
        and inability to act 164
        and 'original choice' 163
        and sense of the possible 160–2
futility, association with sense of
    mortality 271, 277, 280
future, experience of 194
    see also temporal experience

G
gender, and culture 23, 30n18
gender differences
    in bodily experience 77n2
    in depression 29–30